Pediatric and Neonatal Mechanical Ventilation

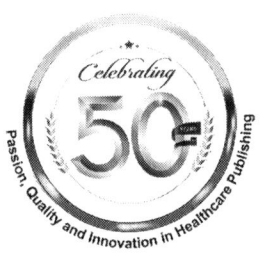

Pediatric and Neonatal Mechanical Ventilation

Third Edition

Editor

Praveen Khilnani MD FAAP MCCM (USA)
American Board Certification in Pediatrics and
Pediatric Critical Care Medicine
Director and Senior Consultant: Pediatric Critical Care,
Pulmonology and Emergency Services
Madhukar Rainbow Children's Hospital, New Delhi
Vice Chancellor, IAP College Council of Pediatric Intensive Care
Chapter, India
Academic Director, Rainbow Group of Hospitals, India

Foreword

RN Srivastav
MBBS DCH MRCP FRCP FIAP FAMS

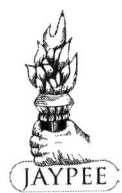

JAYPEE BROTHERS MEDICAL PUBLISHERS
The Health Sciences Publisher
New Delhi | London

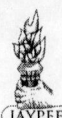

Jaypee Brothers Medical Publishers (P) Ltd

Headquarters

Jaypee Brothers Medical Publishers (P) Ltd
4838/24, Ansari Road, Daryaganj
New Delhi 110 002, India
Phone: +91-11-43574357
Fax: +91-11-43574314
Email: jaypee@jaypeebrothers.com

Overseas Office

J.P. Medical Ltd
83, Victoria Street, London
SW1H 0HW (UK)
Phone: +44 20 3170 8910
Fax: +44 (0)20 3008 6180
E-mail: info@jpmedpub.com

Website: www.jaypeebrothers.com
Website: www.jaypeedigital.com

Inquiries for bulk sales may be solicited at: jaypee@jaypeebrothers.com

Pediatric and Neonatal Mechanical Ventilation

First Edition: 2006
Second Edition: 2011
Third Edition: **2020**

ISBN: 978-93-89587-45-6

Printed at

Contributors

Kumar Ankur MD DNB Neonatology
Director NICU
BLK Superspeciality Hospital
New Delhi, India

Anil Batra DNB (Neonatology)
Senior Consultant
Department of Neonatology and
Perinatology
Madhukar Rainbow Children's
Hospital, New Delhi, India

Shipra Gulati MD IDPCCM
Consultant
Department of Pediatric Critical Care
Max Superspeciality Hospital
New Delhi, India

Naveen Gupta DNB Neonatology
Fellowship in Neonatal critical Care
(Childrens Hospital,
Vancouver BC, Canada)
Senior Consultant and Head
Department of Neonatology and
Perinatology
Madhukar Rainbow Children's
Hospital, New Delhi, India

Ebor Jacob MD
Head Pediatric Critical Care
Unit and Pediatric Critical Care
Fellowship Program
Christian Medical College and Hospital
Vellore, Tamil Nadu, India

Praveen Khilnani MD FAAP MCCM (USA)
American Board Certification in
Pediatrics and Pediatric Critical
Care Medicine
Director and Senior Consultant
Pediatric Critical Care,
Pulmonology and Emergency Services
Madhukar Rainbow Children's
Hospital, New Delhi
Vice Chancellor, IAP College
Council of Pediatric Intensive Care
Chapter, India
Academic Director, Rainbow Group
of Hospitals, India

Navneet Kumar MD
Consultant, Pediatric Critical Care
and Emergency Services
Madhukar Rainbow Children's
Hospital, New Delhi, India

Naresh Lal MD IDPCCM
Senior Consultant PICU
BLK Superspeciality Hospital,
New Delhi, India

Ankur Ohri MD IDPCCM
Consultant, Pediatric Critical Care
and Emergency Services
Madhukar Rainbow Children's
Hospital, New Delhi, India

Madhumati Otiv MD
Head, Pediatric Intensive Care Unit
KEM Hospital
Pune, Maharashtra, India

Mritunjay Pao MD IDPCCM
Senior Consultant
Pediatric Intensivist
Jorhat, Assam, India

VSV Prasad MD Pediatrics (AIIMS, New Delhi)
Fellowship Training in Neonatology
and Pediatric Critical Care—UK & USA
Chief Consultant Neonatologist and
Pediatric Intensivist
Chief Executive Officer
Lotus Hospitals for Women & Children
Hyderabad, Telangana, India

Anil Sachdev DCH MD FICCM
Director Pediatric Emergency,
Critical Care
Pulmonology and Allergic Diseases
Department of Pediatrics
Institute of Child Health
Sir Ganga Ram Hospital
New Delhi, India

Neeraj Sagar MD FNB (Pediatric Critical Care)
Consultant, Pediatric Critical Care
and Emergency Services
Madhukar Rainbow Children's
Hospital, New Delhi, India

Bhaskar Saikia MD IDPCCM
Director PICU and Fellowship
Program
MAX Superspeciality Hospital
New Delhi, India

Romit Saxena MD IDPCCM MRCPCH (UK)
Assistant Professor
Department of Pediatrics
Consultant
Pediatric Intensive Care Unit
MAMC and Associated LNJP Hospital
New Delhi, India

Rachna Sharma MD IDPCCM
Director PICU
BLK Superspeciality Hospital,
New Delhi, India

Abhijit Singh MD
Consultant, Pediatric Critical Care
and Emergency Services
Madhukar Rainbow Children's
Hospital, New Delhi, India

Chandrashekhar Singha MD
Fellowship in Pediatric Critical Care
(Sick Kids Hospital Toronto, Canada)
Senior Consultant: Pediatric Critical
Care and Emergency Services
Madhukar Rainbow Children's
Hospital, New Delhi
Chairman, IAP Pediatric Intensive
Care Chapter, Delhi Branch
New Delhi, India

Rajiv Uttam MRCPCH (UK)
Director and Senior Consultant
Pediatric Critical Care and
Pulmonology
Max Superspeciality Hospital
IP Extension, New Delhi
Director Nayati Health Care
Hospitals, India
Noida, Uttar Pradesh, India

Shekhar Venkataraman MD
Senior Consultant
Pediatric Critical Care and
Director Respiratory Care
Childrens Hospital of Pittsburgh
Pittsburgh School of Medicine
Pittsburgh, Pensylvania, USA

Sanjay Wazir MD DM (Neonatology)
Director and Senior Consultant
Neonatologist
Cloud Nine Hospital
Gurugram, Haryana, India

Foreword

The author of this book, *Pediatric and Neonatal Mechanical Ventilation*, is an experienced Pediatric Intensivist with over 35 years of experience and expertise in the field of Anesthesia, Pediatrics, and Critical Care. He has been involved in training of Pediatric Intensive Care fellows and teaching at various conferences and mechanical ventilation workshops in India as well as at an international level. The text presented is intended to be a practical resource, helpful to beginners and advanced pediatricians who are using mechanical ventilation for newborns and older children.

RN Srivastav
MBBS DCH MRCP FRCP FIAP FAMS
Senior Consultant
Pediatrics and Pediatric Nephrology
Apollo Institute of Pediatrics
Indraprastha Apollo Hospital
New Delhi, India

Preface to the Third Edition

Mechanical ventilation is an age old proven technology commonly used in neonates, infants, and older children in intensive care units for various indications.

It is often confusing for the pediatrician who is starting to learn regarding ventilation to keep up with various technical terms and abbreviations being used by ventilator companies and neonatologist and pediatric intensivists.

This text has been prepared with a view to be simple, practical, concise and easy-to-read for pediatricians, pediatric intensive care unit (PICU) and neonatal intensive care unit (NICU) residents and fellows using conventional mechanical ventilation for commonly seen conditions such as respiratory distress syndrome (RDS), meconium aspiration syndrome (MAS), persistent pulmonary hypertension (PPHN), pneumonia, acute respiratory distress syndrome (ARDS), asthma, and various cardiovascular and neurological conditions.

Standard terminology has been used and defined in the text for convenience of the reader. Ventilation technique specifically applicable to neonate or an older child has been indicated wherever necessary to avoid any confusion.

Some easy-to-read flow diagrams (algorithms) have been used for management of respiratory distress, rapid sequence intubation (RSI), basic mechanical ventilation, and weaning. Noninvasive ventilation modalities such as continuous positive airway pressure (CPAP), biphasic positive airway pressure (BIPAP), and high flow nasal oxygen have also been included. Newer modes such as high frequency ventilation and common ventilator graphics interpretation have also been included for the reader aspiring to learn the newer and advanced modes of ventilation. A chapter on extracorporeal membrane oxygenation has been added to make the reader familiar with technology beyond mechanical ventilation to support patients with refractory hypoxemia. A chapter on how to choose a ventilator has also been included as a guide to new units providing care to neonates and children.

It is hoped that this book would be helpful to the user in management of common conditions requiring CPAP, invasive and noninvasive mechanical ventilation in neonates and older children.

Praveen Khilnani MD FAAP MCCM (USA)

Preface to the First Edition

As the field of pediatric critical care is growing, the need for a simple and focused text of this kind has been felt for past several years in this part of the world for pediatric mechanical ventilation. Effort has been made to present the method and issues related to mechanical ventilation of neonate, infant and the older child. Basic and some advanced modes of mechanical ventilation have been described for advanced readers, topics like high frequency ventilation, ventilator graphics and inhaled nitric oxide have also been included. Finally, some commonly available ventilators and their features and utility in this part of the world have been discussed. I hope this book will be helpful to pediatricians, residents and neonatal pediatric intensivists who are beginning to work independently in an intensive care setting, or have already been involved in care of critically ill neonates and children.

Praveen Khilnani MD IAAP MCCM (USA)

Acknowledgments

I would like to thank all the contributing authors and my Neonatology, Pediatric ICU and anesthesia colleagues in India, UAE and USA for all the shared knowledge and experience. Most importantly I am deeply indebted to all my critically ill patients who needed mechanical ventilatory support to always bring me back to a humbling experience and make all of us intensivists realize how little did we know and that there is a lot more to learn in this vast field of intensive care and field of Medicine at large.

Finally I wish to thank my family for supporting all my publications whole heartedly by constant encouragement and support towards teaching and training juniors to save lives of critically ill neonates and children.

I would like to thank Shri Jitendar P Vij (Group Chairman), Mr Ankit Vij (Managing Director), Mr MS Mani (Group President), Ms Chetna Malhotra Vohra (Associate Director—Content Strategy), Ms Pooja Bhandari (Production Head), Ms Prerna Bajaj (Development Editor) and the publishing staff at Jaypee Brothers Medical Publishers (P) Ltd, New Delhi, India, for their work in completing this book.

Contents

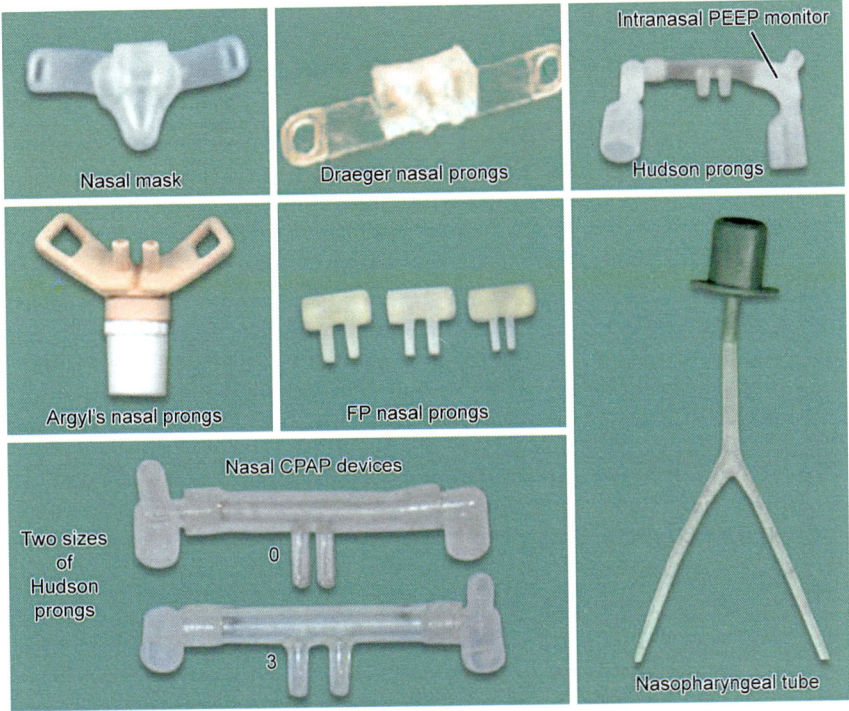

Chapter 5, Fig. 1: Different types of nasal interfaces.

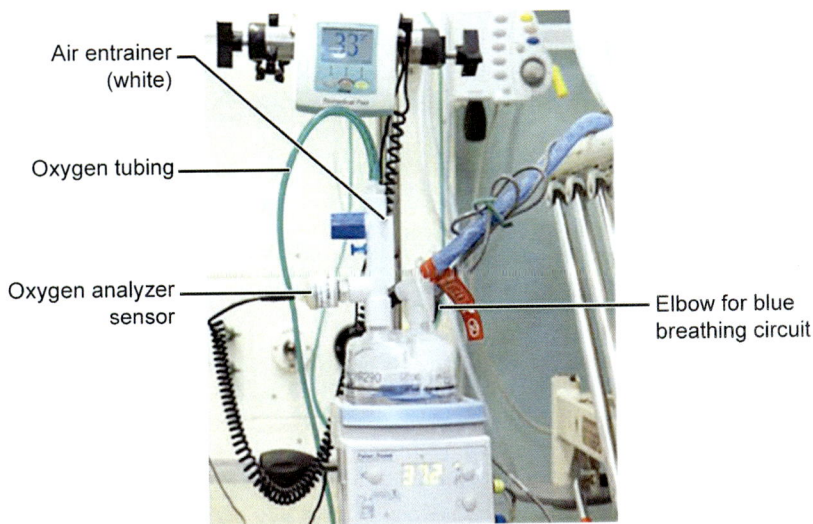

Chapter 6, Fig. 6: Complete oxygen analyzer with air entrainer blender set up.

PLATE 2

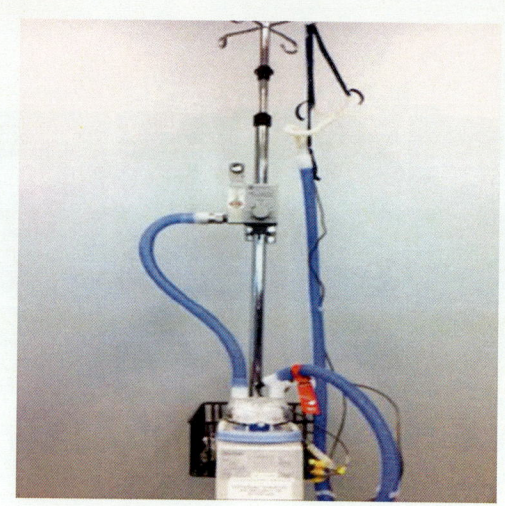

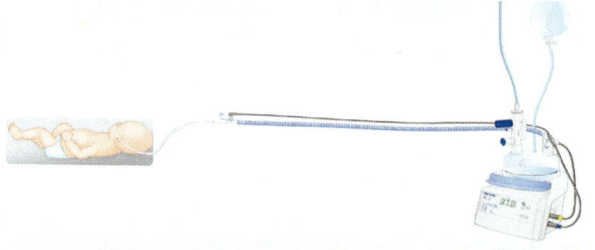

Chapter 6, Fig. 2: Basic set up of high flow nasal cannula (HFNC).

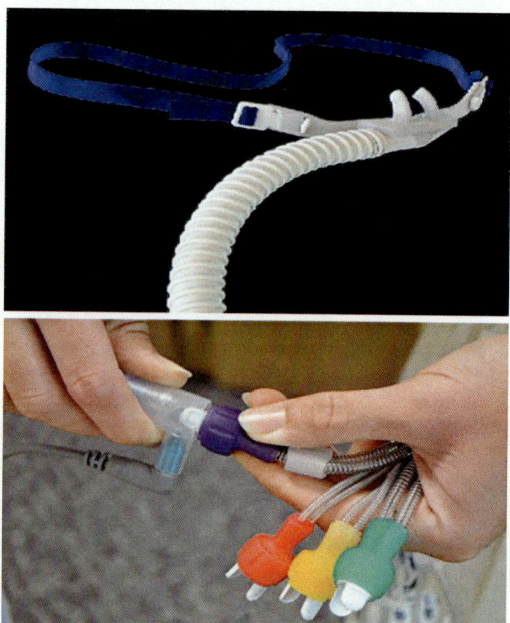

Chapter 6, Fig. 3: Nasal cannula.

PLATE 3

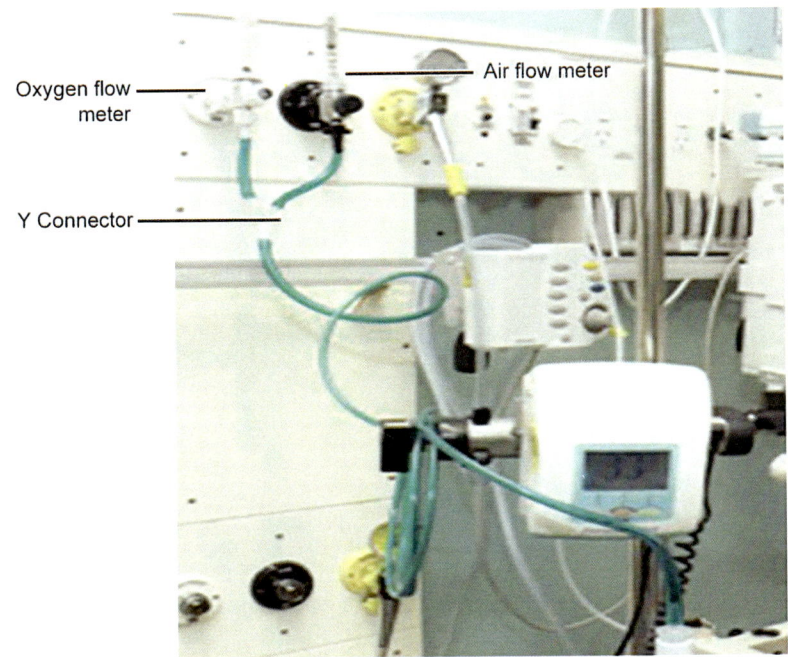

Oxygen flow meter

Air flow meter

Y Connector

Chapter 6, Fig. 4: High-flow air and O_2 flow meters connected via Y connector.

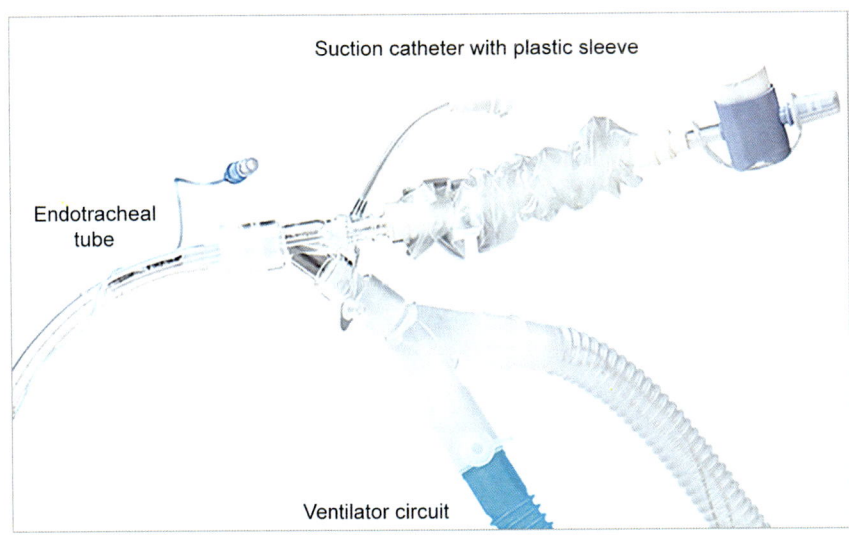

Suction catheter with plastic sleeve

Endotracheal tube

Ventilator circuit

Chapter 14, Fig. 1: Close suction system.

PLATE 4

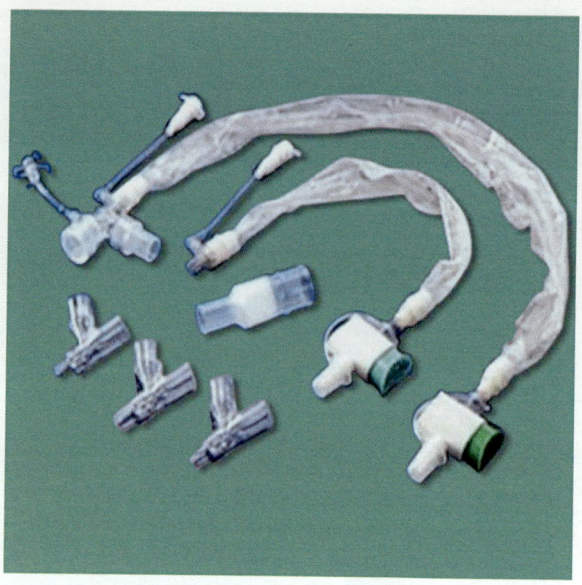

Chapter 14, Fig. 2: Pediatric and neonatal close suction catheters.

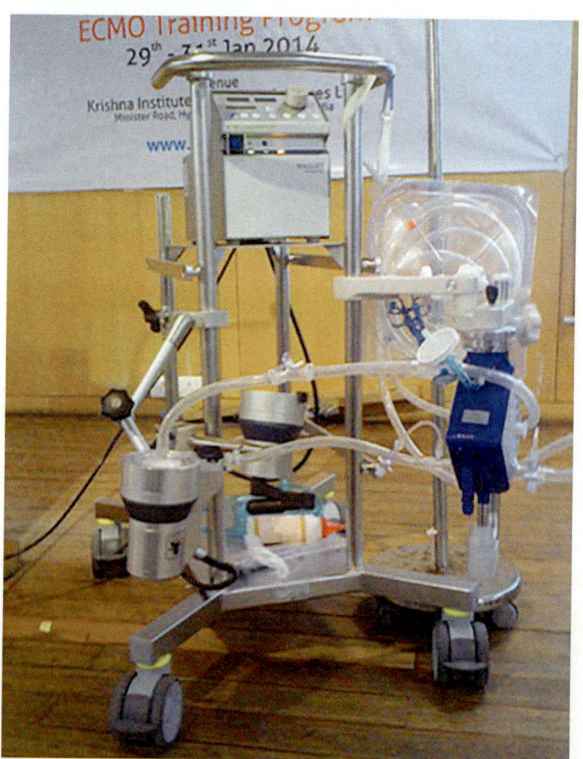

Chapter 16, Fig. 2: Extracorporeal membrane oxygenation (ECMO) equipment in pediatric intensive care unit (PICU).

PLATE 5

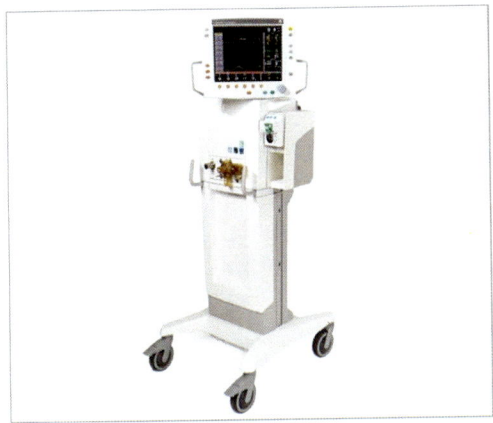

Chapter 17, Fig. 1: Engström ventilator.

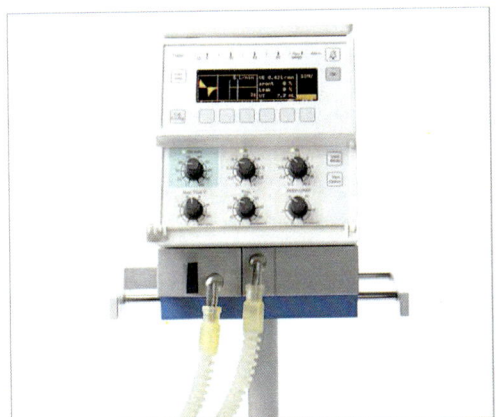

Chapter 17, Fig. 2: Drager Babylog 8000.

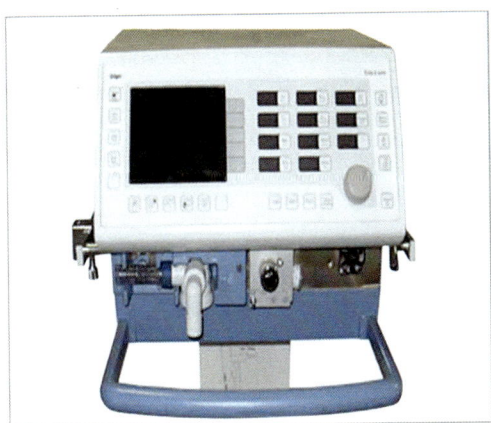

Chapter 17, Fig. 3: Drager Babylog 8000 Plus.

PLATE 6

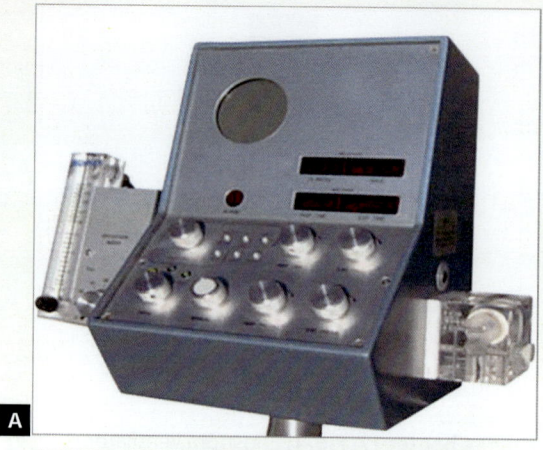

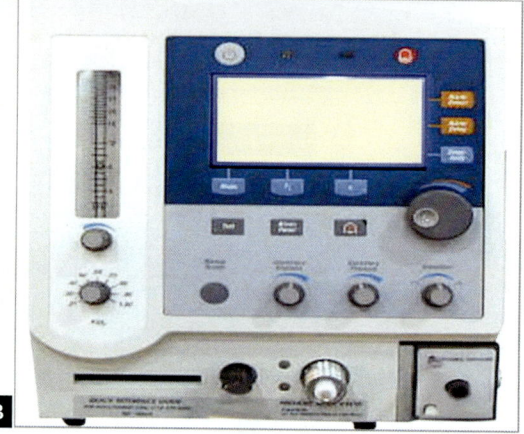

Chapter 17, Figs. 4A and B: Sechrist ventilator: (A) Old and (B) New.

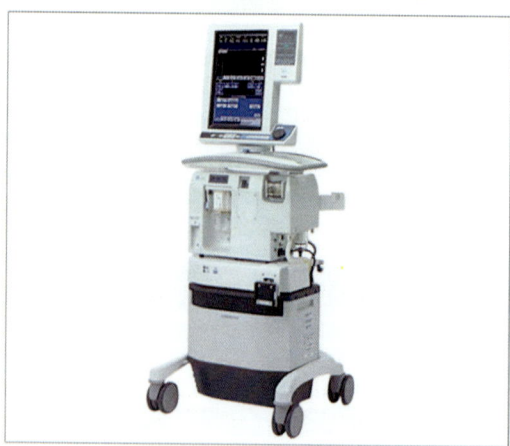

Chapter 17, Fig. 6: Puritan Bennett™ 840 ventilator.

PLATE 7

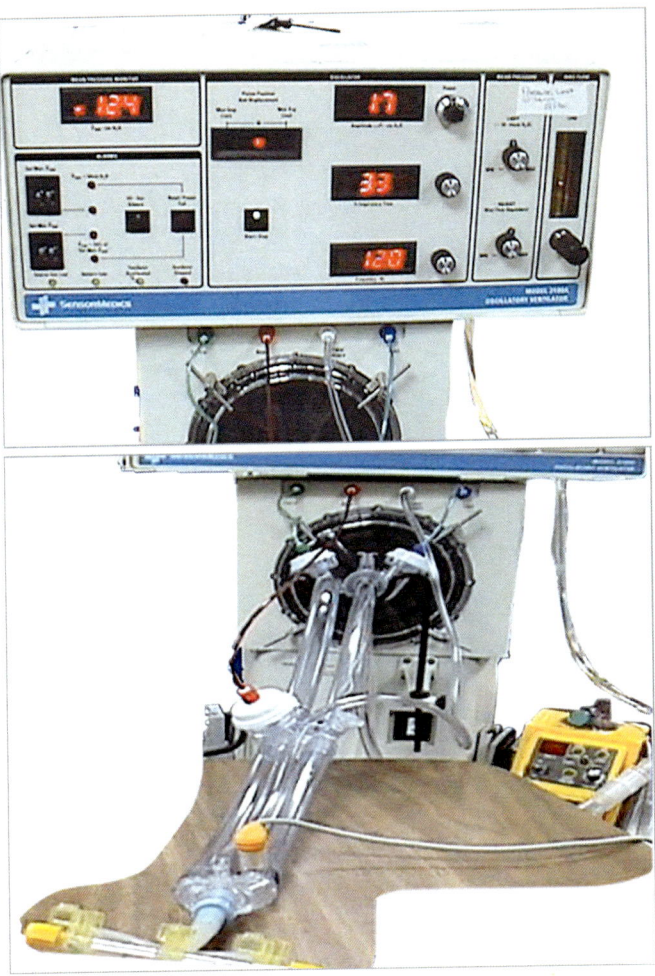

Chapter 17, Figs. 12A and B: SensorMedics 3100A (high frequency oscillator ventilator).

PLATE 8

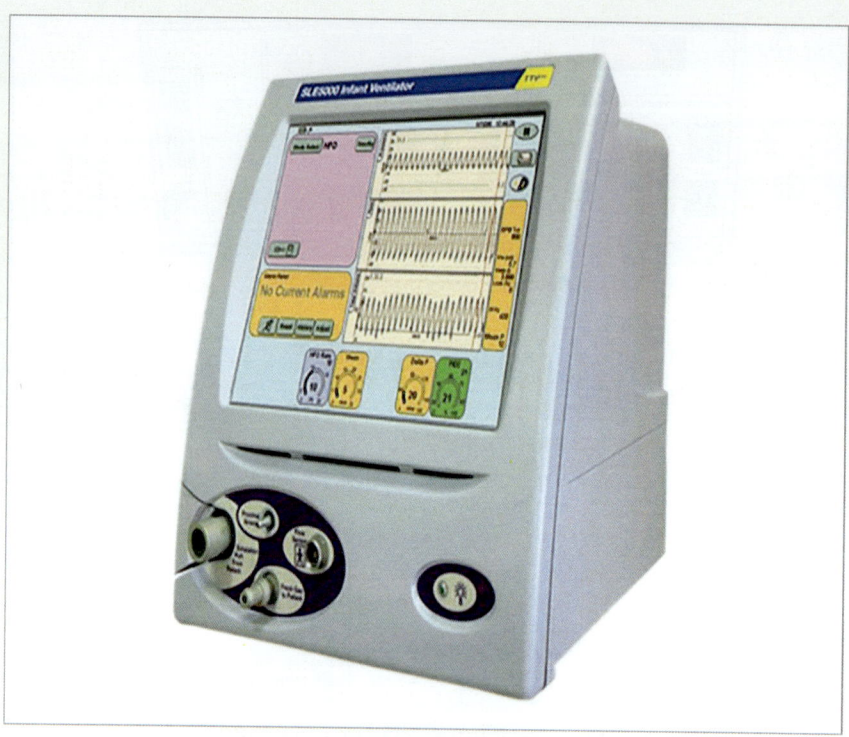

Chapter 17, Fig. 13: SLE5000 ventilator.

Basics of Mechanical Ventilation

Praveen Khilnani

Basic principles of physics and gas flow apply to all age groups; anatomical and physiological differences play a significant role in selecting the type of ventilator as well as the ventilator modes and settings.

Upper airway in children is cephalad, funnel shaped with narrowest area being subglottic (at the level of cricoid ring), as compared to adults where the upper airway is tubular with narrowest part at the vocal cords. Airway resistance increases inversely by 4th power of radius i.e. in an already small airway even one mm of edema or secretions will increase the airway resistance and turbulent flow markedly necessitating treatment of airway edema, suctioning of secretion, measures to control secretions. Low functional residual capacity (*FRC*: Volume of air in the lungs at end of expiration) reduces the oxygen reserve, and reduces the time that apnea can be allowed in a child.

Respirations are shallow and rapid due to predominant diaphragmatic breathing, and inadequate chest expansion due to inadequate costovertebral bucket handle movement in children. Therefore, a child tends to get tachypnea rather than increasing the depth of respiration in response to hypoxemia. Oxygen consumption/kg body weight is higher; therefore, tolerance to hypoxemia is lower.

Susceptibility to bradycardia in response to hypoxemia is also higher due to high vagal tone. Pores of Kohn and channels of Lambert (bronchoalveolar and intermalleolar collaterals) are inadequately developed, making regional atelectasis more frequent. Closing volumes are lower and airway collapse due to inadequate strength of the cartilage in the airways is common, making a child particularly susceptible to laryngomalacia, and tracheobronchomalacia as well as lower airways closure at a higher lung volume.

Therefore, children tend to require smaller tidal volumes, faster respiratory rates, and adequate size endotracheal tubes and adequately suctioned clear airways for proper management of mechanical ventilation. Other important factors for choosing ventilatory settings include the primary pathology i.e. asthma, acute respiratory distress syndrome (ARDS), pneumonia, air leak syndrome, raised intracranial tension, neuromuscular weakness, neonatal hyaline membrane disease, or neonatal persistent pulmonary hypertension (PPHN).

BASIC MECHANICS OF VENTILATION

During spontaneous breathing, pleural pressure is negative. During inspiration active work is done to generate the gradient between the mouth and pleural space as the driving pressure for inspired gases to enter the alveolus, and this gradient is needed to overcome resistance and to maintain the alveolus open, by overcoming elastic recoil forces.

Therefore, a balance between elastic recoil of the chest wall and the lung determines lung volume at any given time. Expiration is passive. During positive pressure ventilation, pressure gradient generated by the ventilator at the mouth (or endotracheal tube) is higher than the pleural pressure which is also positive, however at the end of inspiration, expiration is again passive though it can be manipulated by application of positive pressure to prevent complete deflation at the end of expiration (PEEP: positive end expiratory pressure).

Two main issues are important physiologically during mechanical ventilation: ventilation and oxygenation.

Ventilation

Ventilation washes out carbon dioxide from alveoli keeping arterial $PaCO_2$ between 35 mm of Hg and 45 mm of Hg. Increasing dead space increases the $PaCO_2$.

$$PaCO_2 = k \times \frac{\text{Metabolic production}}{\text{Alveolar minute ventilation (MV)}}$$

Alveolar MV = Respiratory rate × Effective tidal volume

Effective TV = TV – Dead space

Dead space = Anatomic (nose, pharynx, trachea, bronchi) + Physiologic (alveoli that are ventilated but not perfused)

Adequate minute ventilation is essential to keep $PaCO_2$ within normal limits.

Oxygenation

Partial pressure of oxygen in alveolus (PaO_2) is the driving pressure for gas exchange across the alveolar-capillary barrier determining oxygenation.

$PaO_2 = [(\text{Atmospheric pressure} - \text{Water vapor}) \times FiO_2] - PaCO_2/RQ$

RQ = Respiratory quotient

Adequate perfusion to alveoli that are well ventilated improves oxygenation. Hemoglobin is fully saturated 1/3 of the way through the capillary.

Hypoxemia can occur due to:

- Hypoventilation
- V/Q mismatch (V—ventilation, Q—perfusion)
- Shunt (Perfusion of an unventilated alveolus, atelectasis, fluid in the alveolus)
- Diffusion impairments.

Hypercarbia can occur due to:

- Hypoventilation
- V/Q mismatch
- Dead space ventilation.

Gas Exchange

Hypoventilation and V/Q mismatch are the most common causes of abnormal gas exchange in the pediatric intensive care unit (PICU).

Hypoventilation can be corrected by increasing minute ventilation.

V/Q mismatch can be corrected by increasing the amount of lung that is ventilated or by improving perfusion to those areas that are ventilated.

Concept of Time Constant

Time constant is the time required to fill an alveolar space (or empty it). It depends on the resistance and compliance. In the pediatric age group one time constant that fills an alveolar unit to 63% of its capacity is 0.15 seconds. It takes three time constants to achieve greater than 90% capacity of the alveolar unit filled.

$$\text{Time constant} = \text{Resistance (pressure} \times \text{time/volume)} \times \\ \text{Compliance (volume/pressure)}$$

This signifies that a certain minimum inspiratory time (Ti) is required to fill the alveoli adequately which is generally two to three time constants; i.e. 0.3–0.45 seconds. This is important when selecting the Ti on the conventional ventilator.

INDICATIONS OF MECHANICAL VENTILATION

Indications remain essentially clinical and may not be always substantiated by objective parameters such as blood gas analysis.

Common indications include:

- Respiratory failure:
  - Apnea/respiratory arrest
  - Inadequate ventilation
  - Inadequate oxygenation
  - Chronic respiratory insufficiency with failure to thrive
- Cardiac insufficiency/shock:
  - Eliminate work of breathing
  - Reduce oxygen consumption

- Neurologic dysfunction:
  - Central hypoventilation/frequent apnea
  - Patient comatose, Glasgow Coma Score (GCS) ≤8
  - Inability to protect airway
- Postoperative ventilation

COMMONLY USED NOMENCLATURE FOR MECHANICAL VENTILATION (FIGS. 1 TO 7)

- Airway pressures:
  - Peak inspiratory pressure (PIP)
  - Positive end expiratory pressure (PEEP)

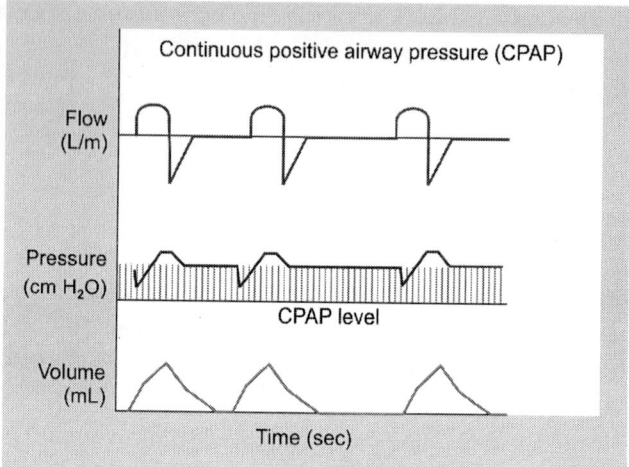

Fig. 1: Graph showing continuous positive airway pressure (CPAP).

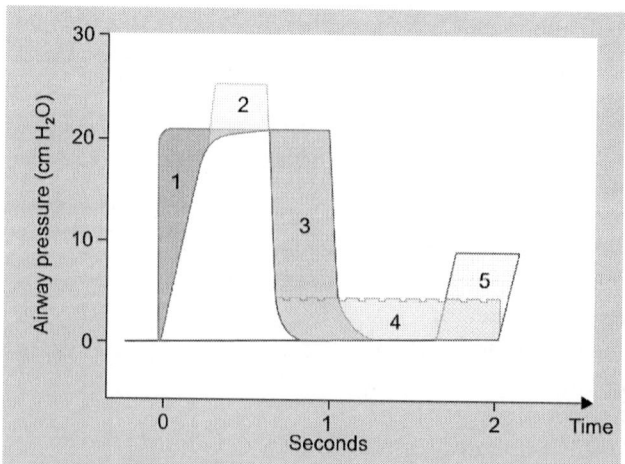

Fig. 2: Graph showing factors affecting mean airway pressure (and oxygenation). 1. Inspiratory time, 2. Peak inspiratory pressure, 3. Expiratory time, 4. Positive end expiratory pressure, and 5. Pause time.

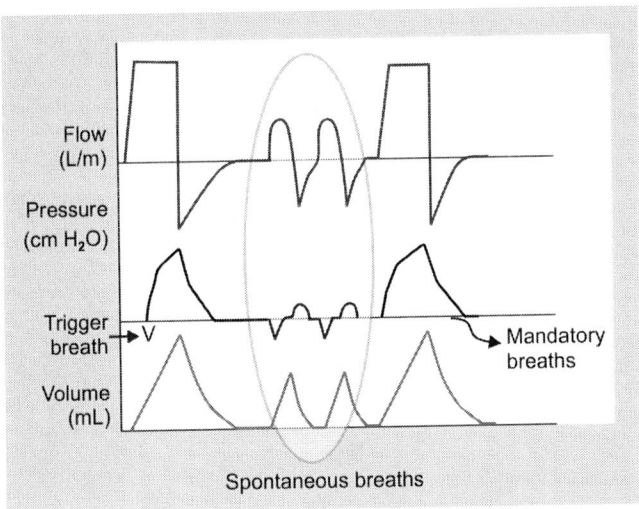

Fig. 3: Synchronized intermittent mandatory ventilation with volume control (SIMV-VC).

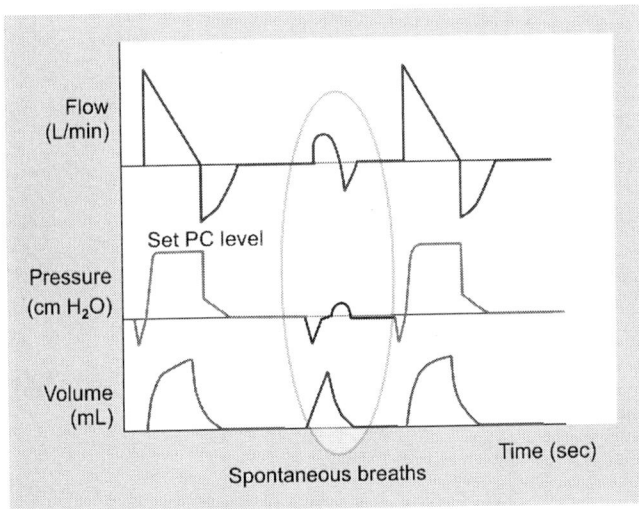

Fig. 4: Synchronized intermittent mandatory ventilation with pressure control (SIMV-PC).

- Pressure above peep (PAP or δp)
- Mean airway pressure (MAP)
- Continuous positive airway pressure (CPAP)
- *Inspiratory time* (Ti)
- *I:E ratio*: Ratio of Ti and expiratory time in seconds
- *Frequency (f)*: Ventilatory rate (breaths/min)
- *Tidal volume (Vt)*: Amount of gas delivered with each breath
- *Expired tidal volume (Ve)*: Amount of gas measured by the machine at expiration.
- *Expired Minute volume (MV)*: Volume of gas in L expired per minute.

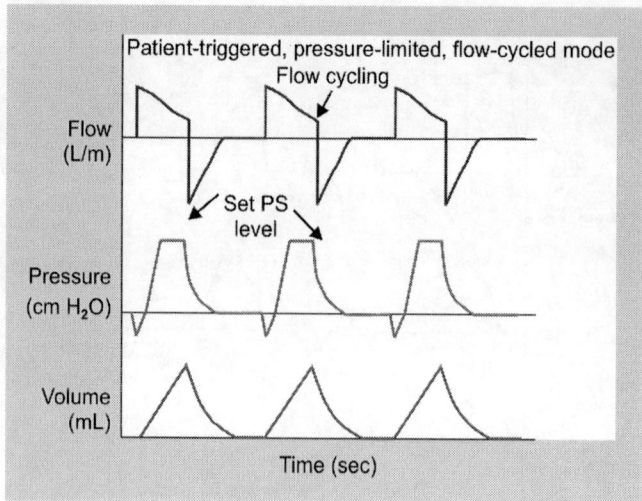

Fig. 5: Patient-triggered, pressure-limited, flow-cycled ventilation.

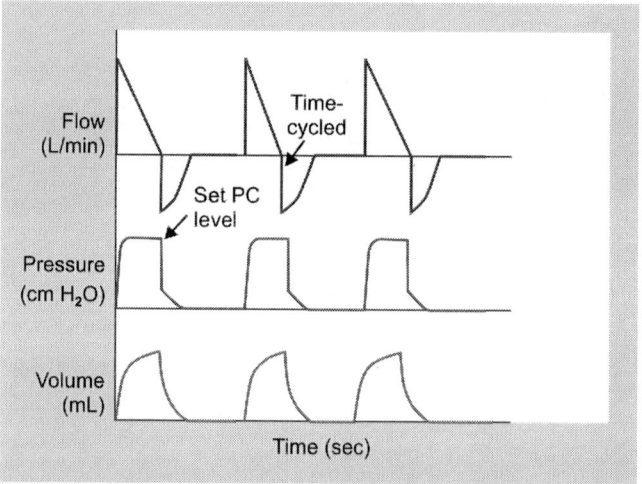

Fig. 6: Time-triggered, pressure-limited, time-cycled ventilation.

MODES OF VENTILATION

Control Modes

In this mode, every breath is fully supported by the ventilator. In classic control modes, patients were unable to breathe except at the controlled set rate. In a conventional controlled mode, weaning is not possible by decreasing rate, the patient may hyperventilate if agitated leading to patient/ ventilator asynchrony. Patients on control modes will need sedation and or paralysis with a muscle relaxant in newer control modes, machines may act

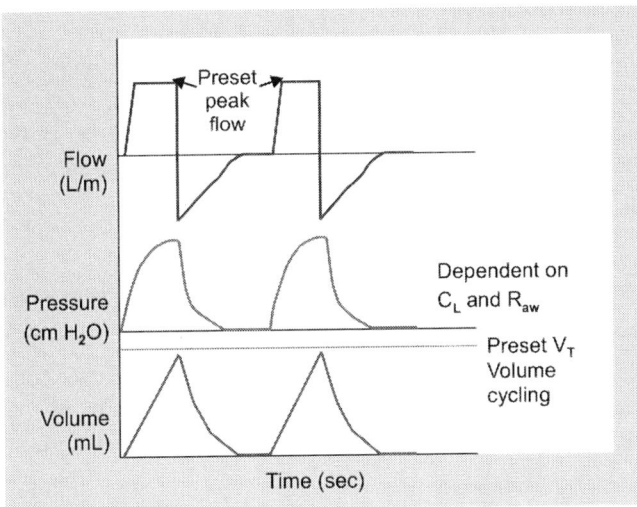

Fig. 7: Time-triggered, volume-limited, time-cycled ventilation.
(C_L: compliance lung; R_{aw}: airway resistance; V_T: volume tidal)

in assist-control, with a minimum set rate and all triggered breaths above that rate are also fully supported.

Intermittent Mandatory Ventilation Modes

In this mode breaths "above" the set rate are not supported. Most modern ventilators have synchronized intermittent mandatory ventilation (SIMV).

Synchronized Intermittent Mandatory Ventilation

Ventilator synchronizes intermittent mandatory ventilation (IMV) "breath" with patient's effort.

Patient takes "own" breaths in between (with or without pressure support) the set SIMV rate. There is a potential for increased work of breathing and patient/ventilator asynchrony, if the ventilator interferes with the patient's effort to breath or if there is insufficient flow for the spontaneous breaths. Ventilators would have an inbuilt latent period of about 25% of the Ti in which to recognize the patient's effort in order to synchronize the mandatory breath in order to reduce asynchrony. SIMV breath can be pressure limited or volume limited.

Support Mode

Pressure Support

Ventilator supplies pressure support (flow) at a preset level but rate is determined by the patient, expiration begins passively when inspiratory flow decreases below a certain level preset in the ventilator (flow cycled). Volume support is also available in Servo 300 ventilators following the principle of pressure support (delivery of the set volume over the patient's natural inspiratory time duration keeping the pressure to a minimum.

Pressure support can decrease work of breathing by providing flow during inspiration for patient triggered breaths. It can be given with spontaneous breaths in IMV modes or as stand-alone mode without set rate as well as for weaning to retrain coordination of respiratory muscles in patients on ventilation for longer than few weeks.

Trigger

Trigger is defined as the variable that initiates the breath from the ventilator. The trigger variable is usually pressure or flow.

Pressure trigger: With pressure triggering, in order to trigger the ventilator and initiate the inspiratory flow, the patient must decrease the pressure in the ventilator circuit to a preset value, which will then open a demand valve.

Flow trigger: With flow triggering, the patient triggers the ventilator when the respiratory muscles generate a certain preset inspiratory flow. It is generally believed that triggering of the ventilator is better with flow than with pressure.

The real clinical significance is unclear in terms of the work of breathing and patient ventilator interaction. Pressure sensors in current ventilators are much improved, reducing any difference between flow and pressure triggering systems. Recent studies in patients with different diseases show that the difference in the work of breathing between flow and pressure triggering is of minimal clinical significance.

Trigger setting: A pressure trigger setting of greater than 0 (cm of water) makes it too sensitive (meaning the triggered breath from the ventilator will be too frequent). A negative setting (negative1 or negative 2) setting is usually acceptable. Too negative setting will increase the work of the patient (to generate a negative pressure) to trigger a ventilator breath.

BASIC FUNDAMENTALS OF VENTILATION

Ventilators deliver gas to the lungs using positive pressure at a certain rate. The amount of gas delivered can be *limited* by time, pressure or volume. The duration can be *cycled* by time, pressure or flow. If volume is set, pressure varies; if pressure is set, volume varies according to the compliance.

$$Compliance = \Delta \text{ volume}/\Delta \text{ pressure}$$

Chest must rise, no matter which mode is chosen.

Following are three main expectations from the ventilator:
1. Ventilator must recognize patient's respiratory efforts (trigger)
2. Ventilator must be able to meet patient's demands (response)
3. Ventilator must not interfere with patient's efforts (synchrony)

Whenever a breath is supported by the ventilator, regardless of the mode, the limit of the support is determined by a preset pressure or volume.

Volume limited: Preset tidal volume

Pressure limited: Preset PIP

Pressure versus Volume Control

Goal is to ventilate and oxygenate adequately. Both pressure and volume control modes can achieve it. Important requirements include adequate movement of the chest, smooth gas flow, and minimal barotrauma or volu-trauma.

One must have a setup of high/low pressure alarms in volume cycling and, low expired tidal volume alarm when using pressure cycling.

Pressure-limited Ventilation

Ventilator stops the inspiratory cycle when set PIP is achieved.

Caution: Tidal volume changes suddenly as patient's compliance changes. Ventilator delivers a decelerating flow pattern (lower PIP for same Vt). This can lead to hypoventilation or overexpansion of the lung. If endotracheal tube is obstructed acutely, delivered tidal volume will decrease. This mode is useful if there is a leak around the endotracheal tube.

For improving oxygenation, one needs to control FiO_2 and MAP, (I-time, PIP, PEEP) and to influence ventilation, one needs to control PIP and respiratory rate.

Volume-limited Ventilation

Ventilator stops the inspiratory cycle when set tidal volume has been delivered. One can control minute ventilation by changing the tidal volume and rate. For improving oxygenation primarily FiO_2, PEEP, I-time can be manipulated. Increasing tidal volume will also increase the PIP, hence affecting the oxygenation by increasing the MAP. It delivers volume in a square wave flow pattern. Square wave (constant) flow pattern results in higher PIP for same tidal volume as compared to pressure modes.

Caution: There is no limit per se on PIP (so ventilator alarm will have to be set for an upper pressure limit to avoid barotrauma). Volume is lost if there is a circuit leak or significant leak around the endotracheal tube, therefore an expired tidal volume needs to be monitored and set. Some ventilators will alarm automatically if the difference between set inspired tidal volume and expired tidal volume is significant (varies between the ventilators).

Initial Ventilator Settings

One should always have the general idea regarding what initial ventilator settings to choose when initiating the ventilation.

Choose the mode: Control every breath (assist control) if planned for heavy sedation and muscle relaxation or use SIMV when patient likely to breath spontaneously.

General parameters to choose will include:

Rate: Start with a rate that is somewhat normal; i.e. 15 for adolescent/child, 20–30 for infant/small child, 30–40 for a neonate, 40–50 for a premature neonate.

FiO$_2$: 1(100%) and quickly wean down to level <0.5. Depending upon oxygen requirement 0.5 may be a starting point for the FiO$_2$.

PEEP: 3–5 cm of H$_2$O (higher to 6–7 if ARDS, or low compliance disease, lower (2–3 cm) if asthma, or high compliance disease.

Inspiratory time (I-time or I:E ratio): 0.3–0.4 sec for neonates, 0.5–0.6 sec for children, 0.7–0.9 in older children. Normal I:E ratio = 1:2–1:3

Then specifically choose if the modality of delivered breath will be pressure controlled or volume controlled (correct term is pressure limited or volume limited).

Pressure limited: Peak inspiratory pressure is set depending upon lung compliance and pathology

Neonates: Apnea 12–14 cm, hyaline membrane disease 18–22 cm H$_2$O

Children: For normal lung 16–18 cm, for low compliance 18–25 cm H$_2$O, severe ARDS 25–35 cm may be required.

Volume Limited

Tidal volume 8–10 mL/kg with a goal to get 6–8 mL/kg expired tidal volume. Initial tidal volume at 10–12 mL/kg may need to be set if leak is present around endotracheal tube; in such patients, pressure limited ventilation may be preferred. Flow in most ventilators is set at 6–10 L for the washout of the CO$_2$ from the internal ventilator circuit, tubing's, etc. Flow less than 4 L/min is not recommended. Following discussion includes cases and principles of ventilation based on disease specific pathophysiology.

Adjustments after Initiation: Usually based on blood gases and oxygen saturations

For oxygenation: FiO$_2$, PEEP, I Time, PIP (tidal volume) can be adjusted (increase MAP)

For ventilation: Respiratory rate, tidal volume (in volume limited) and PIP (in pressure limited mode) can be adjusted.

Positive end expiratory pressure is used to help prevent alveolar collapse at end inspiration; it can also be used to recruit collapsed lung spaces or to stent open floppy airways.

Gas Exchange-related Problems

- Inadequate oxygenation (hypoxemia)
- Inadequate ventilation (hypercarbia)

Inadequate oxygenation: Important guidelines
- Do not just increase FiO_2
- Increase tidal volume if volume limited mode, PEEP, Ti.
- Increase PIP/PEEP/ Ti if pressure limited mode
- If O_2 worse, get chest X-ray to rule out air leak (treat!)/If lung fields show worsening (increase PEEP further)
- Do not forget other measures to improve oxygenation
  - Normalize cardiac output (if low output) by fluids and/inotropes
  - Maintain normal hemoglobin
  - Maintain normothermia
  - Deepen sedation/consider neuromuscular block

High PaCO₂: Common reasons include hypoventilation, dead space ventilation (too high PEEP, decreased cardiac output, pulmonary vasoconstriction), increased CO_2 production, hyperthermia, high carbohydrate diet, and shivering. Inadequate tidal volume delivery (hypoventilation) will occur with endotracheal tube block, malposition, kink, circuit leak, and ventilator malfunction.

Measures for normalizing high $PaCO_2$ guidelines:
- *If volume limited*: Increase tidal volume (Vt), increase frequency (rate) (f).
- *If asthma:* Increase expiratory time, may need to decrease ratio to achieve an I:E ratio >1:3.
- *If pressure limited:* Increase PIP, decrease PEEP, increase frequency (rate).
- Decrease dead space (increase cardiac output, decrease PEEP, vasodilator)
- *Decrease CO_2 production:* Cool, increase sedation, decrease carbohydrate load.
- Change endotracheal tube if blocked, kinked, malplaced or out, check proper placement.
- Fix leaks in the circuit, endotracheal tube cuff, humidifier

Measures to reduce barotrauma and volutrauma: Following concepts are being increasingly followed in most PICUs.
- *Permissive hypercapnia:* Higher $PaCO_2$s are acceptable in exchange for limiting peak airway pressures: as long as pH>7.2.
- *Permissive hypoxemia:* PaO_2 of 55-65; SaO_2 88-90% is acceptable in exchange for limiting FiO_2 (<60) and PEEP, as long as there is no metabolic acidosis. Adequate oxygen content can be maintained by keeping hematocrit >30%.

Patient Ventilator Dyssynchrony

In coordination between the patient and the ventilator: Patient fights the ventilator! Common causes include, hypoventilation, hypoxemia, tube block/kink/malposition, bronchospasm, pneumothorax, silent aspiration, increased oxygen demand/increased CO_2 production (in sepsis), and inadequate sedation.

If patient fighting the ventilator and desaturating: Immediate measures

USE MNEMONIC: D O P E

D: displacement, O; obstruction, P: pneumothorax, E: equipment failure.

- Check tube placement. When in doubt take the endotracheal tube out, start manual ventilation with 100% oxygen.
- *Examine the patient*: Is the chest rising? Breath sounds present and equal? Changes in examination? Atelectasis, treat bronchospasm/tube block/malposition/pneumothorax? (Consider needle thoracentesis.)
- *Examine circulation:* Shock? Sepsis?
- Check arterial blood gas and chest X-ray for worsening lung condition, and for confirming pneumothorax.
- Examine the ventilator, ventilator circuit/humidifier/gas source.

If no other reason for hypoxemia: Increase sedation/muscle relaxation, put back on ventilator.

Sedation and muscle relaxation during ventilation: Most patients can be managed by titration of sedation without muscle relaxation. Midazolam (0.1–0.2 mg/kg/hr) and vecuronium drip (0.1-0.2 mg/kg/hr) is most commonly used. Morphine or fentanyl drip can also be used if painful procedures are anticipated.

Do not use muscle relaxants without adequate sedation.

Routine ventilator management protocol: Following protocol is commonly followed:

- Wean FiO_2 for SpO_2 above 93–94. In ARDS, 89–92 may be acceptable.
- Arterial blood gas (ABG) one hour after intubation, then am pm schedule (12 hourly), and after major ventilator settings change, and 20 minutes after extubation
- Pulse oximetry on all patients, end tidal carbon dioxide ($EtCO_2$)/graphics monitoring, if available
- Frequent clinical examination for respiratory rate, breath sounds, retractions, color
- Chest X-ray every day/alternate day/as needed.

Respiratory care protocol

- Position changes every 2 hourly → right chest tilt/left chest tilt/supine position and try to maintain 30° head up position.
- Suction 4 hourly and as needed (in line suction to avoid derecruitment/loss of PEEP/desaturation if available)
- *Physiotherapy 8 hourly*: Percussion, vibration, and postural drainage. NO physiotherapy if labile oxygenation such as ARDS, PPHN

- *Nebulization*: In line nebulization is preferred over manual bagging. Metered dose inhalers (MDIs) can also be used
- Disposable circuit change, if visible soiling
- Humidification/in line disposable humidifier
  Ventilator care protocols, suctioning, physiotherapy, and positioning should all be under proper protocols for patient safety and to prevent adverse events such as unplanned intubation.

Weaning from Mechanical Ventilation

Process of weaning begins at the time of initiation of ventilation (i.e. minimal ventilatory settings to keep blood gases and clinical parameters within acceptable limits although these settings will be very high).

If such procedure is followed then ventilatory settings would be reduced once the primary pathology/condition that led to ventilation is improving.

How do we know if the condition is improving?

- Improving general condition, fever, etc.
- Decreasing FiO_2 requirement
- Improving breath sounds
- Decreasing endotracheal secretions
- Improving chest X-rays
- Decreased chest tube drainage, bleeding/air bubbles(as the case may be)
- Improved fluid and electrolyte status (no overload or dyselectrolytemia)
- Improving hemodynamic status
- Improving neurological status, muscle power, airway reflexes/control. Described weaning criteria such as maximal negative inspiratory force, vital capacity measurement are usually impractical. In pediatrics and neonatal age group, weaning criteria are generally clinical.

Weaning Methodology

There are no set protocols supported by any pediatric studies. Protocol followed at author's institution is as follows:

When FiO_2 requirement is down to 0.4, improvement in secretions, and chest X rays, improving clinical condition, muscle relaxant drip is stopped and sedation can be slowly weaned. One should change control mode (or PRVC) to SIMV mode with pressure support. Pressure support can be set at 10–15 cm above PEEP so that the spontaneous breaths can be adequately supported. Trigger sensitivity should be 0 to negative one. Then slowly SIMV rate can be weaned, followed by weaning of pressure support while closely monitoring for signs of respiratory distress, restlessness, nasal flaring, accessory muscle use, tachypnea, desaturations, and hemodynamic instability such as tachycardia, hypertension or hypotension.

Following weaning guidelines can be followed:

- Decrease FiO_2 to keep SPO_2 >94
- Decrease the PEEP to 4–5 gradually by decrements of 1–2 cm H_2O

- Decrease the SIMV rate to 5 (by 3-4 breath/min)
- Decrease the PIP (to 20 cm H_2O, by reducing 2 cm H_2O each time/tidal volume, to no less than 5 mL/kg to prevent atelectasis (usually guided by blood gases).
- Ventilator rate and PIP can be changed alternately. If at any point patient's oxygen requirement increases greater than 0.6, or spontaneous ventilation is fast or distressed with accessory muscle use (increased work of breathing), patient gets lethargic, hypercarbia on blood gas, weaning process should be paused and the support level increased. Patient may not be ready. Goal is to decrease what the ventilator does and see if the patient can make up the difference without desaturations/hypercarbia/significant tachypnea, and respiratory distress. (For example, if patient's SIMV was reduced from 20/min to 15/min and the patient's spontaneous rate is increased from 25 to 50, this patient may need more time on the ventilator).
- *Spontaneous breathing trials (SBT)*: A trial for 15-20 minutes may be conducted by connecting the patient to collapsible anesthesia bag (C circuit trial), if no distress, desaturation or excessive tachycardia, sweating or hypertension, consider as readiness of extubation. With or without weaning protocols, most pediatric patients can be extubated successfully. SBT and clinical indicators for extubation readiness may be used in difficult situations of extubation failure; however, none of the pediatric specific weaning protocols and guidelines are able to predict successful extubation.

Extubation

Most patients can be weaned to SIMV of 5 and extubated, some will need pressure support 5-10 above PEEP with CPAP, while others may need CPAP 5 cm H_2O before extubation, with or without SBT with T piece.

Clinical indicators of extubation readiness: Extubation can generally be performed when following criteria are met:

- Control of airway reflexes, minimal secretions
- Patient upper airway (air leak around tube?)
- Good breath sounds
- Minimal oxygen requirement <0.3 with SPO_2 >94
- Minimal rate 5/min
- Minimal pressure support (5-10 above PEEP)
- "Awake" patient

KEY MESSAGES

- Remember shock and post resuscitation are important indications for ventilation, in addition to respiratory failure and neuromuscular disease.
- Clinical monitoring of adequate chest rise and oxygen saturations is very important (regardless of mode volume, pressure or time cycled mode).

- *If ventilator fails, turn FiO$_2$ to 1 (100%) and take over hand bag tube ventilation*: Follow DOPE protocol and correct accordingly.
- *If and when in doubt regarding endotracheal tube status, do not waste time*: Remove endotracheal tube and try bag mask ventilation.
- Low tidal volume is recommended to prevent lung trauma (permissive hypercapnia and permissive hypoxemia).
- Ventilator care protocols, suctioning, physiotherapy, and positioning should all be under proper protocols for patient safety and to prevent adverse events such as unplanned intubation.
- With or without weaning protocols, most pediatric patients can be extubated successfully.
- Spontaneous breathing trial and clinical indicators for extubation readiness may be used in difficult situations of extubation failure; however, none of the pediatric specific weaning protocols and guidelines are able to predict successful extubation.

SUGGESTED READING

1. Chatburn RL, El-Khatib M, Mireles-Cabodevila E. A taxonomy for mechanical ventilation: 10 fundamental maxims. Respir Care. 2014;59:1747-63.
2. Chatburn RL. Classification of ventilator modes: update and proposal for implementation. Respir Care. 2007;52:301-23.
3. Duyndam A, Ista E, Houmes RJ, et al. Invasive ventilation modes in children: a systematic review and meta-analysis. Crit Care. 2011;15(1):R24.
4. Essouri S, Chevret L, Durand P, et al. Noninvasive positive pressure ventilation: five years of experience in a pediatric intensive care unit. Pediatr Crit Care Med. 2006;7(4):329-34.
5. Khilnani P. Pediatric and neonatal mechanical ventilation, 2nd edition. New Delhi: Jaypee Brothers Medical Publishers (P) Ltd; 2011.
6. Kneyber MCJ, de Luca D, Calderini E, on behalf of the section Respiratory Failure of the European Society for Paediatric and Neonatal Intensive Care. Recommendations for mechanical ventilation of critically ill children from the Paediatric Mechanical Ventilation Consensus Conference (PEMVECC). Intensive Care Med. 2017;43(12):1764-80.
7. Levitt MA. A prospective randomized trial of BIPAP in severe acute cardiac heart failure. J Emerg Med. 2001;21:363-9.
8. Marraro GA. Innovative practices of ventilatory support with pediatric patients. Pediatr Crit Care Med. 2003;4:8-20.
9. Ruza F. Noninvasive ventilation in pediatric acute respiratory failure: a challenge in pediatric intensive care units. Pediatr Crit Care Med. 2010;11:750-1.
10. Schultz TR, Costarino AT, Durning SM, et al. Airway pressure release ventilation in pediatrics. Pediatr Crit Care Med. 2001;2:243-6.
11. van Velzen A, De Jaegere A, van der Lee J. Feasibility of weaning and direct extubation from open lung high-frequency ventilation in preterm infants. Pediatr Crit Care Med. 2009;10:71-5.
12. Younes M, Puddy A, Roberts D, et al. Proportional assist ventilation: results of an initial clinical trial. Am Rev Respir Dis. 1992;145:121-9.

2

Applied Respiratory Physiology of Mechanical Ventilation

Shekhar Venkataraman, Praveen Khilnani

PHYSIOLOGY OF INFLATION AND DEFLATION

Impedance to Lung Inflation

Thoracic structures impede lung inflation and a certain amount of force is required to overcome this impedance. Elasticity of the lung and chest wall is a major factor that impedes lung inflation. Elastance is defined as the change in pressure for a unit change in volume. Compliance is the reciprocal of elastance. Lung compliance is defined as the change in lung volume for a unit change in transalveolar pressure (alveolar pressure minus the pleural pressure). Chest wall compliance is the change in thoracic cage volume produced by a unit change in transthoracic pressure (ambient pressure minus the pleural pressure). Total respiratory system compliance is the total change in lung volume (lung and chest) for a unit change in transrespiratory pressure (alveolar pressure minus the ambient pressure). Specific lung compliance refers to lung compliance that is normalized to the lung volume or body weight (similar in children and adults). The pressure required to overcome compliance is:

$$P_{Compliance} = Volume/Compliance \text{ or } Volume \times Elastance$$

Total respiratory system resistance is the second factor that impedes inflation and is defined as the change in transpulmonary pressure (proximal airway pressure minus the alveolar pressure) required to produce a unit flow of gas through the airways of the lung. Total resistance can be partitioned into airway resistance and frictional resistance to deformation of the lungs, chest wall, and abdominal contents. In the infant, the airway resistance is equally distributed between the upper and lower airways. With increasing age, most of the airway resistance resides in the upper airways. Frictional resistance is also known as the nonelastic viscous resistance. In certain pathological conditions, such as pulmonary edema, interstitial lung disease, and pulmonary fibrosis, frictional resistance may be increased. The pressure required to overcome this total resistance can be written as:

$$P_{Total\ Resistance} = P_{Airflow\ Resistance} + P_{Frictional\ Resistance}$$

$$= \text{Total Respiratory Resistance} \times \text{Flow}$$

Inertance of the respiratory gas is another factor that impedes inflation and the pressure required to overcome inertial forces of the gas is normally low and can be omitted. Then, the total pressure (P_{tp}) required to inflate the lung can be mathematically expressed as follows, termed the "Equation of Motion":

$$P_{tp} = P_{Compliance} + P_{Total\ Resistance}$$

LUNG VOLUMES AND CAPACITIES

Air gets in, air gets out; oxygen is taken up, carbon dioxide is eliminated; this is the essence of breathing. Tidal volume is the volume of gas that is moved in and out of the lungs per breath and is normally 6–8 mL/kg for a spontaneous breath, regardless of age. Total lung capacity (TLC) is the volume of gas present in the lung with maximal inflation (60–80 mL/kg). Vital capacity is the volume of gas that can be maximally expired from TLC (40–50 mL/kg). Functional residual capacity (FRC) is the volume of gas that is present in the lung at the end of a normal expiration. FRC results from the balance between forces that favor alveolar collapse and maintain alveolar inflation. The normal FRC is about 30 mL/kg. Residual volume is the volume of gas present in the lung at the end of a maximal expiratory effort. Closing volume refers to the volume of gas present in the lung at which small conducting airways begin to collapse. When FRC exceeds closing volume, the small airways and the alveoli remain open. On the other hand, when closing volume exceeds FRC, the small airways and alveoli tend to collapse. In infants and children younger than 6 years, the closing volume exceeds FRC. This explains the propensity for atelectasis in infants and young children. With development, FRC exceeds closing volume in children older than 6 years.

Concept of Time Constant

With a constant inflation pressure, it takes a finite amount of time to inflate the lung with a given volume of gas. The rate of inflation and deflation of the lung is approximately mono-exponential and is directly proportional to the compliance and the resistance. Time constant is calculated as the product of compliance and resistance. It takes one, 3, and 5 time constants to cause a 63%, 95%, and a 99% change in lung volume, respectively. Normal expiration is passive because of the elastic recoil of the lung, which is attributable to alveolar surface tension and tissue elasticity. Surface tension is greatest at high lung volumes, and lowest at FRC. Elastic recoil of the lung provides most of the force required to expel the gas from the lungs. Inspiratory and expiratory time constants may be different since the inspiratory and expiratory resistances are different.

WORK OF BREATHING

Work of normal breathing is performed entirely by the inspiratory muscles, and almost all of the work is performed during inspiration. Nearly half of the work of breathing during inspiration is dissipated as heat to overcome frictional resistance. The remaining inspiratory work is stored as potential energy that is used to perform the expiratory work. Increased airway resistance and decreased chest and lung compliances would require a greater P_{tp} to inflate the lung to the same lung volume. These changes impose a greater workload on the respiratory muscles and increases the oxygen cost of breathing. When the oxygen supply-demand balance to the respiratory muscles is perturbed, respiratory failure may ensue because of muscle fatigue.

DETERMINANTS OF GAS EXCHANGE

The determinants of systemic arterial oxygenation are inspired oxygen concentration and tension, lung volume, cardiac output, ventilation-perfusion (V/Q) matching, and the magnitude of venous admixture or intrapulmonary shunting. Lung volumes are increased during inspiration and fall during expiration. During expiration, the presence of alveolar surfactant prevents alveolar collapse. A critical opening pressure is required to maintain both the patency of the terminal airways and alveolar volume. When the airway pressure is below the critical opening pressure, the terminal airway closes and the alveoli collapse because of continued absorption of gases into the bloodstream. Surfactant deficiency, loss, or alteration promotes alveolar collapse and increases the critical opening pressure. In parenchymal lung disease, which is characterized by an increased critical closing pressure, alveoli collapse during expiration if the airway pressures cannot be maintained above the critical opening pressure. Alveolar collapse leads to inadequate oxygenation due to increased intrapulmonary shunting resulting from (V/Q) mismatch.

The determinants of systemic arterial carbon dioxide ($PaCO_2$) include the tidal volume and the ventilator rate. $PaCO_2$ reflects the balance between metabolic production of CO_2 and its elimination. Decreased CO_2 elimination usually results from decreased central drive, lower airway obstruction, parenchymal disease, and muscle weakness. Inadequate ventilation causes CO_2 retention when it becomes insufficient to clear metabolic CO_2 production. Increased metabolic production of CO_2 usually results from hypermetabolic states or excessive caloric intake, especially high carbohydrate alimentation.

PRINCIPLES OF MECHANICAL VENTILATION

Although the principles behind mechanical ventilation—an artificial airway, a source of fresh gas, and a power source, the increasing need for ventilation assistance, coupled with ever-improving life support technology, need to under-stand the basic principles and to stay at the cutting edge of this technology.

Ventilator Design Principles—Breath Delivery

A ventilator delivered breath can be described by its trigger, its gas delivery target, and its breath cycling criteria. The trigger is what initiates the breath and is either a timer, which is a controlled breath or an effort, which is an assisted breath. The second component of breath is the gas delivery target or limit. On most ventilators, it is either a set flow or a set pressure that governs gas flow. Then there is the cycle—that is what turns the breath off.

The controlled breath is initiated by machine timer whereas the assisted or supported breath is initiated by patient effort.

There are two ways to trigger the assisted or supported breath: the pressure trigger and the flow trigger. Originally, ventilators used the pressure trigger. The patient effort would produce a pressure drop in the ventilator circuit, which the ventilator responded to by supplying the gas. However, the original machines were not very sensitive. In the late 1980s, the flow trigger was introduced. With the flow trigger, there is a continuous flow of gas running through the ventilator circuit, typically 5–20 L/min. If patient makes an effort, some of that flow is delivered into the patient, which is sensed by the ventilator to trigger the breath. However, in today's microprocessor-based ventilators, the pressure trigger and the flow trigger have comparable sensitivity. Indeed, many ventilators have both, and whichever one activates first is the one that is used first.

There is no inherent difference in the amount of gas or tidal volume these two types of breaths can give except the flow behavior.

There are three common types of breath cycles. The breath reaches a set volume (i.e. a volume cycle breath, a set time (i.e. a time cycle breath) or a certain flow reduction (i.e. a flow cycle breath). Airway pressure usually function as a backup cycle, which means that if the pressure exceeds certain limits, usually under the condition of an airway occlusion or active exhalation, the breath cycle off to prevent over pressurization. Newer ventilators have pressure release mechanism, so that if pressure start to increase because the patient starts forcefully exhale, for example, then instead of the breath turning off, the machine will allow the patient to exhale, thus providing relief.

Basic Respiratory System Mechanics

The respiratory system consists of the tracheobronchial tree and 300 million alveoli enclosed by the thoracic cage. Pressures are usually measured in the ventilator circuit (often referred to as airway pressure). This pressure is determined by gas flow and volume interacting with airway resistance and respiratory system compliance. By stopping flow, this circuit pressure equilibrates with alveolar pressure. This stop flow is commonly done at end inspiration and the resulting circuit pressure (alveolar pressure) is known as plateau pressure. When the stop flow is used at end expiration, the alveolar pressure reflects intrinsic positive end expiratory pressure (PEEPi).

The pleural pressure can also be estimated with use of an esophageal balloon, although it is very rarely used.

Pressure, Flow, and Volume

During a spontaneous breath, the inspiratory muscles are pulling the chest wall out and the lung open. Consequently, the pleural pressure is negative while the ventilator applies positive airway pressure, causing the alveolus to expand and push the chest wall outward. As a result, the pleural pressure becomes positive.

If this patient develops pulmonary edema, the lung will stiffen. It will not affect the flow or the chest wall. There will be high peak and plateau pressures, but the pleural pressure will not change. So this elevation in plateau pressure reflects an increase in lung stiffness, not chest wall stiffness.

Interestingly, stiff chest wall, not a stiff lung can be responsible for driving up the plateau pressure. Anasarca, ascites, obesity or chest bandages could be the cause of low chest wall compliance. Putting the patient in the prone position can also cause a bit of this effect.

DESIGN AND FUNCTIONAL CHARACTERISTICS OF VENTILATORS

Ventilator as a Machine

The concept is a simple one—a ventilator is simply a machine that performs external work. This requires energy to be applied to the device which is then altered, transmitted, and directed in a predetermined manner to perform the work of breathing. This work can either replace the patient's work of breathing completely or partially, or augment a patient's breathing efforts. Therefore, a ventilator is a mechanical device that is used to move gas into the lungs by increasing P_{tp}. Positive pressure ventilators create P_{tp} by raising the airway pressure (Paw) above the intrapleural pressure (P_{pl}), whereas negative pressure ventilators create P_{tp} by decreasing P_{pl} below Paw.

The pressure generated within the ventilator can be thought of as the driving pressure that forces the gas into the lungs through the conducting system involving the ventilator circuit and the patient's airways. During mechanical ventilation, for a single breath, P_{tp} may be generated either by the ventilator or a spontaneous breath or a combination of both. Therefore, the equation of motion can be re-expressed as:

$$P_{tp} = P_{mus} + P_{vent} = (\text{Volume} \times \text{Elastance}) + (\text{Total Resistance} \times \text{Flow}), \text{ where}$$

P_{mus} is the pressure exerted by the respiratory muscles and P_{vent} is the pressure exerted by the ventilator.

A ventilator can also be viewed as a form of mechanical controller that "controls" either pressure (in a pressure generator) or flow (in a flow generator). A pressure generator is a ventilator that generates a fixed pattern of pressure within the ventilator and at the mouth, regardless of the lung conditions whereas the flow waveform is free to vary. This occurs when the generated pressure is low (generally between 20 cm H_2O and 50 cm H_2O), which results in a high initial flow rate that decays to zero as the alveolar pressure approaches the generated pressure. The generated pressure can be constant, nonconstant, increasing, or decreasing. The Hand-E-Vent (Ohio Medical Products), Bird Asthmatik (Bird Corporation), the Bennett PR-1, and the Bennett PR-2 ventilators are examples of pressure generators. A flow generator is a ventilator that generates a high driving pressure (3–50 psig corresponding to 200–3,500 cm H_2O) and controls the inspiratory flow of gas into the patient by interposing a high series resistance system between the generated pressure and the patient. The flow generated may be constant, nonconstant, increasing, or decreasing.

Patterns of Gas Flow

The pattern of gas flow from the ventilator to the patient depends on the driving mechanism and the driving pressure in the ventilator. Four distinct flow patterns can be recognized: (1) a constant flow, (2) a decelerating flow, (3) an accelerating flow, and (4) a sinusoidal or sine-wave flow. A constant inspiratory flow is generated when the driving pressure is very high (e.g. 50 psig) relative to the airway pressure. The drive mechanism is usually a high-pressure gas system (compressed air or oxygen at 10–50 psig). The driving force generally exceeds 1,000 cm H_2O and is many times higher than the typical proximal airway pressure required to inflate the lungs. An adjustable resistance controls the pressure and the flow to the proximal airway. The airway pressure and lung volume increase linearly until inspiration is terminated. Constant flow can also be generated by a linear-driven piston, which moves at a constant rate of speed during inspiration. A decelerating inspiratory flow is created when the driving pressure is relatively low (<60 cm H_2O). In this case, a pressure-reducing valve controls the driving pressure to the desired level. As the airway pressure and lung volume increase during inspiration, the pressure gradient between the drive mechanism and the proximal airway decreases. Consequently, as inspiration progresses, the inspiratory flow from the ventilator decreases and finally stops at the end of inspiration. A sine-wave or sinusoidal inspiratory flow is created when the drive mechanism is a rotary-wheel driven piston. As the rotary wheel turns, the piston is moved to and fro in the cylinder in an accelerating and then a decelerating fashion. The inspiratory flow produced also has a similar profile. The notion that one specific flow pattern is more beneficial than the others is controversial. A detailed description of this topic is beyond the scope of this chapter, and the reader is referred to several excellent reviews. Ventilators can also be classified as a single-circuit or a double-circuit device. A single-circuit device refers to a ventilator in which the gases go directly from the drive mechanism to the patient. On the other hand, a double-circuit device refers to a system in which the drive mechanism is used to compress another system that then delivers the tidal volume.

Mechanism of Gas Flow in High-Frequency Ventilation in the Normal Lung

The exact mechanism of gas transport in high-frequency ventilation (HFV) is currently not clear. It is possible that each mode of ventilation may have differing mechanisms of gas flow from the proximal airway to the alveoli. If gas flow to the lungs is increased more than 200 times the minute volume of oxygen demand, the lung parenchyma can be made to oscillate. At ventilatory frequencies less than 7 Hz, regional alveolar ventilation depends on segmental compliance and airway resistance. At a ventilatory frequency greater than 7 Hz, a frequency-dependent excitation of the lung parenchyma and airway conduits occurs, and at frequencies greater than 10 Hz, ventilation becomes independent of regional compliance. When the gas in the airways is oscillated at high frequency, the airways begin to undergo spatial oscillation inside the chest. These oscillations are composed of periodic changes in length and width, movements of curved or angular bronchi, and wave motions in the bronchi. When the frequency of oscillation approaches the natural resonant frequency of the lung structures, the oscillations of the airways and the lung parenchyma are amplified. These result in shaking and squeezing of the neighboring parenchyma, resulting in intraparenchymal and interparenchymal gas mixing. Other mechanisms involved in gas transport during HFV include accelerated axial dispersion, increased collateral flow through pores of Kohn, intersegmental gas mixing or Pendelluft phenomenon, Taylor dispersion, asymmetrical gas flow profiles, and gas mixing within the airway due to the nonlinear pressure-diameter relationship of the bronchi.

Initial Ventilator Settings

One should always have the general idea regarding what initial ventilatory settings to choose when initiating the ventilation. Parameters to choose include:

Rate: Start with a rate that is somewhat normal, i.e. 15 for adolescent/child, 20–30 for infant/small child, 30–40 for a neonate, 40–50 for a premature neonate.

FiO$_2$: 1(100%) and quickly wean down to level <0.5. Depending upon oxygen requirement 0.5 may be a starting point for the FiO$_2$.

Positive end expiratory pressure: 3–5 cm of H$_2$O [higher to 6–7 if acute respiratory distress syndrome (ARDS), or low compliance disease, lower (2–3 cm) if asthma, or high compliance disease].

Inspiratory time (I-time or I:E ratio): 0.3–0.4 sec for neonates, 0.5–0.6 sec for children, 0.7–0.9 in older children. Normal I:E ratio = 1:2–1:3.

Choose the mode: Control every breath (assist control) if planned for heavy sedation and muscle relaxation or use synchronized intermittent mandatory ventilation (SIMV) when patient likely to breath spontaneously.

Pressure Limited

Peak inspiratory pressure (PIP) is set depending upon lung compliance and pathology.

Neonates: Apnea 12–14 cm, hyaline membrane disease 18–22 cm H_2O

Children: For normal lung 16–18 cm, for low compliance 18–25 cm H_2O, severe ARDS 25–35 cm may be required.

Volume Limited

Tidal volume 8–10 mL/kg with a goal to get 6–8 mL/kg expired tidal volume. Initial tidal volume at 10–12 mL/kg may need to be set if leak present around endotracheal tube; in such patients, pressure limited ventilation may be preferred.

Flow in most ventilators is set at 6–10 L for the washout of the CO_2 from the internal ventilator circuit, tubings, etc. Flow less than 4 L/min is not recommended. Following discussion includes cases and principles of ventilation based on disease-specific pathophysiology.

PATHOPHYSIOLOGICAL BASIS FOR INDICATIONS FOR MECHANICAL VENTILATION

Respiratory Failure

The primary indication for institution of assisted ventilation is respiratory failure. Respiratory failure is generally defined as the presence of (1) inadequate oxygenation, (2) inadequate ventilation, or (3) both. Apnea or respiratory arrest is an extreme form of respiratory failure and prolonged apnea is usually an indication for immediate mechanical ventilation. *Inadequate oxygenation*, objectively, is defined as partial pressure of arterial oxygen (PaO_2) less than 60 torr or an arterial hemoglobin oxygen saturation of <90% in room air. Oxygenation can also be expressed as the ratio of PaO_2 to fractional concentration of oxygen in inspired gas (FiO_2). *Inadequate oxygenation* can also be defined as a PaO_2-FiO_2 ratio of less than 300. Other indices include an alveolar-to-arterial oxygen gradient of more than 300 torr with a FiO_2 of 1.0. Inadequate oxygenation due to intrapulmonary shunting can be overcome with the addition of increased inspired oxygen concentration, provided the magnitude of the shunt is less than 15%. Intrapulmonary shunt can be decreased by with the re-expansion of collapsed alveoli or with the decrease in the fraction of pulmonary blood flow going to the collapsed/consolidated alveolar segments. *Inadequate ventilation* is defined as a $PaCO_2$ greater than 45 torr with an arterial pH of less than 7.35 in the absence of chronic hypercapnia. Acute-on-chronic ventilatory failure is defined as a change in $PaCO_2$ of at least 20 torr with a corresponding decrease in arterial pH. Impending respiratory failure, characterized by rapidly rising $PaCO_2$, progressive respiratory distress, $PaCO_2$ out of proportion to the respiratory effort, or fatigue of respiratory muscles, is a relative indication for mechanical ventilation. Intubation and institution of mechanical ventilation in impending respiratory failure are likely to be more controlled than when full-blown respiratory failure develops. Therefore, in critically-ill children, establishing mechanical ventilation before respiratory failure develops is preferable. Chronic respiratory failure is defined as requirement for mechanical ventilation for more than 28 days. Children with chronic lung disease often fail to grow despite adequate caloric intake. In these patients, mechanical ventilation may decrease the work of breathing enough to allow the child to grow.

Cardiovascular Dysfunction and Shock

Moderate to severe cardiovascular dysfunction is another major indication for mechanical ventilation. The cardiovascular and respiratory systems must act in concert to maintain adequate gas exchange and thereby meet the metabolic demands of the whole body. Therefore, the two systems cannot be functionally divorced from each other. Cardiovascular dysfunction can result in a decrease in respiratory reserve, increase in respiratory work, and may ultimately result in respiratory failure. Positive pressure ventilation decreases lactic acid production by respiratory muscles during circulatory shock, and withdrawal of ventilatory support results in a marked increase in cardiac work with poor cardiac reserve.

Neurological and Neuromuscular Disorders

Acute neurological disorders may require mechanical ventilation for many reasons. First, neurological disorders may result in decreased ventilatory drive and therefore result in acute hypercapnia. Second, loss of airway protective reflexes may require an artificial airway for maintaining airway integrity and for providing an access for suctioning pooled secretions. Third, mechanical ventilation may be instituted to deliberately cause hyperventilation in disorders associated with intracranial hypertension to produce hypocapnia and respiratory alkalosis. Fourth, certain acute neuromuscular disorders such as Guillain-Barré syndrome, transverse myelitis, botulism, and drugs may result in decreased ventilatory effort because of muscle weakness and may result in hypoventilation and hypercarbia. Mechanical ventilation is usually instituted under these circumstances until the patient recovers from the primary disorder. Mechanical ventilation is also instituted for various chronic neuromuscular disorders such as muscular dystrophy and for permanent neurological disorders such as spinal cord transection for prolonged home ventilator support.

VENTILATION FOR SELECTED UNDERLYING PATHOPHYSIOLOGY

Please also refer to chapter 4 on disease specific ventilation for detailed discussion.

Primary Respiratory Muscle Failure ("Respiratory Pump Failure")

The primary difficulty in these disorders is inadequate ventilation due to weakness of the respiratory muscles (pump failure). Tidal volumes and ventilatory rates are set to provide normal minute ventilation to maintain normocarbia. Complete control of ventilation may result in disuse muscle atrophy and complicate weaning from mechanical ventilation. Therefore, spontaneous breathing should be encouraged as much as possible. Assisted ventilation is a useful mode of ventilation in these disorders because the trigger sensitivity can be adjusted to encourage spontaneous breathing on the one hand and prevent muscle fatigue on the other. FiO_2 is usually kept to a minimum (≤ 0.3) because these disorders are not associated with inadequate oxygenation. In chronic hypoventilation, hypercarbia is often acceptable, provided the arterial pH is within the normal range. PEEP is usually set at a relatively low level (3–5 cm H_2O).

Disorders with Airway Obstruction

Provision of an artificial airway relieves respiratory distress due to upper airway obstruction (e.g. epiglottitis, croup). Respiratory failure due to lower airway obstruction poses a special problem during mechanical ventilation. Depression of cardiac output and hypotension may occur during intubation because of the institution of positive airway pressure to already hyperinflated lungs. This causes further impedance to venous return and increased pulmonary vascular resistance. Volume-controlled ventilation is the preferred mode of ventilation. Inspiratory-expiratory ratio should be at least 1:2. The expiratory time required depends on the severity of the lower airway obstruction. If the expiratory time is inadequate to empty the lung, "auto-PEEP" or "inadvertent PEEP" will result. Inadvertent PEEP results in air-trapping and hyperinflation with its attendant complications. The level of PEEP selected for patients with lower airway obstruction is controversial. There are two schools of thought: "low PEEP" and "high PEEP." Low PEEP advocates usually apply a PEEP of 3–5 cm H_2O because of the concern for pulmonary barotrauma from air-trapping and alveolar hyperinflation. In lower airway disease, air-trapping often results in an end-expiratory alveolar pressure that is higher than the proximal airway pressure because of incomplete emptying of the alveoli. This results in "auto-PEEP" or "inadvertent PEEP." End-expiratory lung volume and therefore the level of alveolar inflation will not be affected by the level of proximal set PEEP as long as it is less than the amount of auto-PEEP. In adults with severe asthma, high levels of PEEP, which is closer to the level of auto-PEEP, have been shown to decrease the magnitude of air-trapping and work of breathing without significant complications. In children with tracheomalacia or bronchomalacia, PEEP decreases the airway resistance by distending the airways and preventing dynamic compression during expiration. The use of low levels of PEEP compared with high levels has been described previously.

Parenchymal Lung Disease

Acute respiratory distress syndrome, hyaline membrane disease of the newborn, and interstitial pneumonias are examples of parenchymal lung disorders that are characterized by a reduction in FRC, an increase in closing volume above FRC, and diffuse subsegmental atelectasis. These diseases are characterized primarily by inadequate oxygenation due to V/Q mismatching and intrapulmonary shunting. Therapy should be directed toward maintaining lung volumes above closing volume throughout the respiratory cycle, increasing FRC above closing volume, and reducing V/Q mismatching and intrapulmonary shunting. The most effective method of achieving these goals is with an increase of mean lung volume, which is usually obtained with an increase of the mean airway pressure. During spontaneous breathing without any ventilatory assistance, continuous positive airway pressure (CPAP) is the most reliable method to increase lung volume. CPAP is effective in improving oxygenation in hyaline membrane disease and ARDS. During positive-pressure breathing, the level of PEEP required to maintain adequate oxygenation primarily depends on the severity of the underlying lung disease. The degree of intrapulmonary shunting, ventilation-perfusion mismatching, alveolar edema, alveolar collapse, and decreased compliance is directly proportional to the severity of lung disease. As the severity of lung disease increases, the airway pressures required to maintain adequate gas exchange also increase. Therefore, arbitrary limits cannot be placed on the level of PEEP or mean airway pressure that will be necessary to maintain adequate gas exchange. Tidal volumes should be limited to 6–8 mL/kg. Studies in adults, including the ARDS network study, have demonstrated that using high tidal volumes of 12 mL/kg is detrimental to patient outcome. When high levels of PEEP are used, PIP may reach levels that contribute to pulmonary air leak and barotrauma. Attempts to decrease PIP with the reduction of tidal volume will result in decreased mean airway pressure, mean lung volume, and decreased minute ventilation. With a high airway pressure maintained throughout inspiration, pressure-control ventilation may provide higher mean airway pressure and maintain a higher mean lung volume compared with volume-control ventilation. A general rule of thumb is to consider switching to pressure-limited time-cycled ventilation when PEEP requirement is more than 10 cm H_2O. For hyperinflation to be avoided, the end-inspiratory pause pressure should not exceed 35 cm H_2O. Hypercapnia may be permitted under these circumstances provided arterial pH is adequate (permissive hypercapnia). It has been recommended that the optimal PEEP should be set above the critical closing or critical opening pressure of the airways. This can be deduced by the lower inflection point generated with static pressure-volume loops. As the lung is inflated from zero end-expiratory pressure, in many lungs there is an abrupt change in compliance as denoted by the "lower inflection point." It is generally thought that this is the critical opening pressure of the airways above which the alveoli and airways remain open. As the lung is further inflated in increments, the pressure-volume slope increases and then abruptly changes direction as the "upper inflection point." It is generally thought that the upper inflection point reflects overdistension of the alveoli. The general recommendation is to keep the PEEP level above the lower inflection point and to keep the end-inspiratory pause pressure below the upper inflection point. Currently, bedside use of static pressure-volume loops to set PEEP is not a standard practice in infants and children. Therefore, the level of PEEP should be set by titrating the level of PEEP and selecting the level by the maximal level of improvement in oxygenation compliance seen without affecting systemic hemodynamics. The repeated collapse and reopening of the lung units at low lung volume have been shown to contribute to ventilation-induced lung injury. A strategy combining recruitment maneuvers, low-tidal volume, and higher PEEP has been shown to decrease the incidence of barotrauma or volutrauma.

Alveolar Recruitment and Derecruitment

Alveolar recruitment, by definition, means opening up of closed alveoli. In ARDS and other parenchymal lung diseases, atelectasis and consolidation are common pathological features which results in intrapulmonary shunting. The goals of positive pressure support in ARDS are to recruit closed alveoli and present derecruitment of open alveoli. The benefits of optimal lung recruitment and prevention of derecruitment are: (1) a reduction in the intrapulmonary shunt fraction and venous admixture resulting in an improvement in arterial oxygenation; (2) improvement in lung compliance; and (3) prevention of repeated alveolar collapse and reopening, which may ameliorate or prevent ventilator-induced lung injury. The primary determinants of alveolar recruitment and derecruitment are transpulmonary pressure and PEEP both of which increase mean airway pressure. Mean lung volume depends on mean alveolar pressure. Mean airway pressure has been shown to be an excellent marker of mean alveolar pressure. Increasing mean airway pressure will improve oxygenation if there is alveolar recruitment.

Currently, several techniques of alveolar recruitment have been described in the literature. These include manual inflation to high airway pressures, the increase of PEEP in a stepwise manner, application of a sign maneuver, the use of pressure-limited time-cycled ventilation with a high peak inspiratory pressure, and the combination of titrated levels of PEEP with increased inflation pressures. Ventilatory sighs are effective in recruiting alveoli in ARDS. They are effective, however, only from an optimal level of PEEP that does not result in derecruitment. At optimal PEEP, a sigh maneuver increases end-expiratory lung volume and improves oxygenation.

Heart Failure

The goals in respiratory management in congestive heart failure are prevention and relief of alveolar collapse from alveolar and interstitial edema due to pulmonary vascular congestion, as well as decreased oxygen demand on the heart with a reduction in the work of breathing. CPAP/PEEP will provide relief of atelectasis. Hyperinflation should be avoided because it may increase pulmonary vascular resistance and increase right ventricular afterload. The oxygen cost of breathing can be reduced with a decrease in the work of breathing. This can be provided by a judicious combination of controlled ventilation and sedation. By unloading the respiratory muscles, mechanical ventilation can also reduce the work of breathing. In extreme cases, muscle relaxation by neuromuscular blockers may provide additional reduction in oxygen cost of breathing. As a general principle, the greater the inotropic support a heart needs, the greater should be the respiratory support provided. Tidal volumes should be generally maintained on the lower range (8–10 mL/kg). In adults with congestive heart failure, positive intrathoracic pressure has been shown to improve cardiac output. This effect has been attributed to decreased left ventricular afterload provided by positive airway pressure.

Postoperative Management after Repair of Congenital Heart Disease

After open heart surgery, many infants and children require mechanical ventilation during the postoperative period. The duration of requirement of mechanical ventilation depends on several factors such as age of the patient, complexity of the cardiac lesion, complexity of the operative procedure, duration of bypass, duration of circulatory arrest, and postoperative cardiopulmonary status. Prolonged intubation and mechanical ventilation are more likely in children younger than 1 year of age, with more complex heart lesions, prolonged bypass and prolonged circulatory arrest times, and postoperative respiratory failure and hemodynamic instability. In the immediate postoperative period, patients should be supported with controlled mechanical ventilation until hemodynamic functions improve. Adequate PEEP should be applied to prevent and relieve atelectasis. Initially, the ventilator rate should be appropriate for the age. As the hemodynamic function improves, the rate can be weaned, as dictated by the clinical status. The choice of ventilatory parameters depends on the goals for each patient. In patients with pulmonary hypertension or pulmonary vascular disease, hyperventilation to provide respiratory alkalosis will decrease pulmonary vascular resistance and right ventricular afterload. In patients with marginal cardiac output, high airway pressures are to be avoided. In patients who have undergone a Fontan procedure, early extubation is desirable, and if that is not possible, then spontaneous ventilation should be encouraged. Because these patients are totally dependent on venous return for their cardiac output, airway pressures must be kept at a minimum. High intrathoracic pressure may not only impede venous return, but also decrease pulmonary blood flow from increased pulmonary vascular resistance.

Diseases with Abdominal Distention

The presence of abdominal distention poses a special problem. Positive intra-abdominal pressure tends to elevate the diaphragm, decrease P_{tp} (total pressure) in the lung bases, and decrease alveolar lung volumes in the lung bases. For normal lung volumes to be maintained, a greater P_{tp} has to be generated. This increases the airway pressures during positive pressure ventilation and increases work of breathing during spontaneous breathing. During positive pressure ventilation, a higher P_{tp} may cause hyperinflation of the apical regions while restoring normal volumes in the bases. Therapy should be directed primarily toward reducing the intra-abdominal pressure.

Neurological and Neuromuscular Diseases

Hyperventilation with respiratory alkalosis is an effective method of reducing intracranial pressure. High intrathoracic pressure may impede venous return from the brain by increasing central venous pressures. Therefore, high levels of PEEP are to be avoided. The goals of respiratory support in patients with acute neuromuscular diseases that are self-limiting are: (1) provision of respiratory assistance to maintain adequate minute ventilation, and (2) avoidance of disuse muscle atrophy from mechanical ventilation. Spontaneous breathing must be encouraged as much as possible. Neuromuscular blockade must be avoided.

KEY MESSAGES

- A good working knowledge of respiratory physiology is important to understand the basic mechanism of airflow to and from the lungs including resistance and compliance.
- Understanding disease pathophysiology is important and is closely related to the specific ventilator settings required for ventilating a child requiring mechanical ventilation.
- In patients with pulmonary hypertension or pulmonary vascular disease, hyperventilation to provide respiratory alkalosis will decrease pulmonary vascular resistance and right ventricular afterload. In patients with marginal cardiac output, high airway pressures are to be avoided.

- For neuromuscular conditions minimal settings are sufficient considering lung mechanics are normal and the ventilator compensates for muscular weakness by simply providing mechanical support.
- Central nervous system indications such as traumatic brain injury or raised intracranial tension due to other causes require specific ventilator settings to avoid hypercarbia and hypoxemia to continue optimal cerebral blood flow without raising the intracranial pressure.
- *All ventilator strategies* have *a common goal*: lung protective ventilation with minimal patient ventilator asynchrony.

SUGGESTED READING

1. Bhalla A, Khemani RG, Newth CJL. Pediatric applied respiratory physiology–the essentials. Paediatrics and Child Health. 2017;27(7):301-10.
2. Fuhrman BP, Zimmerman JJ, Clark RSB, et al. Pediatric Critical Care, 5th edition. Philadelphia: Elsevier; 2017.
3. Lumb A. Nunn's Applied Respiratory Physiology, 8th edition. Philadelphia: Elsevier; 2016.
4. West JB, Luks AM. West's Respiratory Physiology: The Essentials, 10th edition. Philadelphia: Wolters Kluwer; 2015.

3

Pediatric Intensive Care Unit Algorithms

Mritunjay Pao

Time is of essence while treating a child with respiratory distress or respiratory failure to prevent cardiorespiratory arrest due to severe hypoxemia or hypercarbia. For any child with respiratory distress or failure, a quick algorithmic approach is important for effective and safe outcome. Initial approach, a rapid cardiopulmonary assessment to reach a clinical diagnosis and further interventions including endotracheal intubation (rapid sequence intubation) and initiation of mechanical ventilation for patients with acute respiratory failure are lifesaving interventions.

Common pediatric intensive care unit algorithms as they relate to children with life-threatening respiratory distress or failure requiring mechanical ventilatory support have been shown in Flowcharts 1 to 3.

Flowchart 1: Management algorithm of respiratory distress/failure.

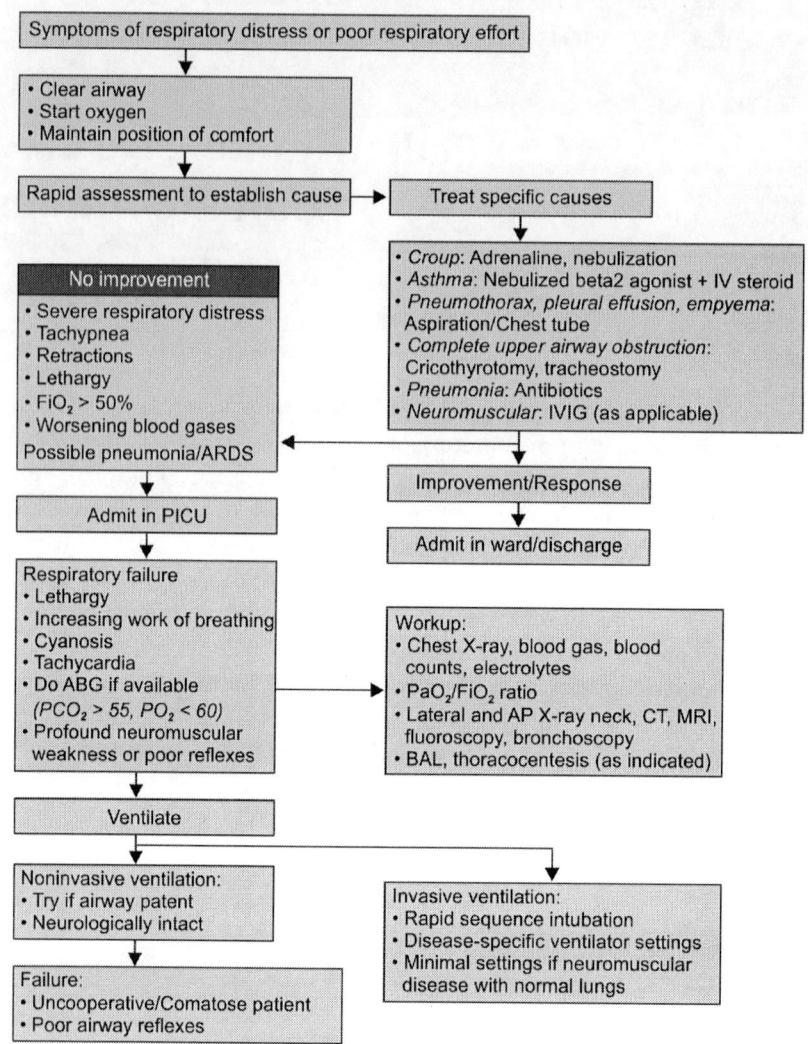

Flowchart 2: Rapid sequence intubation.

Rapid sequence intubation

Objective: To secure the airway rapidly and prevent aspiration of gastric contents

Steps:

• Preparation
• Preoxygenation
• Pretreatment
• Paralysis with induction
• Protection and positioning
• Placement with proof
• Postintubation management

Preparation

• Assess patient: anatomy (short neck, micrognathia), habitus, injuries
• Establish IV
• Monitor SpO_2
• Monitor ECG, BP continuously
• Assemble equipment: Tube and stylet, test cuff
• Choose laryngoscope blade, test light

Preoxygenation

Preoxygenate for a full 3 minutes, to wash all of the nitrogen out of the lungs and create a reservoir of O_2

Pretreatment:

• Often optional step
• Mitigate adverse reactions
• Lidocaine: 1 mg/kg
• Opioids
• Atropine for children < 8 years
• Defasciculating dose of paralytics

Paralysis with induction

• Rapidly acting induction agent:
  - Midazolam: 0.1–0.5 mg/kg
  - Ketamine: 1–3 mg/kg
• Rapidly acting neuro-muscular paralytic:
  - Succinylcholine: 1–2 mg/kg
  - Rocuronium: 1 mg/kg

Protection and positioning
Watch for apnea within 20 seconds

• Bag mask ventilation
• Sellick's maneuver
  - Cricoid cartilage pressure
  - Helps prevent aspiration
  - Continue until tube is placed or paralysis worn off
  - No bagging during rapid sequence intubation (RSI) after induction

Placement with proof

• Tube placement:
  - Test jaw for flaccidity 45 seconds after succinylcholine
  - Insert ETT
  - Sellick's maneuver discontinued after cuff inflated
• Confirm tube placement:
  - $ETCO_2$
  - Breath sounds
  - Chest rise
  - Chest X-ray

Postintubation management
• Secure tube
• Recheck vital signs
  - Heart rate
  - Blood pressure

Postintubation management
Medications:
• Continued paralysis
    Vecuronium: 0.1 mg/kg
• Sedation
  - Benzodiazepines
  - Opioids

Flowchart 3: Respiratory failure—mechanical ventilation.

Indications for mechanical ventilation
1. Respiratory failure:
   • Apnea, respiratory arrest
   • Inadequate ventilation: $PCO_2 > 55$
   • Inadequate oxygenation: $PO_2 < 60$
   • Chronic respiratory failure + FTT
2. Cardiac insufficiency/shock
3. Neurologic dysfunction:
   • Central hypoventilation/ frequent apnea
   • GCS < 8
   • Inability to protect airway

Rapid sequence intubation
Secure the airway rapidly and prevent aspiration of gastric contents.

Steps
• Preparation
• Preoxygenation
• Pretreatment
• Paralysis with induction
• Protection and positioning
• Placement with proof
• Postintubation management

Tube placement
Use *Sellick's maneuver*
Confirm tube placement:
• $ETCO_2$/Breath sounds
• Adequate chest rise
• Secure tube
• Chest X-ray
Recheck vital signs:
• Heart rate
• Blood pressure
Medications:
• Continued paralysis
  - Vecuronium: 0.1 mg/kg/hour
• Sedation
  - Benzodiazepines/Opioids

Initial ventilator settings
FiO_2: 100%
Rate: 30–40 neonates, 20–30 for infants and small children, older children and for adolescents
Inspiratory time: (I:E: 1:2–1:3)
   Neonates: 0.3–0.4 sec
   Small children: 0.5–0.6 sec
   Older children: 0.7–0.9 sec
PEEP: 3–5 cm H_2O
Pressure control:
   PIP: Neonates: 18–22 cm H_2O, children: 18–25 cm H_2O (Adequate chest rise)
Volume control:
   Tidal volume: 6–10 mL/kg (Adequate chest rise)

Adjustments after initiation
Remember: Tidal volume or PIP should be sufficient to make the chest move adequately
Check for adequate:
   Bilateral air entry
   Chest rise and SpO_2
Check ABG:
To improve oxygenation:
   Adjust: FiO_2, PEEP, inspiratory time, PIP, VT (Rapidly bring down to lowest tolerable level)
To improve ventilation:
   Adjust: Respiratory rate, tidal volume, PIP

Management of low PAO_2
Do not just increase FiO_2
Increase inspiratory time, increase VT/PIP
If O_2 worsens get CXR to rule out air leak/pneumothorax

Optimize cardiac output— fluid/Inotrope

Keep hemoglobin > 9 mg/dL

Maintain normothermia

Rule out tube obstruction/ suction
Deepen sedation/consider paralysis

Management of high $PACO_2$
Increase PIP/volume
Increase frequency

Decrease dead space: decrease PEEP, increase cardiac output

Decrease CO_2 production: bring down temperature, sedate, decrease carbohydrate load

Rule out blocked/misplaced endotracheal tube, fix leaks in the circuit, endotracheal tube cuff, humidifier

Measures to minimize barotrauma
Permissive hypercapnia:
Tolerate higher pCO_2 to limit PIP as long as pH > 7.2

Permissive hypoxia:
Tolerate PaO_2 of 55–65, SaO_2 88–90% in exchange for limiting FiO_2 < 60% and to minimize PEEP requirements, as long as there is no metabolic acidosis

Sudden desaturation/patient-ventilator asynchrony
Use "DOPE" mnemonic:
D: displacement of tube
O: obstruction of tube
P: pneumothorax
E: equipment failure
Check tube placement if in doubt take tube out and ventilate manually with 100% O_2
Examine patient: is the chest rising? Breath sounds present and equal?
Look for atelectasis, bronchospasm, pneumothorax

($ETCO_2$: end-tidal CO_2; FTT: failure to thrive; GCS: Glasgow coma scale; PaO_2: partial pressure of oxygen; pCO_2: partial pressure of CO_2; PIP: peak inspiratory pressure; SaO_2: arterial oxygen saturation; VT: tidal volume)

Disease Specific Mechanical Ventilation

Praveen Khilnani, Bhaskar Saikia , Ankur Ohri

In this chapter we will discuss case-based approach to use ventilation strategies in different diseases requiring ventilator support.

- Acute respiratory distress syndrome (ARDS) and pneumonia
- Severe asthma
- Cardiovascular illness
- Postoperative case of congenital heart disease
- Neurological illness and neuromuscular disease
- Neonatal respiratory distress syndrome
- Meconium aspiration and persistent pulmonary hypertension (PPHN)

MECHANICAL VENTILATION STRATEGIES

Acute Respiratory Distress Syndrome and Pneumonia

Case 1: A 5-year-old, premorbidly well child weighing 15 kg comes to emergency with 3 days of moderate to high grade fever and cough. He has been lethargic for the past 1 day and is not feeding well. Mother noticed that he is breathing fast since morning and has become dusky and unresponsive for the past 10 minutes. On examination, he is unresponsive with a heart rate of 140/min, respiratory rate 60/min with retractions and head bobbing. He is peripherally cyanosed, saturating 80% in air and oxyhemoglobin saturations slowly increasing to 88% in 100% oxygen. Auscultation reveals bilateral extensive crepitations. The chest X-ray is suggestive of ARDS with bilateral diffuse infiltrates in lungs with no cardiac enlargement. Liver was not enlarged.

He was intubated and ventilated on pressure regulated volume control mode (PRVC). His initial settings were:

- Tidal volume 90 mL (6 mL/kg expired tidal volume), set tidal volume of 120 mL (8 mL/kg)
- FiO_2: 1 (100%)
- Rate: 25/min
- I:E ratio 1:2
- Positive end expiratory pressure (PEEP) 6 cm of H_2O
- On these settings, his peak pressures were 36 cm.

His saturations improved to 85% on the above settings and an ABG done showed pH 7.30, PCO_2 45 mm Hg, PO_2 47 mm Hg, HCO_3 20.4, BE –5, and O_2 saturation 85%. To improve his oxygenation, his PEEP was increased to 8 cm H_2O and I:E ratio to 1:1. Following the intervention, his O_2 saturations improved to 89%. Two hours later, his O_2 saturations were gradually down to 84%. ABG revealed pH 7.25, PCO_2 52 mm Hg, PO_2 42 mm Hg, HCO_3 19, B.E –5. A repeat chest X-ray was obtained revealing bilateral diffuse infiltrates. PEEP was further titrated in increments of 2–12 cm H_2O over next 2 hours. His saturations improved to 95%. At this point his FiO_2 was decreased to (0.9) 90%. His ABG revealed pH 7.29, PCO_2 49 mm Hg, PO_2 63 mm Hg, HCO_3 22 B.E 2.

Twenty four hours later, he had sudden deterioration with desaturation to 75% persistently despite 100% oxygen on the ventilator. Endotracheal tube was checked to be properly placed and not displaced or obstructed. Ventilator was working, but chest movement was less on the right side, with diminished breath sounds. At this point hand ventilation with C circuit bag (anesthesia bag) with PEEP was started with 100% oxygen. O_2 Saturations momentarily came up to 80 but then deteriorated again. His blood pressure was 80 mm Hg, fluid bolus was given and dopamine was started immediately with mild improvement only to 85 mm Hg. A tamponade situation such as tension pneumothorax was suspected and stat chest X-ray revealed right tension pneumothorax. Right thoracostomy tube was placed. In these emergency situations chest needling in 2nd intercostals space mid-clavicular line anteriorly can be tried if chest X-ray is not immediately available (Which is a common scenario!).

Goals of Ventilation in Acute Respiratory Distress Syndrome

Ventilation should be delivered with minimal volutrauma to lungs (using low tidal volume: 6–7 mL/kg), minimal tolerable inspired oxygen with PEEP to achieve PaO_2 55–80 mm Hg and maximal tolerable arterial PCO_2 (50–60 mm Hg) with arterial pH >7.25 (permissive hypercapnia) and absence of metabolic acidosis. Conventional ventilation is the most readily available modality. Earlier standard approach used to be: Volume ventilation with tidal volume 10–15 mL/kg with PEEP, adequate filling pressures with use of fluid, and good cardiac contractility with inotropic support to prevent low cardiac output.

Problems with conventional 10–15 mL/kg tidal volume and PEEP are as follows:

Barotrauma, volutrauma, air leak (pneumothorax), chronic lung disease, delayed recovery, poor cardiac output, prolonged ventilation, and nosocomial infections.

In view of problems with conventional tidal volume ventilation: Low tidal volume strategy is recommended (NIH ARDS Network study).

This was a prospective randomized multicenter trial of 240 patients with two groups using 12 mL/kg vs. 6 mL/kg tidal volume, PEEP 5–18 cm of H_2O, FiO_2 0.3–1, showed 25% reduction in mortality in 6 mL/kg group. In another study, use of higher PEEP with lower tidal volumes (Open lung approach) has been used with improved results. It is also important to note that without specific practices or strategies for initiating mechanical ventilation (MV) in young children, clinicians look to the above mentioned study, which provides a protocol for use of a low tidal volume (V_T), permissive hypercapnia, and FiO_2 and PEEP, despite the fact that children have not been studied by the ARDS Net.

Gattinoni et al. in adults and Marraro in pediatrics ARDS patient showed benefits of prone positioning in patients with ARDS with underventilated posterior zones. Prone positioning is being recommended in patients with severe hypoxemia after low tidal volume ventilation is instituted and PEEP has been titrated and despite that patients oxygenation is not improving. In some patients immediate improvement in oxygenation occurs but in other patients it may take few hours to see the effect of improving oxygenation. If improvement is observed, up to 12 to 18 hours a day of prone positioning has been used. It is believed that prone positioning helps by improving recruitement of collapsed alveoli which were earlier in dependent positions as well as by getting the weight of heart and anterior mediastinal structures away from lungs to prevent lung compression. These maneuvers improve ventilation perfusion mismatch and oxygenation. A survival benefit has also been shown in adults with ARDS with use of prone positioning by Guerin et al. in 2014. Problems associated with prone positioning include difficulty in nursing management and monitoring (chances of accidental extubation, especially during X-ray examination, and physiotherapy).

Currently, no specific pediatric studies are available on use of prone positioning in ARDS patients and the effect on outcomes, however in view of benefits proven in adults prone ventilation is being recommended in pediatric patients with severe hypoxemia on conventional ventilation with low tidal volumes who are unresponsive to PEEP titration. Prone positioning may also be used while the patient is on high frequency ventilation.

Ventilation in Severe Asthma

Case 2: A 6-year male child presented with cough for 2 days, gradually worsening along with respiratory distress. On examination, child has altered sensorium, SpO_2 83% in room air. History of multiple episodes of wheezing with relief after nebulization. Mother had history of asthma. During this episode of wheezing, there was no significant improvement in clinical condition with conventional medical management including continuous albuterol, steroids, magnesium, and intravenous terbutaline. Subsequently, child was intubated and started on mechanical ventilation. Initial arterial blood gas revealed pH 7.00, PCO_2 85, PO_2 43, and lactate 4.5.

Most children with status asthmaticus respond to medical therapy, and only 2–6% of those admitted to the hospital require care in an intensive care unit. Out of these patients, 8.5–33% requires intubation and mechanical ventilation.

Indication of intubation and mechanical ventilation:
- Altered sensorium/coma
- Increasing and decreasing pulsus paradoxus
- Respiratory and cardiac arrest
- Acute barotrauma
- Severe lactic acidosis (especially in infants)
- Refractory hypoxemia with increasing $PaCO_2$

The goals of mechanical ventilation are:
- To decrease the work of breathing and allow respiratory muscle rest.
- To insure sufficient (not necessarily "normal") gas exchange until airway obstruction can be reversed.

Strategies of Ventilatory Support in Childhood Asthma

Major pathophysiology in asthma is inflammation, lower airway mucosal edema and mucous plugging as well as severe bronchospasm leading to increased airway resistance and expiratory obstruction, causing alveolar overdistension (dynamic hyperinflation) and generation of auto PEEP (also known as intrinsic PEEP), therefore increasing susceptibility to airleak syndrome (pneumomediastinum and pneumothorax) as well as pulsus paradoxus due to increased intrathoracic pressure producing a tamponade effect on the heart.

There is no uniform agreement about which ventilation strategies are optimal. Pressure-control mode or volume-control mode both can be used judiciously. Gentle ventilation with plateau pressure under 30 cm water is preferred with a long expiratory time, because it is capable of maintaining more consistent alveolar ventilation in the face of high and potentially changing airways resistance giving ample time for air to move out during expiration. Auto PEEP should be monitored and PEEP level should be kept less than the level of auto PEEP. Essential principle is that lung hyperinflation should be avoided (seen as beaking pointing to right on pressure volume curve on ventilator graphics (Figure 1).

Recommended initial ventilator settings include:
- *Mode*: Controlled
- Inspired oxygen fraction = 1.0.
  Tidal volume 6–8 mL/kg or Peak pressure 28–35 cm of water in pressure control mode (enough to move chest) as long as plateau pressures are below

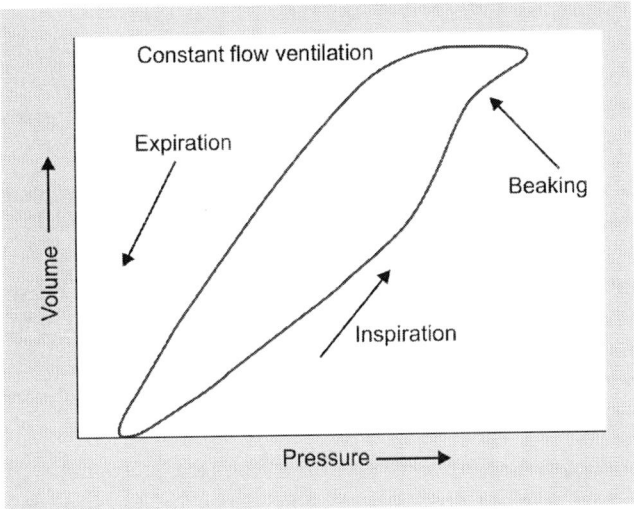

Fig. 1: Pressure–volume loop: overdistension of the lung seen as beaking.

30 cm water . Both volume and pressures need to be monitored closely, depending on the ventilator mode used.

- Respiratory rate 8–16 breaths per minute
- Inspiratory to expiratory (I:E) times should range from 1:3 to 1:5.

Positive end-expiratory pressure (PEEP) should be generally about 2–4 cm H_2O (to target to be less than the Auto PEEP measured during end expiration). Measured pressure targets during mechanical ventilation include:

- Peak airway pressure less than 35 cm H_2O
- Plateau airway pressure less than 30 cm H_2O.

Mean airway pressure (MAP) less than 25 cm H_2O. In our patient child was placed on volume cycle ventilation with tidal volume of 6 mL/kg, respiratory rate 14, PEEP of 4, plateau pressure less than 30 cm H_2O. Along with maximum medical therapy with bronchodilators and steroids, subsequent improvement was seen with ABG showing pH 7.28, PCO_2 65, PO_2 90, and lactate 2.3.

Permissive Hypercapnia

Persistent hyperinflation and high levels of airway pressure lead to pneumothorax and decreased cardiac output. To circumvent these adverse effects, strategies are aimed at intentional hypoventilation. Increased levels of $PaCO_2$ (up to 90 mm Hg) are tolerated as long as levels do not increase rapidly and with acceptable pH $\geq$ 7.2. The overall strategy of permissive hypercapnia has not been well studied in children, and its use cannot be unequivocally recommended without controlled studies.

Use of Positive End-Expiratory Pressure

Positive end expiratory pressure is generally kept to a minimum during the acute phase of mechanical ventilation in order to avoid dynamic hyperinflation and development of excessive auto-PEEP (intrinsic PEEP). However, there are two situations in which the addition of PEEP is beneficial:

- During the recovery phase, when intrinsic PEEP lessens, potentially resulting in hypoxemia from worsened V/Q mismatch and/or atelectasis.
- When "auto-PEEP" results in dynamic airways compression and inequality of ventilation. In this situation, extrinsic PEEP evens out the distribution of ventilation and improves the efficiency of pulmonary gas exchange.

Refractory Hypoxemia

In occasional patients with severe asthma, hypoxemia is a more problematic issue than hypercarbia. Readily treatable causes of hypoxemia should be sought, such as atelectasis, pneumothorax, frequent beta-2-agonist therapy, and hypovolemia.

Mechanical Ventilation for Cardiovascular Illness

Case 3: An 18-month-old boy presented with history of upper respiratory infection for 3 days with respiratory distress and poor feeding. He was diagnosed with cardiogenic shock with cardiomyopathy, presumably secondary to acute myocarditis. An echocardiogram revealed severely depressed left ventricular (LV) function and evidence of bilateral hazy lung fields with cardiomegaly. The patient was orotracheally intubated and mechanically ventilated, initial settings on the ventilator were FiO_2 of 0.6, tidal volume of 7 mL/kg (PIP of 25 mm) and PEEP of 5 cm of H_2O, rate of 22/min, inspiratory time of 0.8 sec and milrinone and epinephrine infusions were initiated. Over the next 5 days later, the patient's condition improved gradually. The epinephrine infusion discontinued. A follow-up echocardiogram demonstrated moderately depressed LV function-clearly improved from the initial study. The decision was made to extubate the patient. Two hours after extubation, the patient developed hypotension, tachycardia, and poor peripheral perfusion.

Cardiorespiratory Interactions: The Heart

Preload and afterload can be affected by fluid administration and vasoactive agents, but they can also be significantly affected by MV.

The right side of the heart obtains its blood from outside the thorax and pumps it within the thorax. As the thorax is pressurized with positive pressure ventilation (PPV), the mean intrathoracic pressure in the chest increased. This can make it more difficult for the blood from the systemic venous circulation to return through the superior and inferior vena cava to the right atrium. The higher the mean intrathoracic pressure, the more difficult it is for blood to return to the right side of the heart. PPV will always decrease right ventricular (RV) preload; however, this effect is mostly not clinically significant.

In the majority of patients whose cardiac status is otherwise reasonably healthy, compensation for the decreased RV preload is fairly good. However, this is not necessarily so in critically-ill patients. Those patients with significant lung injury requiring elevated PEEP or high MAP during high frequency oscillatory ventilation (HFOV) must be monitored closely for signs of right side heart dysfunction related to decrease preload.

The left side of the heart obtains its blood from within the thorax and pumps it outside the thorax.

Consequently, the effects of PPV on the left ventricle are the opposite of those on the right ventricle. As the thorax and lung pressurize, the lung may open to such a degree that blood is physically pushed forward into the left atrium, thus augmenting LV preload.

As the case mentioned above, deterioration after extubation is best explained by an increase in LV after load and patient with already depressed left ventricle had to generate a higher pressure to obtain the same systemic output. However, the patient's left ventricle was unable to maintain against that increase in afterload and resulted in poor cardiac output as demonstrated by hypotension and poor peripheral perfusion.

Unlike the effects of PPV on LV afterload, the effects of PPV on LV preload beyond the concept of thoracic pump augmentation can be somewhat variable because the effects of PPV on LV preload is generally based on the patient's intravascular volume status and on what has happened on the right side of the heart. If PPV is decreasing venous return to the right side of the heart, it is obviously going to decrease LV preload as well. The effects of this change in LV preload may be good or bad depending on the patient's place on the Frank-Starling curve. Thus, LV preload is complex as it can be largely affected by ventricular independence.

Cardiorespiratory Interactions: The Lungs

When the lungs are atelectatic, the large pulmonary vessels become tortuous and the resistance in the large vessels is elevated. As the lung is opened, these large vessels straighten and the resistance decreases. As the lung expands to normal lung volume and then becomes overdistended, the resistance in the large vessels is minimal.

When the lung collapsed, the resistance in the small vessels is very low. However, as the lung volume increases and the lungs overdistended, the resultant overdistended alveoli compress the surrounding capillaries, causing an elevation in the pulmonary vascular resistance (PVR) and a subsequent increase in RV afterload.

The total PVR will be highest at the extremes of alveolar over distension and lung collapse and lowest at an optimal lung volume, which is approximated by functional residual capacity (FRC). The goals are to maintain an optimal lung volume and to avoid overdistension and collapse.

Ventilator Management in Postoperative Cardiac Patient

Due to lack of randomized or nonrandomized controlled trials, examining various ventilator strategies of mechanical ventilation in the postoperative cardiac patient remains challenging. Clinicians are forced to extrapolate from animal models, case series, or individual experiences. The ventilatory management of these patients requires an individualized approach.

The application of end-expiratory pressure to the postoperative cardiac patient can have a significant negative effect on the circulatory state. However, the application of an "appropriate" level of end-expiratory pressure has substantial beneficial effects, especially in Fontan physiology. The level of "appropriate" PEEP for lung disease in the Fontan patient remains unknown. Howell et al. demonstrated that in the non-Fontan patient, PVR may fall at low levels of PEEP with subsequent increases at higher levels of PEEP. In contrast, Williams et al. demonstrated in Fontan patients that PVR is increased at all levels of PEEP (3–12 cm H_2O), and the cardiac index is decreased at high levels of PEEP (9–12 cm H_2O). PEEP maintains FRC and increases PaO_2 after the Fontan procedure and also it has been demonstrated to have beneficial effects on arterial oxygenation, atelectasis, and right-to-left shunting in children after a variety of cardiac operations.

Mechanical Ventilation in the Neurologically-Ill Patient

Neurologically ill patients not only have the potential for primary lung pathology but also predominantly neurological concerns necessitate endotracheal intubation and mechanical ventilation. These include the following:

- An adequate level of consciousness to demonstrate a central drive to breathe
- Neuromuscular strength to maintain adequate ventilation and cough to clear the airway
- An ability to swallow to manage the secretions, i.e. airway protection.

The Glasgow coma scale (GCS) is a rapid bedside tool to assess level of consciousness. Intubation is typically necessary when GCS is 8 or less especially with traumatic brain injury (TBI). Patients with an inadequate ventilator effort, impending loss of airway due to neck or pharyngeal injury, or neurological deterioration should be intubated.

Approximately, 10–20% of people with acute spinal cord injury die before reaching medical care. About 3% of patients die during acute hospitalization. Cervical spine injuries represent approximately 55% of all spinal cord injuries.

The diaphragm is innervated from the levels of C3 through C5. For this reason, a common misconception is that respiratory failure does not occur if the cord injury is below the C5 level. The musculature of the chest wall, innervated at the thoracic level, assist in a cough and deep inspiration by splinting the ribcage. Normally, the diaphragm descends and the abdomen and chest wall should rise. Without intercostals innervations, during deep inspiration when the diaphragm descends and the abdomen rises, the chest wall will collapse. As a result, the patient is unable to deep breathe or cough effectively for adequate pulmonary toilet. Patients even with high thoracic levels injury, especially if there is an accompanying aspiration or pre-existing pulmonary disease that requires clearance of secretions, may require early elective intubation.

Basic Premises of Intracranial Pressure

To understand the impact of mechanical ventilation on the brain, it is important to be familiar with the basic premises of ICP. The Monro-Kellie hypothesis maintains that within the skull, a semi-closed box, are the brain, fluid (i.e. interstitial fluid, cerebrospinal fluid), and blood. Efforts to decrease the intracranial pressure include maneuvers to decrease the intracranial volume. Acutely, these include hyperventilation, which causes vasoconstriction and thereby blood volume; sedation, and osmotic therapy with mannitol or hypertonic saline, which draw the interstitial fluid from the brain. The extent to which these maneuvers decrease the pressure depends upon the intracranial compliance.

Another basic premise in dealing with brain injury is that the difference of mean arterial pressure and ICP is cerebral perfusion pressure. Adequate CPP is between 50 mm Hg and 60 mm Hg. TBI showed that a CPP less than 60 mm Hg is predictive of poor outcome.

Oxygenation

In neurologically-injured patients, ventilator management strategies often include maintaining a partial pressure of arterial oxygen (PaO_2) 90 mm Hg or higher. In patients with high ICP and steepened cerebral compliance curves, episodes of desaturation and hypoxia are not well-tolerated. Even incrementally small changes in cerebral blood flow may increase the blood volume and are associated with elevated spikes in intracranial pressure.

Hypercarbia and Hypocarbia

Hyperventilation to $PaCO_2$ of 25–30 mm Hg can cause significant vasoconstriction and a reduction in cerebral blood flow. As a reminder, cerebral autoregulation occur in relatively intact brain, not in contusional or ischemic tissue. Vasoconstriction associated with hyperventilation may induce ischemia in areas. In one trial, patients with severe head injury were randomized to either empiric hyperventilation of $PaCO_2$ of 25 mm Hg or ventilated to a $PaCO_2$ of 35 mm Hg. Patients kept normocapnic had better outcome as measured by GCS outcome score at 3 and 6 months although these differences equalized after 1 year. Secondary cerebral ischemia may occur with hyperventilation and should be avoided. Guidelines recommend against empiric hyperventilation and avoid $PaCO_2$ <30 if hyperventilation is necessary.

Temperature

While normalizing $PaCO_2$, it is essential to remember that muscle activity and warmer temperatures are associated with increase in metabolism and higher CO_2 production. Each increase of 1°C increases the cerebral metabolic rate by 7%. If the cerebral metabolic rate goes up, so follows cerebral blood flow, blood volume, ICP, and blood pressure. Consequently, in patients with fever or hypothermic, close attention to minute ventilation is essential ventilator management in patients whom ICP is being managed.

The same principle regarding CO_2 applies to shivering. Shivering increases the metabolic rate of the muscles and so the CO_2 production. Sometimes, shivering itself will increase the ICP and CO_2 as well.

Effects of PEEP on the Brain

The effect of PEEP is relevant to ICP when it increases the right atrial pressure and superior vena cava pressure subsequently decreasing the venous outflow of the brain. When the central venous pressure (CVP) is higher than the ICP, then CVP rather than ICP becomes the determinant pressure for CPP. PEEP also affects CPP when the PEEP decreases venous return to the heart and decreases the mean arterial pressure which is subsequently decreases CPP.

Impact of Ventilation Modes

The different modes of ventilation can also affect the brain. For example, HFOV decouples oxygenation and ventilation. When using HFOV, oxygenation is determined by the MAP and the FiO_2. Lower oscillatory frequency and higher pressure amplitudes results in lower $PaCO_2$.

The effect of HFOV on ICP has been subject of a couple of studies. MAP >30 cm H_2O appears increased ICP. Higher airway pressures decrease the MAP, which will decrease the CPP.

Neuromuscular Disease: Ventilation Strategy

Case 4: A 13-year-old immunized female child weighing 30 kg was admitted with complaints of sudden onset weakness of lower limbs with inability to stand and bear weight for 2 days. The next day she developed weakness of both upper limbs such that she could only move her arms in the bed. She started to have decreased volume of voice and complained of some tingling sensation in both legs. There was no history of fever, cough, loose stools, trauma, and alteration in sensorium or seizures. She had an episode of fever with cough 2 weeks back which lasted for 3–4 days.

On examination she was alert, conscious, and oriented. Her Heart rate was 110/min and respiratory rate 30/min. She had shallow respiratory efforts with paradoxical respiration. CNS examination revealed quadriparesis with power in both lower limbs and upper limbs being 1/5 and 2/5 respectively. She had global areflexia. There was no objective sensory loss and no other focal deficits. She was diagnosed to have Guillain-Barre syndrome with respiratory muscle weakness supported by nerve conduction velocity (NCV) findings. She was ventilated for neurogenic cause of respiratory failure on SIMV mode of ventilation with the following settings:

- Tidal volume: 200 mL (6–7 mL/kg)
- Rate: 15/min
- FiO_2: 0.4 (40% O_2)
- PEEP: 3 cm H_2O
- I: E ratio 1: 2

Her ABG on the above settings was within normal limits.

Chronic/Progressive Neuromuscular Disorder—Home Ventilation

Most children with neuromuscular disease eventually require assistance with airway clearance and with breathing, especially during sleep. Techniques and devices for airway clearance and noninvasive ventilation (NIV) that are commonly used in adults have been successfully adapted for use in infants and young children. Both physiological differences and small size of young patients with neuromuscular disease, however, can limit the applicability of such interventions or require special consideration. The appropriate time to begin airway clearance assistance is lacking for young children, and the role of early introduction of NIV to preserve or enhance lung growth and chest-wall mobility remains to be elucidated. Despite these issues, a greater number of children with neuromuscular diseases are living well past their second decade.

There is a typical sequence of events that leads to respiratory insufficiency and ultimately to respiratory failure in cases like Duchenne muscular dystrophy, spinal muscular atrophy, etc. Initially respiratory muscle weakness leads to impaired cough and airway clearance, so these patients are prone to recurrent atelectasis and chest infections. Progressive inspiratory muscle weakness first causes nocturnal respiratory dysfunction, which is manifested by frequent arousals, sleep fragmentation, and sleep-related hypoventilation. Subsequently, hypercapnia extends into the day time and frank respiratory failure ensues. The duration of this timeline can be expanded by interventions such as assistance with clearance of respiratory secretions and nocturnal mechanical ventilation, or it can be compressed by acute respiratory illnesses.

Airway Clearance in Children with Neuromuscular Weakness

Assistance with airway clearance is a critical component in the care of children with neuromuscular disease, because of their propensity to develop mucus plugging and atelectasis with chest infections, and their greater exposure to common viral respiratory illnesses. In fact, acute respiratory illness leading to respiratory compromise was found to be the most common cause of unplanned admission to a pediatric intensive care unit among children with neuromuscular disease. Manual assisted cough, breath stacking, manual and mechanical insufflation, and mechanical exsufflation with negative pressure have all been used to treat pediatric patients with neuromuscular disease. The common goal of all of these interventions, used alone or in combination, is to increase the velocity of expiratory flow during a cough maneuver.

Mechanical Ventilatory Support

American and European guidelines suggest that patients with neuromuscular disease should receive ventilatory support when daytime hypercapnia ($PCO_2 > 50$ mm Hg) exists. Others have instituted nocturnal mechanical ventilation when the patient has sleep hypoventilation ($PCO_2 > 50$ mm Hg) accompanied by oxyhemoglobin desaturation (< 92%) or a history of recurrent hospitalization for pneumonia or atelectasis. Nocturnal noninvasive positive-pressure ventilation (NPPV) improves survival and reduces the frequency of hospitalization, even in children with progressive neuromuscular diseases. Nocturnal NPPV also improves diurnal gas exchange and normalizes sleep-disordered breathing. Nevertheless, the timing of institution of NPPV remains controversial. The role of mechanical ventilation in promoting lung growth, or at least preventing decline in function, in children with respiratory muscle weakness has not been fully explored. A multicenter study of the role of "preventive" NPPV in boys with Duchenne muscular dystrophy disappointingly found no evidence for preservation of lung function in those patients treated with NPPV.

Two important factors in patient adherence with NPPV are patient-ventilator synchrony and the fit and comfort of the interface. Aside from the usual possible complications related to nasal mask ventilation described in adults, including skin irritation or breakdown, sinus and ear pain, eye irritation, gastric distention and excessive leak leading to inadequate ventilation, certain problems and complications are unique to infants and small children that can undermine adherence with therapy. There is a paucity of nasal interfaces commercially available for infants and toddlers. Often, nasal prong systems are adapted for use, but they leak around the prongs, and the resistance across their narrow orifices reduces or eliminates small and weak children's ability to trigger and cycle assisted breaths, so patient-ventilator synchrony is compromised. The resistance across small prongs, coupled with the leak, can also simulate patient effort, causing some bi-level generators to auto-trigger when set in spontaneous/timed mode. For such children, a common practice is to wait for the child to fall asleep and then set the ventilator in a timed or control mode at a rate that overrides the patient's respiratory drive.[30]

Noninvasive ventilation and acute hypoxic respiratory failure (AHRF): Patients with varying comorbidities like immune compromised and status asthmaticus—in a prospective, randomized trial conducted by Hilbert and colleague, intermittent NIV was compared to standard medical treatment for patients with AHRF who were immunecompromised. The study included 52 immunosuppressed patients in the early stage of AHRF with bilateral pulmonary infiltrates and fever. Patients were randomized into one of two groups. Group 1 received NIV via a full face mask with alternating 3 hours periods 3 hours of spontaneous breathing. Group 2 received the standard medical treatment as per the institution which consists of supplemental O_2 without any ventilator support. The primary end points were rate of intubation, serious adverse events, ICU, and hospital death. Results showed the group with NIV had a decrease rate of intubation (12 NIV patient vs. 20 standard therapy patients), serious complications (13 vs. 21), fewer ICU deaths (10 vs. 18), and fewer hospital death (13 vs. 21). Therefore, the patients in this study with AHRF who were immunecompromised did benefit from NIV.

Patients with severe asthma present in extreme respiratory distress; the use of invasive artificial airways and MV in this population can be especially problematic. Patients with asthma are poor candidates for intubation since manipulation of the airway may exacerbate the airway inflammation already existing in population. Meduri and colleagues provide a descriptive report of 17 adult inpatients with status asthmaticus treated over a 3 years period. All of the patients received NIV with an acute care ventilator via full face mask. Their head of bed was elevated ≥45°, NIV pressure was set to deliver 7 mL/kg of tidal volume. Patients were given a "rest" period with no NIV every 4–6 hours. Their average length of NIV was 16 ± 2 hours. Only two patients required sedation, none required endotracheal intubation, and all survived, suggesting NIV may prove beneficial for treating patients with status asthmaticus.

Issues in Prolonged Mechanical Ventilation—Tracheostomy

Tracheostomy to be considered when it becomes apparent that the patient will require prolong mechanical ventilatory assistance after an initial period of stabilization. The patient should also be evaluated to determine if he/she will likely benefit from one of the following additional benefits associated with having a tracheostomy:

- Need for less sedation than with a translaryngeal tube
- Potential for improved respiratory mechanics as may result from decreased dead space
- Potential for psychological benefit from the ability to eat, speak, communicate, improve mobility or participate in physical therapy.

Previously, the best time to perform a tracheostomy in a patient receiving MV was controversial. The general consensus was that it was best to wait 21 days to do a tracheostomy. Today, with the availability and ease of performing a percutaneous tracheostomy and the psychological benefit to patients having one, tracheostomies are being performed earlier in the care process. One of the benefits of having a tracheostomy in place for prolonged ventilatory support is that weaning is much easier because the biggest fear of not having an airway.

Neonatal Ventilation

Ventilation in a neonate is needed for following commonly seen conditions: Apnea, hyaline membrane disease (HMD), pneumonia, congestive cardiac failure, meconium aspiration, PPHN, and postoperative ventilation. To-date, a pressure limited time cycled mode is preferred by most neonatologists. A discussion on continuous positive airway pressure (CPAP) has also been included as it remains the most frequently used mode for respiratory distress syndrome in neonates.

Continuous positive airway pressure: A continuous flow of heated humidified gas is circulated past the infants' airway at a set pressure of 3–8 cm of H_2O maintaining an elevated end expiratory lung volume while the infant breathes spontaneously. CPAP is usually delivered by means of nasal prongs or nasopharyngeal tube. It improves oxygenation by an increase in the FRC. However, over reliance on CPAP may be dangerous and it should only be used if infants show adequate respiratory effort, appear to be tolerating the procedure well and maintain adequate arterial blood (PCO_2 <50 mm Hg, pH >7.25, PaO_2 >50 mm Hg).

With all CPAP devices, some air may get into the gut and cause gastric distension. This can be prevented by using an open-ended orogastric tube in-situ. CPAP effectively splints the chest wall, keeps the airways patent; thereby, preventing obstructive apneas and atelectasis. Various studies have documented the efficacy of CPAP in respiratory distress (HMD) of mild to moderate degree. Recently, trials have been conducted on using nasal intermittent positive pressure (NIPPV) and it has been found to have similar results as CPAP. Individual CPAP machines are available. CPAP can also be delivered via nasopharyngeal route using an endotracheal tube at the level where it is just beyond the soft palate (distance of nares to angle of mandible may be used as a guide).

Conventional neonatal ventilation

Pressure limited time cycled ventilation: The most common type of ventilation used for neonates is pressure limited, time cycled ventilation where a peak inspiratory pressure (PIP) is set and gas is delivered to achieve that target pressure. In pressure limited, time cycled continuous flow ventilators following parameters are set at the outset:

- Peak inspiratory pressure
- Positive end expiratory pressure
- Inspiratory time (T_i)
- Rate/frequency (f)

This system is relatively simple and maintains good control over respiratory pressures.

Respiratory Distress Syndrome

Case 5: Respiratory Distress Syndrome (Neonatal RDS)

A neonate is born to a 24-year-old primigravida with pregnancy-induced hypertension (PIH) through lower segment cesarean section due to uncontrolled hypertension at 34 weeks of gestation. He had a birth weight of 1.8 kg. He was tachypneic at birth with a rate of 68/min and subcostal, intercostal and sternal retractions. He had grunting and had pulse oximeter saturations at 85% in room air which picked to 94% in oxygen. The chest X-ray revealed bilateral homogenous opacities suggestive of HMD. He was intubated and ventilated on pressure limited time cycled mode of ventilation with the following settings:

- PIP: 22 cm H_2O
- PEEP: 4 cm H_2O
- FiO_2: 1 (100% O_2)
- Rate: 50/min
- Inspiratory time: 0.4 sec

Optimal management of mechanical ventilation requires astute bedside clinical assessment and accurate interpretation of blood gas data and chest radiographs.

Recommended Initial Settings

- Always give fair trial of NIV--nasal CPAP (Bubble or ventilator CPAP)
  - Set flow rate
  - Set FiO_2 with blender as per target SPO_2
  - Target SPO_2
    - Preterm: 88–92%
    - Term: > 90%
  - Attach with humidifier
  - Set PEEP (5 cm or more)
  - If you are using bubble CPAP:
    - Look for bubbling and set flow rate accordingly (Note: PEEP also increases if you increase the flow rate)
    - *If no bubbling or ventilator showing leak:* Look for any leak in tubing's or from mouth, so if possible wrap mouth with splint.
  - Look for work of breathing, SPO_2, chest X-ray, ABG
  - Now how to proceed:

➤ *Step 1*: If distress is still there and FiO_2 requirement is increasing and chest X-ray revealed low FRC and white lung then increase the vPEEP up-to 8 cm of H_2O to *recruit* the lung.

➤ Signs of adequate recruitment:
- Decreased work of breathing (RR, grunting, and subcostal retraction)
- Gradual decrease in FiO_2 requirement to 21% over few minutes
- Gradual decrease in PEEP from 8 cm of H_2O to 5 cm of H_2O over few hours
- *Chest X-ray*: Good FRC

After fair trial of CPAP (PEEP is >7 cm of H_2O along with FiO_2 requirement >40%) if work of breathing is still there and baby is barely maintaining SPO_2 then consider for intubation and surfactant administration.

- *Invasive ventilation*: Conventional mechanical ventilation
  - Intubate the patient
  - Consider for Surfactant-INSURE
  - *Mode:* SIMV, SIMV + PC (PSV), PSV or volume guarantee mode as per your ventilator
  - Set parameter:
    - ➤ *Flow*: 6–8 L/min
    - ➤ *PEEP*: > 5 cm of H_2O (change as *chest X-ray –FRC*)
    - ➤ *PIP*: Look for chest rise during inspiration
    - ➤ *Rate*: If SIMV/SIMV+PC: 30–50/min. *If PSV*: Only purpose of setting is back-up rate.
    - ➤ *FiO_2*: As per your target SPO_2
    - ➤ *Ti*: 0.3–0.4 second
    - ➤ If you are using SIMV, SIMV+PC, PSV; then regulate PIP and PEEP till you to achieve the target Vt.
    - ➤ If you are using volume guarantee mode; then set target Vt and ventilator will achieve with change in pressure.
    - ➤ Always *look for*:
      - Work of breathing (RR and retraction)
      - *SPO_2*: Decrease or increase FiO_2
      - If spontaneous breathing rate is very high then most of the time it appears that you are not giving adequate pressure.
      - *Target tidal volume(Vt)*: 4–6 mL/kg
      - *Do not* give any sedation even if RR is very high, provided if tidal volume, SPO_2 and ABG is within *acceptable* range.

Inspiratory time: Adjust the I time so that there is minimal gap between inspiratory and expiratory flow waveforms. Ti is usually kept short in HMD (close to 0.25 sec) and little longer in MAS (0.35 sec). In normal lung ventilation, Ti may be as high as 0.5 sec. It is better to look at flow waveforms for final adjustment or switch to PSV mode.

Rationale for these settings is derived from clinical trials and physiologic principles.

Rapid ventilator rates and short Ti values are generally tolerated because of the characteristically low pulmonary compliance and short time constant in neonatal RDS. Always try to avoid volutrauma, as it is most dangerous.

Situation I

- Baby stable on ventilator. *Chest X-ray:* Good FRC. *ABG:* pH: 7.25, PCO_2-up to 65 mm.

  In this condition, tolerate hypercapnia if pH is ≥ 7.2 and baby is hemodynamically stable.

  If one targets to correct hypercapnia, that means peak inspiratory pressure may need to be increased leading to higher tidal volume delivery causing volutrauma and barotrauma.

Situation II

- Baby stable but blood gas is showing hypocapnia, then reduce PIP first and use high rates to maintain adequate minute ventilation. Also, tolerate permissive hypercapnia means PCO_2 in range of 55–65 cm H_2O as long as pH remains above 7.25.

Situation III

Post surfactant: After surfactant delivery, reduce their settings fast especially PIP and try to shift them to nasal CPAP. This technique is known as INSURE meaning Intubation, Surfactant administration and Rapid extubation. Our ultimate aim is to reduce the lung injury and in other way to prevent development of bronchopulmonary dysplasia.

Meconium Aspiration Syndrome

Case 6: Meconium Aspiration PPHN

A 29-year-old 2nd gravida mother delivered at 38 weeks of gestation by lower segment cesarean section in view of Meconium stained liquor (MSL). At birth, the baby was crying vigorously. He developed respiratory distress soon after birth. He was breathing at a rate of 80/min with severe retractions and was saturating 88% in 100% oxygen. His chest X-ray was suggestive of meconium aspiration syndrome (MAS). He was ventilated due to persistent hypoxia on the following settings:

- Mode: Pressure limited time cycled
- PIP: 26 cm H_2O
- PEEP: 3 cm H_2O
- Rate: 60/min
- FiO_2: 1 (100% O_2)
- I:E ratio 1:3

His post-ventilation ABG was: pH 7.18, PCO_2 56 mm Hg, PO_2 40 mm Hg, HCO_3 16.2, BE –7.5, and oxyhemoglobin saturation at 86%. An echocardiogram was done on suspicion of PPHN which showed pulmonary pressures of 90 mm Hg with systemic pressure being 82/40 mm Hg. He was started on dopamine to increase the systemic pressure and milrinone for pulmonary vasodilation. Sodium bicarbonate was given to correct acidosis and PIP was increased to 28 cm H_2O. I:E ratio was not increased due to a high risk of air leaks in MAS. After these interventions the ABG improved to pH 7.24, PCO_2 45 mm Hg, HCO_3 19.6, BE –2.6 but PO_2 remained low on 45 mm Hg. Sildenafil was administered and he was given a trial of high frequency ventilation on which his hypoxia slowly improved.

Meconium Aspiration Syndrome

Pathophysiology:
- Airway obstruction
- Chemical pneumonitis
- Surfactant inactivation
- Increased PVR

In infants with MAS without PPHN:
- Maintain pH between 7.3 and 7.4
- PaO_2 60–80 mm Hg
- $PaCO_2$ 40–50 mm Hg
- Use minimum effective PIP for adequate chest rise
- Low to moderate PEEP (3–5 cm H_2O)
- Adequate T_e, usually 0.5–0.7 sec (as both inspiratory and expiratory time constant increases in MAS) required to prevent gas trapping and air leaks.

Note: Some infants with MAS, especially those who are fighting with the ventilator, may benefit from sedation with narcotics and muscle relaxants.

In infants with PPHN:
- Ventilatory strategies differ
- Maintain high PaO_2
- Increase FiO_2 before increasing MAP
- If hypoxia persists, use high frequency ventilation

Goals of treatment:
- To maintain adequate oxygenation:
  - These babies are extremely sensitive
  - Handling them might cause a decrease in PaO_2 and hypoxia
  - Crying also causes a decrease in PaO_2. So sedate the baby or paralyze as required
- Decrease pulmonary pressure and increase systemic pressure so as to decrease the shunting and in turn maintaining good oxygenation.
  - Dilate pulmonary arteries (NO, sildenafil)
- Optimize perfusion (fluids, vasopressors)
- Oxygenate but minimize barotrauma

- Surfactant, high frequency ventilation, extracorporeal membrane oxygenation (ECMO).

Proposed ventilatory strategies in PPHN:
- *Ventilatory settings:* Recruit lung use HFOV, preferably sedate or paralyze the child.
  - *Decrease pulmonary pressure:* Hypoxia and acidosis are potent pulmonary vasoconstrictors
    - Prevent hypoxia (maintain PO_2 in range of 70–100 mm Hg, we can do it by keeping saturations of baby above 95%)
    - Prevent acidosis (try to maintain pH between 7.4 and 7.5. This can be done by inducing respiratory or metabolic alkalosis)
    - Nitric oxide, sildenafil, high frequency ventilation, ECMO.

KEY MESSAGES

- Almost all neonates can be ventilated using pressure limited time cycled ventilation. Infants under 1-2 years of age can be ventilated using pressure control.
- *For PPHN decrease pulmonary pressure:* Hypoxia and acidosis are potent pulmonary vasoconstrictors. Prevent hypoxia (maintain PO_2 in range of 70–100 mm Hg, we can do it by keeping saturations of baby above 95%)
- Volume control may be required if there is severe ARDS. Use 7–9 mL/kg tidal volume (6–8 mL expired tidal volume)
- Patients with asthma may be ventilated with pressure control with pressure support and low PEEP with higher expiratory times to avoid dynamic hyperinflation and auto PEEP.
- Patients with neuromuscular weakness (GBS) and raised ICP will require minimal settings to maintain normal ABGs and maintain PCO_2 30–35 mm Hg.

SUGGESTED READING

1. Acute Respiratory Distress Syndrome Network, Brower RG, Matthay MA, et al. Ventilation with lower tidal volumes as compared with traditional tidal volumes of acute lung injury and the acute respiratory distress syndrome. N Eng J Med. 2000;342.1301-8.
2. Amato MB, Barbas CS, Medeiros DM, et al. Effects of protective ventilation strategy in the acute respiratory distress syndrome. N Eng J Med. 1998;338:347-54.
3. Bach JR, Niranjan V, Weaver B. Spinal muscular atrophy type I: a noninvasive respiratory management approach. Chest. 2000;117(4):1100-5.
4. Bernstein G, Mannino FL, Heldtt GP, et al. Randomized multicenter trial comparing synchronized and conventional intermittent mandatory ventilation in neonates. J Pediatr. 1996;128:453-63.
5. Brain trauma Foundation, American Association of Neurological Surgeons, Joint Section on Neurotrauma and Critical Care. Guidelines for the management of severe traumatic brain injury. J Neurotrauma. 2000;17:457-554.

6. Chatwin M, Ross E, Hart N, et al. Cough augmentation with mechanical insufflation/exsufflation in patients with neuromuscular weakness. Eur Respir J. 2003;21(3):502-8.

7. Coles JP, Minhas PS, Fryer TD, et al. Effect of Hyperventilation on cerebral blood flow in traumatic head injury: clinical relevance and monitoring correlates. Crit Care Med. 2002;30:1950-9.

8. Cox RG, Barker GA, Bohn DJ. Efficacy, results and complications of mechanical ventilation in children with status asthmaticus. Pediatr Pulmonol. 1991;11:120-6.

9. DeNicola LK, Monem GF, Gayle MO, et al. Treatment of critical status asthmaticus in children. Pediatr Clin North Am. 1994;41:1293-324.

10. De Vivo MJ, Krause MJ, Lammertse DP. Recent trends in mortality and causes of death among persons with spinal cord injury. Arch Phys Med Rehabil. 1999;80:1411-9.

11. Do Boer RC, Jones A, Ward PS, et al. Long term trigger ventilation in neonatal respiratory distress syndrome. Arch Dis Child. 1993;68:308-11.

12. Dworkin G, Kattan M. Mechanical ventilation for status asthmaticus in children. J Pediatr. 1989;114:545-9.

13. Finder JD, Birnkrant D, Carl J, et al. Respiratory care of the patient with Duchenne muscular dystrophy: ATS consensus statement. Am J Respir Crit Care Med. 2004;170(4):456-565.

14. Gattinoni L, Togononi G, Pesenti A, et al. Effects of prone positioning on the survival of patients with acute respiratory failure. N Eng J Med. 2001;345:568-73.

15. Guérin C. Prone ventilation in acute respiratory distress syndrome. European Respiratory Review. 2014;23:249-57.

16. Hilbert G, Gruson D, Gargas F, et al. Noninvasive ventilation in immunosuppressed patients with pulmonary infiltrates, fever, and acute respiratory failure. N Eng J Med. 2001;344:481-7.

17. Howell JBL, Permutt S, Proctor DF, et al. Effect of inflation of the lung on different parts of the pulmonary vascular bed. J Appl Physiol. 1961;16:71-6.

18. Kattwinkel J, Nearman HS, Franoff AA, et al. Apnea of prematurity. Comparative Therapeutic effects of cutaneous stimulation and nasal continuous positive airway pressure. J Pediatr. 1975;86:588-92.

19. Katz S, Selvadurai H, Keilty K, et al. Outcome of non-invasive positive pressure ventilation in paediatric neuromuscular disease. Arch Dis Child. 2004;89(2):121-4.

20. Khilnani P. Pediatric and Neonatal Mechanical Ventilation, 2nd edition. New Delhi: Jaypee Brothers Medical Publishers (P) Ltd; 2011.

21. Luce JM, Husbey JS, Kirk W, et al. Mechanism by which positive end-expiratory pressure increases cerebrospinal fluid pressure in dogs. J Appl Physiol Respir Environ Exerc Physiol. 1982;52:231-5.

22. Marraro GA. Innovative practices of ventilatory support with pediatric patients. Pediatr Crit Care Med. 2003; 4:8-20.

23. Meduri GU, Cook TR, Turner RE, et al. Noninvasive positive pressure ventilation in status asthmaticus. Chest. 1996;110:767-74.

24. Muizelaar JP, Marmarou A, Ward JD, et al. Adverse effect of prolonged hyperventilation in patients with severe head injury: a randomized clinical trial. J Neurosurg. 1991;75:731-9.

25. Osundwa VM, Dawod S. Four-year experience with bronchial asthma in a pediatric intensive care unit. Ann Allergy. 1992;69:518.

26. O'Rourke J, Sheeran P, Heaney M, et al. Effects of sequential changes from conventional ventilation to high-frequency oscillatory ventilation at increasing mean airway pressures in an ovine model of combined lung and head injury. Eur J Anaesthesiol. 2007;24:454-63.

27. Pediatric acute respiratory distress syndrome: consensus recommendations from the pediatric acute lung injury consensus conference: The Pediatric Acute Lung Injury Consensus Conference Group. Pediatr Crit Care Med. 2015;16(5): 428-39.

28. Petty T. CO_2 can be good for you. Respir management. 1987;17:7.

29. Raphael JC, Chevret S, Chastang C, et al. Randomized trial of preventative nasal ventilation in Duchenne muscular dystrophy. French Multicentre Cooperative Group on Home Mechanical Ventilation Assistance in Duchenne de Boulogne Muscular Dystrophy. Lancet. 1994;343(8913):1600-4.

30. Rossi A, Santos C, Roca J, et al. Effects of PEEP on V/Q mismatching in ventilated patients with chronic airflow obstruction. Am J Respir Crit Care Med. 1994;149:1077.

31. Rutgers M, Lucassen H, Kesteren RV, et al. Respiratory insufficiency and ventilatory support. 39th ENMC International Workshop, Naarden, The Netherlands, 26–28 January 1996. European Consortium on Chronic Respiratory Insufficiency. Neuromuscul Disord. 1996;6(6):431-5.

32. Simonds AK, Ward S, Heather S, et al. Outcome of paediatric domiciliary mask ventilation in neuromuscular and skeletal disease. Eur Respir J. 2000;16(3): 476-81.

33. Simonds AK. Paediatric non-invasive ventilation. In: Simonds AK, (Ed). Non-invasive respiratory support, 2nd edition. London: Arnold; 2001. pp. 177-202.

34. Stein R, Canny GJ, Bohn DJ, et al. Severe acute asthma in a pediatric intensive care unit: Six years' experience. Pediatrics. 1989;83:1023-8.

35. Teague WG. Long-term mechanical ventilation in infants and children. In: Hill NS, (Ed). Long-term mechanical ventilation. New York: Marcel Dekker; 2001. pp. 177-213.

36. Tuxen DV. Detrimental effects of positive end-expiratory pressure during controlled mechanical ventilation of patients with severe airflow obstruction. Am Rev Respir Dis. 1989;140:5-9.

37. Venkataraman ST, Orr RA. Mechanical ventilation and respiratory care. In: Fuhrman BP, Zimmerman JJ (Eds). Pediatric Critical Care. St.Louis: Mosby; 2011.

38. Vianello A, Bevilacqua M, Salvador V, et al. Long-term nasal intermittent positive pressure ventilation in advanced Duchenne's muscular dystrophy. Chest. 1994;105(2):445-8.

39. Williams DB, Kiernan PD, Mctke MP, et al. Hemodynamic response to positive end-expiratory pressure following right atrium-pulmonary artery bypass (Fontan procedure). J Thorac Cardiovasc Surg. 1984;87:856-61.

5

Neonatal Continuous Positive Airway Pressure and Nasal Intermittent Positive Pressure Ventilation

Kumar Ankur, Naveen Gupta, Anil Batra

Continuous positive airway pressure (CPAP) is positive pressure applied to the airways of a spontaneously breathing baby throughout the respiratory cycle. Advocates of noninvasive ventilation cite the reduced risk of trauma to the larynx and trachea, infection and acute and chronic lung disease with this form of support. The rationale for use of CPAP is to support the airways and avoid alveolar collapse to a level below functional residual capacity (FRC).

How does CPAP work?

Continuous positive airway pressure supports the breathing of premature infants in a number of ways. The upper airway of the preterm infant is very compliant and therefore prone to collapse. CPAP splints the upper airway and therefore reduces obstruction and apnea. CPAP assists expansion of the lungs and prevents alveolar collapse. In doing so, it reduces protein leak and conserves surfactant.

Physiology and how CPAP helps

Preterm: Inability to maintain FRC due to various reasons:

- Not able to generate enough negative pressure to achieve an effective FRC
- Has low laryngeal tone to maintain positive end expiratory pressure (PEEP) by grunting
- Fluid clearance from lung depends on gestational age of baby because of immature amiloride-sensitive Na channel
- Lack of fat laden superficial fascia in the neck → which stabilize the airway
- Not able to mobilize the genioglossus muscle effectively which normally stabilizes the pharynx
- Insufficient numbers of alveolar channels for collateral ventilation
- Chest wall is soft and horizontal ribs are flatter, reducing the potential for lung expansion
- During rapid eye movement (REM) sleep, intercostal muscle activity may be lost
- Patent ductus arteriosus (PDA) predisposing to pulmonary edema
- Deficient surfactant.

EFFECTS OF CONTINUOUS POSITIVE AIRWAY PRESSURE IN THE INFANT WITH RESPIRATORY DISTRESS

- Reduces upper airway occlusion by decreasing upper airway resistance and increasing the pharyngeal cross-sectional area.
- Increases the FRC.
- Reduces inspiratory resistance by dilating the airways. This permits a larger tidal volume for a given pressure, reducing the work of breathing.
- Increases the compliance and tidal volume of stiff lungs with a low FRC by stabilizing the chest wall and counteracting the paradoxical movements.
- Regularizes and slows the respiratory rate.
- Reduces the incidence of apnea.
- Increases the mean airway pressure and improves ventilation perfusion mismatch.
- By diminishing alveolar edema conserves surfactant on the alveolar surface.

Components of Continuous Positive Airway Pressure System (Table 1)

Continuous Positive Airway Pressure Delivery

Continuous Positive Airway Pressure Interfaces: Nasal continuous positive airway pressure devices (Fig. 1) fall into four groups:

1. A long nasopharyngeal tube
2. A single nasal prong
3. Nose masks
4. Short binasal prongs.

Table 1: Components of a CPAP system.	
Factor	*Relevance*
Pressure-generating device	• Constant vs variable pressure influencing potential for gas exchange and airway recruitment • Constant vs variable flow influencing work of breathing
Heated and humidified circuit	Delivery of appropriate gas energy and saturation content at high flow to avoid mucosal injury and avoidance of condensation
Blended gas source	Avoidance of hyperoxia/hypoxia
Patient interface	Influences ease of application, rebreathing, extrinsic work of breathing and potential for local injury
Safety pressure release and alarm	• Avoidance of over pressurization with obstruction of expiratory tubing • Alert carer to potential deprivation of fresh gas associated with inspiratory limb obstruction

(CPAP: continuous positive airway pressure)

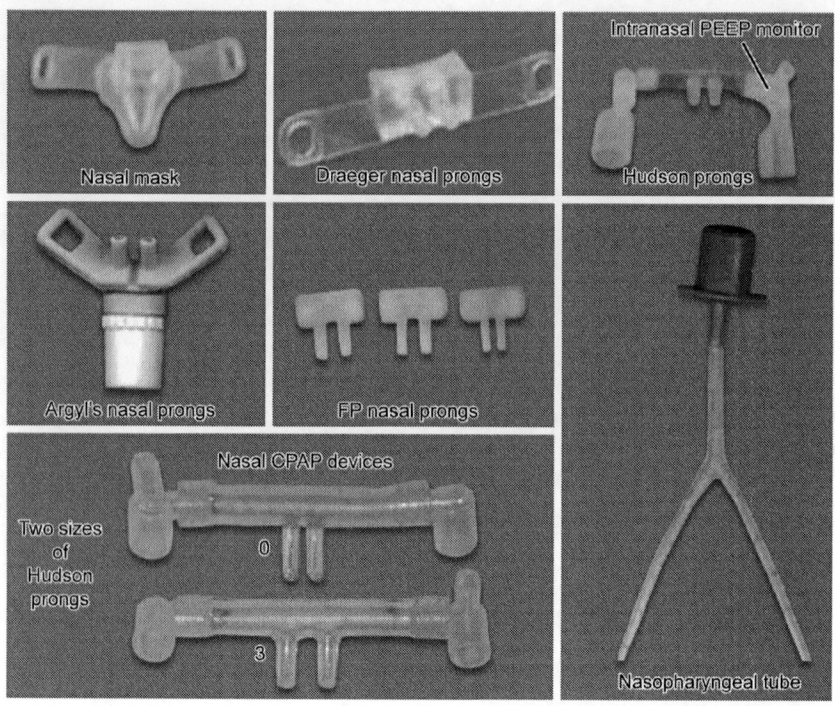

Fig. 1: Different types of nasal interfaces. (*For color version see Plate 1*)
(CPAP: continuous positive airway pressure; PEEP: positive end expiratory pressure)

Short binasal prongs are more effective at preventing reintubation than single nasal prong.

The way CPAP pressure is generated is distinct from the interface device. There are four techniques for generating NCPAP.

1. *Bubble NCPAP (Fig. 2):* With this technique, gas flows past the nasal device and the pressure is generated in the circuit by placing the distal limb of the CPAP circuit under a known depth of water. Gas flow is increased until continuous bubbling is achieved.

2. *Ventilator CPAP:* The ventilator PEEP (positive end expiratory pressure) valve controls the CPAP delivered.

3. *Variable flow NCPAP devices (Fig. 3):* These devices have an integrated nasal interface and pressure generator. They use a higher gas flow than other devices and pressure is generated by increased resistance as the gas leaves the nasal device. The pressure is determined by altering the flow of gas into the device.

4. *High flow nasal cannulae:* High flow cannulae deliver gas flows >2 L/min into the nostrils through small prongs which are loose in the nostrils. Low flow cannulae are used to deliver supplemental oxygen whereas high flow cannulae are used because it is thought that they provide some CPAP.

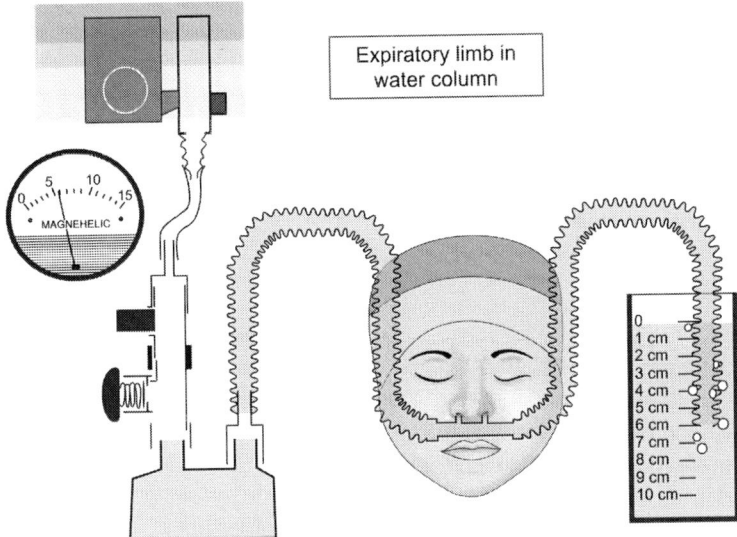

Fig. 2: Bubble nasal continuous positive airway pressure (NCPAP).

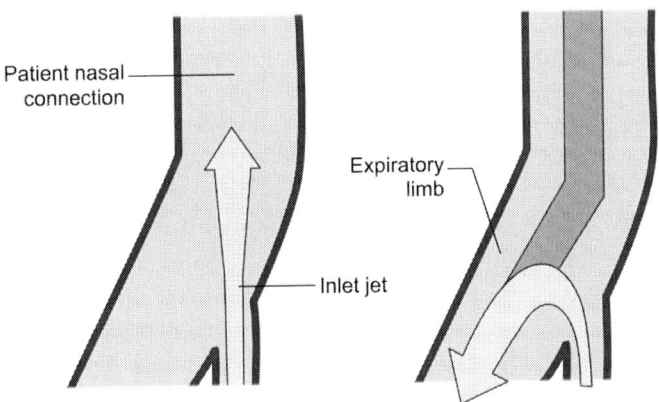

Fig. 3: Variable flow/fluidic flip.

Problems of Nasal Continuous Positive Airway Pressure

- *Leak at the nose and mouth:* It has been reported that the pharyngeal pressure drops markedly when the CPAP supported infant opens his mouth. The use of chin strap or pacifier is recommended to reduce mouth leak for effective CPAP support. However, it should not be so tight as to prevent the infant from yawning or crying but tight enough to prevent leaking at rest.
- *Nasal trauma:* It is mostly caused by incorrect positioning of the prongs. To prevent injury, the nasal device must not be pushed up against the columella. Injury can also *occur inside the* nose and erode the nasal septum if the prongs are not positioned straight into the nostrils.

- *Gastric distension*: Gastric distension is common in the CPAP supported infant (CPAP Belly Syndrome). Frequent decompression of the stomach with an oro-gastric tube is necessary to promote comfort, preventing the distended stomach from splinting the diaphragm and compromising respiration.

How to prevent nasal septal injury?

Nasal septal injury is absolutely preventable by checking following things:
- Snugly fitting nasal prongs
- Secure caps
- Lightweight interface
- Correct positioning and attachment of corrugated tubing (bubble)
- Velcro moustache (Hudson prong, bubble CPAP)
- *Careful, frequent observation*: give rest
- Careful positioning of the infant

Indications for Nasal Continuous Positive Airway Pressure

- Delivery room NCPAP
- Respiratory distress syndrome
- Prophylactic CPAP for very preterm
- Post-extubation

NASAL INTERMITTENT POSITIVE PRESSURE VENTILATION

Any mode of assisted ventilation that delivers positive pressure throughout the respiratory cycle with additional phasic increases in airway pressure, without the presence of an endotracheal tube. These additional phasic increases in airway pressure may be either synchronized or nonsynchronized depending on the delivery system used. Nasal intermittent positive pressure ventilation (NIPPV) provides the benefits of CPAP with the addition of positive pressure breaths.

How does NIPPV work?

The mechanism of action of NIPPV remains uncertain. It is unclear whether mechanical inflations during NIPPV are transmitted to the lungs. Moretti showed that some synchronized breaths were transmitted, but asynchronous breaths were not.

Delivery of Nasal Intermittent Positive Pressure Ventilation

Devices to generate NIPPV: Ventilators can be used to deliver nonsynchronized nasal intermittent mandatory ventilation (NIMV). The only specialized devices which attempt to provide synchronized NIPPV are the Infant Flow SiPAP and Infant Flow Advance–IFDa (Viasys Healthcare, Conshohocken, PA, USA).

Nasal interface: Mask or Prong

How to start NIMV: Ventilator settings

- Changed from CPAP mode to intermittent mandatory ventilation (IMV) mode
- *Positive end expiratory pressure*: 5 or more as determined by lung disease
- *Peak inspiratory pressure*: 2–4 cm H_2O higher than pre-extubation PIP "to see the chest rise" or specific target pressures (16–20 cm H_2O)
- *Rate*: 35–50/min
- *I time*: According to diseased lung
- Monitor work of breathing, apnea, SPO_2, PCO_2 (if required), Chest X-ray

However, the delivered pressure may be lower than the set pressure due to leak at the nose and mouth.

Indications:

- Respiratory distress syndrome (RDS) as a primary treatment
- Apnea of prematurity
- Post-extubation

Criteria to discontinue NIMV:

- *Blood gas*: if pH <7.2 and PCO_2 >65 mm
- Inability to improve gas exchange or increased work of breathing
- Hemodynamic instability

Initiation of Nasal Continuous Positive Airway Pressure

- Try to put baby on CPAP as early as possible, before marked atelectasis sets in. A preterm neonate with RDS is better started on CPAP, right at delivery area and transported to neonatal intensive care unit (NICU) on same mode, as waiting for CPAP till arrival to NICU may cause unnecessarily delay and alveolar collapse.
- Do not rely on oxygen delivery tubing sets for CPAP. Use conventional CPAP circuits, either bubble CPAP or ventilator driven CPAP. Preferably use binasal short prongs.
- Start with PEEP 6–8 cm of H_2O and adjust FiO_2 to maintain SPO_2 in target range (85–95%).
- Success of CPAP is defined by decrease in work of breathing (WOB) to acceptable level, which is usually noticed within 30–60 minutes. Grunting should disappear and retractions should decrease to acceptable limits.

Maintaining and Weaning from Continuous Positive Airway Pressure

- If baby stabilizes on CPAP with acceptable WOB and FiO_2 <50%, CPAP may be continued.
- Pressure and FiO_2 may be reduced gradually as per clinical condition and response.

- Once FiO_2 is <25–30% and CPAP level <5, baby may be weaned off CPAP to O_2 by nasal cannula, though many wait till baby come to 21% FiO_2 before weaning off.
- Duration of CPAP may be as short as couple of hours in mild disease to as long as several weeks in severe lung disease.
- While ventilating the neonate, take care that baby is not too agitated. It may induce pneumothorax. Try to eliminate the reason of irritation and pacify the baby.

Failure of Continuous Positive Airway Pressure

- Persistent severe retractions and/or grunting or FiO_2 need >40–50% even after 30 minutes of CPAP may be considered as indications of intubation and mechanical ventilation. Other indications of intubation are repeated episodes of apnea (despite xanthenes), or marked acidosis (pH <7.2). Failure of CPAP is as follows:
  - Persistently high WOB despite adequate CPAP (6–8)
  - FiO_2 need >40–50%
  - Repeated episodes of apnea, nonresponsive to xanthine therapy (caffeine citrate or theophylline)
  - Severe acidosis (pH <7.2)
- Before declaring failure of CPAP, check whether CPAP is being delivered effectively. If baby is too agitated or there is significant leak of flow through mouth, enough pressure will not be generated. Try to pacify the baby by massaging/stroking/caressing. Look if nasal prongs/assembly is hurting the baby. May consider soother or gentle strapping of chin.
- If baby gets repeatedly apneic on CPAP:
  - Look for airway obstruction
  - Start/escalate xanthines if apnea of prematurity
  - Rule out other causes of apneas.

KEY MESSAGES

- Continuous positive airway pressure is positive pressure applied to the airways of a spontaneously breathing baby throughout the respiratory cycle. CPAP assists expansion of the lungs and prevents alveolar collapse. In doing so, it reduces protein leak and conserves surfactant.
- Persistent severe retractions and/or grunting or FiO_2 need >40–50% even after 30 minutes of CPAP may be considered as indications of intubation and mechanical ventilation. Other indications of intubation are repeated episodes of apnea (despite xanthenes), or marked acidosis (pH <7.2).
- In NIPPV mode, assembly is same as for nasal CPAP, only difference is that on top of PEEP, positive breaths are added at a certain rate. This further augments infants spontaneous efforts and NIPPV has been shown to reduce the intubation rate in infants who were failing on CPAP.

SUGGESTED READING

1. Behnke J, Lemyre B, Czernik C, et al. Non-Invasive Ventilation in Neonatology. Dtsch Arztebl Int. 2019;116(11):177-83.
2. Dewez JE, van den Broek N. Continuous positive airway pressure (CPAP) to treat respiratory distress in newborns in low- and middle-income countries. Trop Doct. 2017;47(1):19-22.
3. Duke T. CPAP: a guide for clinicians in developing countries. Paediatr Int Child Health. 2014;34:3-11.
4. Edwards MO, Kotecha SJ, Kotecha S. Respiratory distress of the term newborn infant. Paediatr Respir Rev. 2013;14:29-36.
5. Ho JJ, Subramaniam P, Henderson-Smart DJ, et al. Continuous distending pressure for respiratory distress syndrome in preterm infants. Cochrane Database Syst Rev. 2015;7:CD002271.
6. Lemyre B, Davis PG, De Paoli AG, et al. Nasal intermittent positive pressure ventilation (NIPPV) versus nasal continuous positive airway pressure (NCPAP) for preterm neonates after extubation. Cochrane Database Syst Rev. 2017;2:CD003212.
7. Lemyre B, Laughon M, Bose C, et al. Early nasal intermittent positive pressure ventilation (NIPPV) versus early nasal continuous positive airway pressure (NCPAP) for preterm infants. Cochrane Database Syst Rev. 2016;2016(12): CD005384.
8. Martin S, Duke T, Davis P. Efficacy and safety of bubble CPAP in neonatal care in low and middle income countries: a systematic review. Arch Dis Child Fetal Neonatal Ed. 2014;99:F495-504.
9. Permall DL, Pasha AB, Chen XQ. Current insights in non-invasive ventilation for the treatment of neonatal respiratory disease. Ital J Pediatr. 2019;45:105.
10. Shi Y, De Luca D, for the NASal OscillatioN post-Extubation (NASONE) study group. Continuous positive airway pressure (CPAP) vs noninvasive positive pressure ventilation (NIPPV) vs noninvasive high frequency oscillation ventilation (NHFOV) as post-extubation support in preterm neonates: protocol for an assessor-blinded, multicenter, randomized controlled trial. BMC Pediatr. 2019;19:256.
11. Tapia JL, Urzua S, Bancalari A, et al. Randomized trial of early bubble continuous positive airway pressure for very low birth weight infants. J Pediatr. 2012;161:75-80.

High Flow Nasal Cannula Oxygen Therapy

Ebor Jacob, Neeraj Sagar, Abhijit Singh

High flow nasal cannula (HFNC) therapy is a relatively new entrant and one of the most important developments in respiratory medicine since the introduction of noninvasive ventilation over 25 years ago. Heated, humidified, HFNC therapy is a method for providing oxygen and a high flow which generates a continuous airway pressure to children with respiratory distress. This provides a valuable triad of warming, humidification, and high flow which ends up in improved patient compliance. It is designed to deliver conditioned gas, flows in an open system via simple nasal cannula-set prongs and not designed to deliver set pressure.

Traditional oxygen flow devices include:

- *Low-flow devices:* Oxygen at flow rates that are lower than patients' inspiratory demands; when the total ventilation exceeds the capacity of the oxygen reservoir, room air is entrained.
- *High-flow devices:* Constant FiO_2 by delivering the gas at flow rates that exceed the patient's peak inspiratory flow rate and by using devices that entrain a fixed proportion of room air (NRBM, Venturi mask, etc.).

In the year 1993, Locke first described it; initial systems were nonheated. In the year 2001, Sreenan coined term "HFNC." In the past decade, widespread worldwide acceptance in neonatal intensive care unit (NICU)'s, pediatric intensive care unit (PICU)'s and now even in adults. Term "heated humidified high flow nasal cannula (HHHFNC) system" is also commonly used.

CURRENTLY AVAILABLE DEVICES IN THE MARKET

Air/oxygen blender—humidifier: Optiflow System (Fisher and Paykel, New Zealand) (Fig. 1A), Precision Flow (Vapotherm, Exeter, UK), and Comfort-Flo (Teleflex Medical, Durham, NC, USA). Airvo2 (Fig. 1B), Fisher and Paykel, New Zealand uses a turbine + humidifier (Table 1). This system has the advantage of not requiring an external source of gas, except oxygen.

COMPONENTS OF THE HHHFNC SYSTEM

- Humidifier breathing circuit (one limb)
  - Infant/Pediatric Respiratory Care System—use with infant/pediatric size cannula

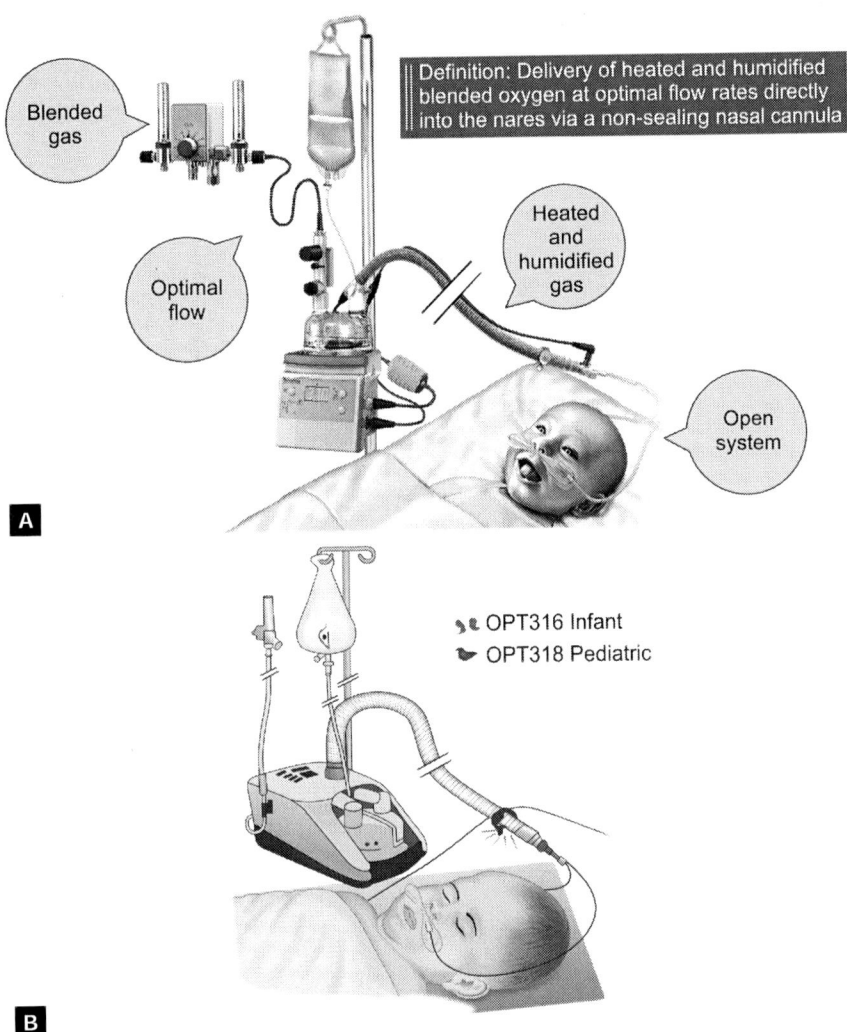

Figs. 1 A and B: (A) Optiflow and (B) AIRVO 2 (Fischer & Paykel).

Table 1: Differences between OPTIFLOW and AIRVO 2.	
OPTIFLOW	*AIRVO 2*
• Needs compressed wall air, oxygen and flow meters	• No compressed gas or flow meter needed
• Blender and humidifier	• Inbuilt blender, humidifier
• No oxygen analyzer	• Inbuilt oxygen analyzer
• Circuits marginally cheaper	• Equipment and circuits more expensive

- Adult Respiratory Care System—use with adult-size cannula and trache-interface
■ Nasal cannula sizes
■ Humidifier base

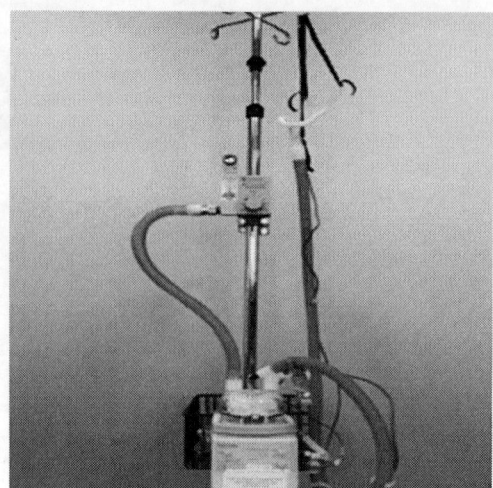

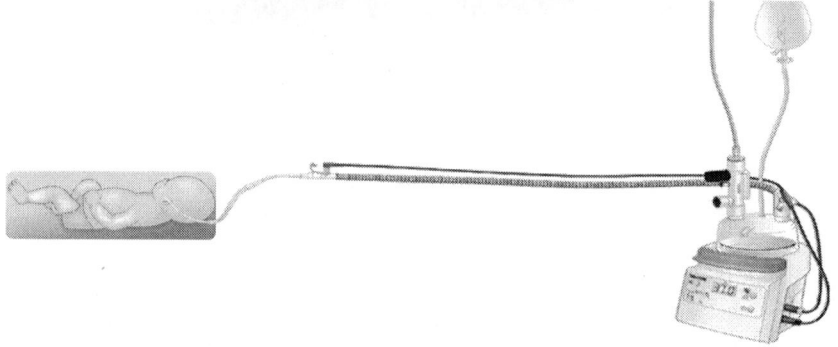

Fig. 2: Basic set up of high flow nasal cannula (HFNC). (*For color version see Plate 2*)

- Oxygen flow meter (older children—high flow)
- Sterile 1 Le water bag/or bottle of sterile water

Basic Set up of HFNC

The basic set up of HFNC is given in Figure 2.

Nasal cannula (high flow) (Fig. 3 and Table 2):

- Soft, flexible, wide bore cannula
- Specifically designed to deliver heated and humidified gas
- Combination of a nasal cannula and optimal humidity enables comfortable delivery of a wide range of flows.

How is different from standard nasal cannula oxygen (Table 3)?

Indications

- High flow can be tried if there is hypoxemia (SPO_2 <94%) and signs of moderate to severe respiratory distress despite standard flow

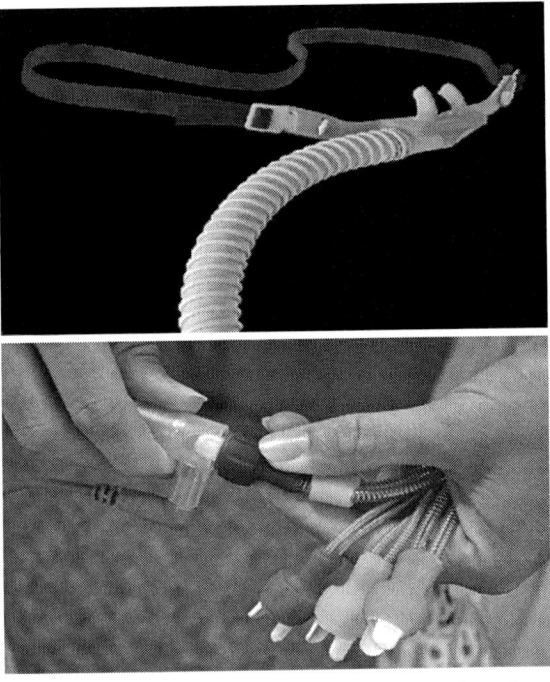

Fig. 3: Nasal cannula. (*For color version see Plate 2*)

Table 2: Nasal cannula sizes.				
F & P optiflow junior				
Product	*Item code*	*Approx. weight range*	*Max. flow rate (L/ Min)*	*Spare wigglepads*
Optiflow junior nasal cannula				
Premature size	OPT312	<2 kg	8	OPT010
Neonatal size	OPT314	1–8 kg	8	OPT012
Infant size	OPT316	3–15 kg	20	OPT012
Pediatric size	OPT318	12–22 kg	25	OPT012
Optiflow junior tubing kit	RT330 for MR850, 900PTS31 for AIRVO 2	N/A	Refer to optiflow Junior nasal	N/A

- Respiratory distress due to bronchiolitis, pneumonia, congestive heart failure, etc.
- Respiratory support in post-extubation
- Weaning therapy from mask continuous positive airway pressure (CPAP)/ bilevel positive airway pressure (BIPAP)
- Apnea of prematurity

Table 3: Difference between low-flow nasal cannula (LFNC), high flow nasal cannula (HFNC), and continuous positive airway pressure (CPAP).

	LFNC	HFNC	CPAP
Delivery	Nasal cannulae	Nasal cannulae	Nasal prongs/masks
Flow	<2 LPM	>4 LPM	Variable
Gas	Unblended oxygen	Unblended oxygen or blended oxygen + air	Unblended oxygen or blended oxygen + air
Temperature	Unheated	Heated	Heated
Humidification	Non-humidified	Humidified	Humidified
Pressure	Minimal	Variable, unregulated	Variable, regulated

Contraindications

- Blocked nasal passages/choanal atresia
- Respiratory failure with low sensorium
- Low sensorium with inability to protect airway
- Trauma/surgery to nasopharynx

HOW DOES IT WORK? MECHANISMS OF HIGH FLOW NASAL CANNULA

In order to understand the mechanisms behind HFNC, it is helpful to review some fundamental respiratory physiology.

- Normally,~ 30% of an inspired tidal volume represents anatomical dead space
- Start of inspiration—dead space is filled with end-expiratory gas
- Dead space volume is essential to:
  - Inspiratory gas warming and humidifying
  - Conducting gas to the thorax and dispersing to lung regions, the contribution of dead-space (end-expiratory gas) to a new breath does impact breathing efficiency.

In a healthy person, alveolar oxygen concentrations are lower than ambient air and alveolar carbon dioxide concentrations are greater than ambient air.

This difference is a function of alveolar ventilation as well as blood gas content. Dead space volume directly impacts tidal volume and/or respiratory rate requirements, and thus breathing effort, even in healthy people.

In this regard, HFNC via cannula can enhance respiratory efficiency by flushing nasopharyngeal anatomical dead space and supporting respiratory work. But, ideal gas conditioning must be achieved.

Washout of Anatomical Dead Space

Flushing the dead space of nasopharyngeal cavity reduces overall dead space, improves alveolar ventilation, and improves respiratory effort.

This washout effect aims to:

- Reduce re-breathing of expired CO_2
- Create a reservoir of fresh gas in the upper airway, ready for the next inspiration
- Allow for better ventilation and oxygenation.

It is believed that this continuous flow of gas through the nasopharynx washes out the oxygen-depleted air so that the upper airway in effect becomes a reservoir of oxygen-enriched gas. Thereby, reducing overall dead space resulting in alveolar ventilation as a greater fraction of minute ventilation.

Humidity

- Humidity is water vapor in a gas
- It is expressed in terms of:
  - Absolute humidity
  - Relative humidity
  - Dew point
- Because high flows are used, heated water humidification is necessary to avoid drying of respiratory secretions and for maintaining nasal cilia function.
- Set humidifier at 37°C.

Importance of Gas Warming and Humidification

- Mucosal tissue of the nasopharyngeal space designed to warm and humidify breathing gas prior to entering the lower respiratory tract
- Done by achieving a large surface area to interact with inspiratory gas
- Exposing the nasopharyngeal tissues to greater than a normal MV rate flow of gas (below body temperature and the water vapor saturation point) overload these tissues
- *Result*: Significant dysfunction, drying, and damage to the nasal mucosa
- Ideally, inspiratory gas should be warmed to body temperature (37ºC) and humidified to 100% relative humidity
- Humidification with vapor is least likely to cause airway and lung injury by latent heat loss and deposition of water droplets
- We better understand the importance of optimal humidification for mucociliary function. The warming of the gas increases its capacity to hold water

Benefits of gas warming and humidification:

- Preserves airway function
- Prevent airway drying
- Clear retained secretions
- Increase sputum clearance
- Allows ease of suctioning
- Maintains patent airway
- Prevents atelectasis/pulmonary infection.

Optimized Mucociliary Clearance

- Delivering optimal humidity (37°C, 44 mg/L) optimizes mucociliary clearance
- Improves secretion quality
- Maintains mobility of secretions for transport out of the airway
- Reduces the risk of respiratory infection

Accurate Oxygen Delivery

Traditionally, the patient is prescribed an oxygen concentration and flow rate. If this flow rate is less than the patient's inspiratory flow demand, any entrainment of room air may dilute the delivered oxygen concentration. The percentage of oxygen the patient actually receives is often unknown through face mask or other low flow devices.

- High flow nasal cannula can deliver enough flow to meet or exceed the patient's inspiratory flow demand
- This enables the delivery of a set FiO_2, even when a patient's inspiratory demand changes

Reduction of Inspiratory Resistance and Work of Breathing

- Nasopharynx—dispensability that contributes to variable resistance, especially inspiratory (UA resistance constitutes 50% of total airway resistance)
- Nasopharyngeal CPAP (NP-CPAP) reduces this supraglottic resistance by 60%
- Reducing work of breathing (WOB) may be due to:
  - Mechanically stenting of the airway
  - Provides gas flow that exceed patient's peak inspiratory flow flushing the dead space—enhances alveolar ventilation.

Improved Lung Mechanics

Five minutes of respiratory support with ambient gas (*not* warmed or humidified) decreases pulmonary compliance and conductance. There is good compliance with standard humidification.

Does HFNC Provide Positive-Distending Pressure? CPAP Effect

- Mechanical splinting of the nasopharynx prevents supraglottic collapse and decreases nasopharyngeal resistance
- Low levels of PEEP (3–6 cm of H_2O) may contribute to alveolar recruitment (decreased dead space), improved compliance and decreased WOB (to overcome iPEEP). This mechanism for HFNC remains poorly understood.
- *High flow nasal cannula pressure is directly related to*:
  - Leak presence at nares and mouth

- Flow rate
- Weight of the infant

■ *Leak magnitude is related to*:
  - Cannula/prong size
  - Infant's mouth being opened or closed

How to initiate HFNC?

■ Select appropriate cannulae and circuit for patient size
■ Circuit tubing to attach to humidifier:
  - *Children <12.5 kg*: Small volume circuit tubing (RT 329)
  - *Children ≥12.5 kg*: Adult oxygen therapy circuit tubing (RT203)
■ Connect bag of sterile water to heater/humidifier
■ Turn on heater/humidifier and allow to warm up before use
■ Select noninvasive mode and set temperature (T37C)
■ Always use a blender, never use flow meter off wall delivering FiO_2 100%
■ Set oxygen flow rate (up to 8 L/min on pediatric tubing, up to 60 L/min in adults)
  - <10 kg 2 L/kg/minute
  - >10 kg 2 L/kg/minute for 1st 10 kg + 0.5 L/kg/min for every kg beyond 10 kg (max 50 LPM)— start off at 6 L/min and increase up to goal flow rate over a few minutes to allow patient to adjust to high flow
■ Set FiO_2 (from 21% to 100%)
■ Place nasal cannulae on patient—ensure there is cannulae NOT totally occluding patient's nares; there should be some space and leak nasal cannula (prongs) to attach to humidifier circuit tubing (size to fit nares comfortably)
  - *Newborn*: OPT312 Premature or OPT314 Neonatal (maximum flow 8 L/min)
  - *Infants and children up to 10 kg*: OPT316 Infant (max flow 20 L/min) or up to 12.5 kg: OPT318 Pediatric cannula (max flow 25 L/min)
  - *Children >10 kg*: Adult cannula size S OPT542, size M OPT544, size L OPT546
■ Titrate FiO_2 and flow rate as required
■ Monitor closely
■ Separate high-flow air and O_2 flow meters (Fig. 4) can be connected via a "Y-piece" adapter.
■ To allow more convenient application, high-flow air/O_2 proportioner valve blenders or high-flow "Venturi" air mixing valves can be used
■ With either approach, an oxygen analyzer or oxygen concentration chart as shown in Figure 5 is needed to confirm accurate air/O_2 mixing.

Oxygen concentration chart (used if oxygen blender or analyzer is not used) (Fig. 5)

There is a pressure relief valve used in the pediatric system as a safety mechanism. Figure 6 shows a complete set up of oxygen analyzer with air entrainer blender with digital display of FiO_2.

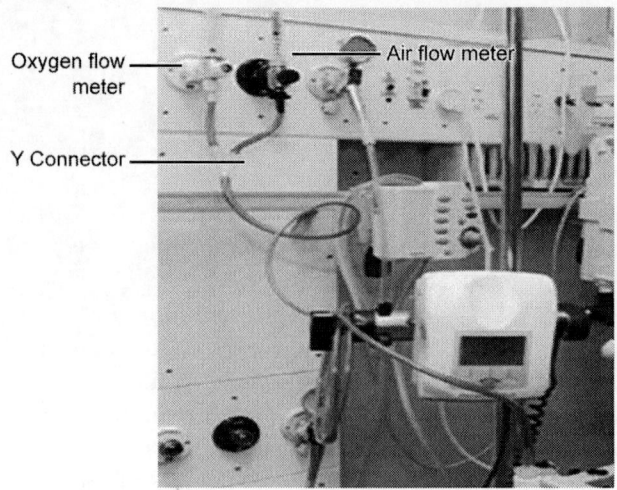

Oxygen flow meter

Air flow meter

Y Connector

Fig. 4: High-flow air and O_2 flow meters connected via Y connector. (*For color version see Plate 3*)

Oxygen Concentration

Medical Air (LPM)

Oxygen (LPM)	1	2	3	4	5	6	7	8	9	10
1	2/61	3/47	4/41	5/37	6/34	7/32	8/31	9/30	10/29	11/28
2	3/74	4/61	5/53	6/47	7/44	8/41	9/39	10/37	11/35	12/34
3	4/80	5/68	6/61	7/55	8/51	9/47	10/45	11/43	12/41	13/39
4	5/84	6/74	7/66	8/61	9/56	10/53	11/50	12/47	13/45	14/44
5	6/87	7/77	8/70	9/65	10/61	11/57	12/54	13/51	14/49	15/47
6	7/89	8/80	9/74	10/68	11/64	12/61	13/57	14/55	15/53	16/51
7	8/90	9/82	10/76	11/71	12/67	13/64	14/61	15/58	16/56	17/54
8	9/91	10/84	11/78	12/74	13/70	14/66	15/63	16/61	17/58	18/56
9	10/92	11/86	12/80	13/76	14/72	15/68	16/65	17/63	18/61	19/60
10	11/93	12/87	13/82	14/77	15/74	16/70	17/67	18/65	19/63	20/61

Fig. 5: Oxygen concentration chart (may be used if oxygen analyzer not available).

Complications:

- Maxillofacial trauma
- Nasal obstruction e.g. choanal atresia, nasal polyps
- Presence of suspected base of skull fracture
- Reduced level of consciousness
- Life-threatening hypoxia
- Foreign body aspiration
- Open chest wound/chest trauma
- Other contradictions for CPAP
- Barotrauma including pneumothorax
- Pressure areas around the nares

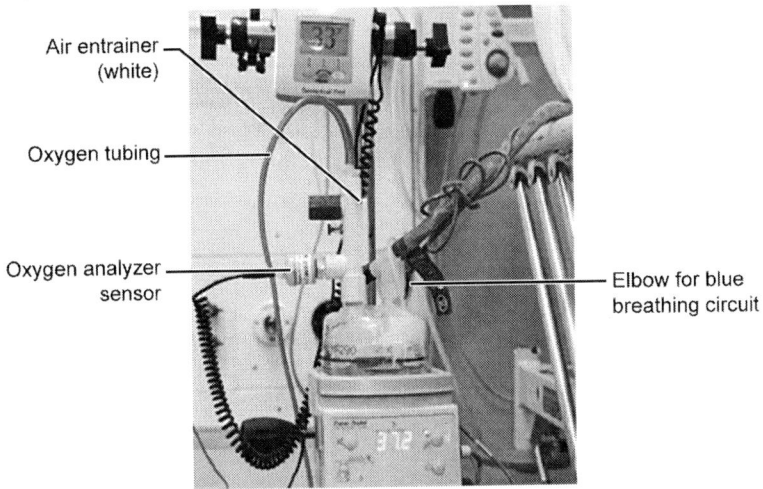

Fig. 6: Complete oxygen analyzer with air entrainer blender set up. (*For color version see Plate 1*)

Caution:

- The humidified tubing—below the height of the patients' airway (water condensation)
- Frequent monitoring
- Check nasal prong position as dislodgement may occur
- Nasal secretions block airways; 0.9% saline drops can be administered intranasally and suctioning done
- Not to use as transport device

Patient monitoring:

- Monitor—respiratory rate (RR), heart rate (HR), degree of chest indrawing, and SPO_2
- Titrate FiO_2
- Heart rate, RR should reduce by 20%
- All infants should have nasogastric tube *in situ*
- Gentle suction to clear nostrils
- Oral and nasal care must be performed 2–4 hourly
- Consult with senior doctor on floor before weaning

In conclusion, HHHFNC is noninvasive respiratory support providing delivery of prescribed FiO_2 with humidification (≥95%) and low-level CPAP. While neonatal studies are limited to premature infants, pediatric studies have examined the use of HFNC, with most focusing on this modality for viral bronchiolitis. It has excellent patient tolerance and has a definite place in the pyramid of respiratory care if used appropriately to right patients at right time with proper monitoring.

KEY MESSAGES

- High flow nasal cannula oxygen therapy is a form of respiratory support which provides heated, humidified flow of air-oxygen mixture to increase oxygen delivery, washing out of the anatomical dead space, prevents drying of upper airway mucosa, and provides some continuous positive airway effect with improved patient comfort.
- There is increasing evidence for its use in acute respiratory distress as an aid to oxygenation and possible avoidance of invasive mechanical ventilation.
- There are few noted complications and caution to be taken while using HFNC and a close monitoring of the patient is necessary.

SUGGESTED READING

1. Beggs S, Wong ZH, Kaul S, et al. High-flow nasal cannula therapy for infants with bronchiolitis. Cochrane Database Syst Rev. 2014;(1):CD009609.
2. Franklin D, Babl FE, Schlapbach LJ, et al. Randomized Trial of High-Flow Oxygen Therapy in Infants with Bronchiolitis. N Engl J Med. 2018;378:1121-31.
3. Ganu SS, Gautam A, Wilkins B, et al. Increase in use of noninvasive ventilation for infants with severe bronchiolitis is associated with decline in intubation rates over a decade. Intensive Care Med. 2012;38(7):1177-83.
4. Hernández G, Roca O, Colinas L. High-flow nasal cannula support therapy: new insights and improving performance. Crit Care. 2017;21:62.
5. Lee JH, Rehder KJ, Williford L, et al. Use of high flow nasal cannula in critically ill infants, children, and adults: a critical review of the literature. Intensive Care Med. 2013;39(2):247-57.
6. Mayfield S, Jauncey-Cooke J, Hough JL, et al. High-flow nasal cannula therapy for respiratory support in children (Review). Cochrane Database Syst Rev. 2014;(3):CD009850.
7. Miguel-Montanes R, Hajage D, Messika J, et al. Use of high-flow nasal cannula oxygen therapy to prevent desaturation during tracheal intubation of intensive care patients with mild-to-moderate hypoxemia. Crit Care Med. 2015;43(3):574-83.
8. Patel A, Nouraei SA. Transnasal Humidified Rapid-Insufflation Ventilatory Exchange (THRIVE): a physiological method of increasing apnoea time in patients with difficult airways. Anaesthesia. 2015;70(3):323-9.
9. Rat JP, Thille AW, Mercat A, et al. High-flow oxygen through nasal cannula in acute hypoxemic respiratory failure. N Engl J Med. 2015;372(23):2185-96.
10. Ricard JD. High flow nasal oxygen in acute respiratory failure. Minerva Anestesiol. 2012;78(7):836-41.
11. Roked F, Samar S, Jyothish D. 4-year (2014-2017) experience of using high flow nasal cannula (HFNC) oxygen therapy on pediatric wards: incremental expansion of the use of HFNC.
12. Ward JJ. High-flow oxygen administration by nasal cannula for adult and perinatal patients. Respir Care. 2013;58(1):98-122.

Mechanical Ventilation in a Neonate

Naveen Gupta, Kumar Ankur, Anil Batra

In most neonates with respiratory distress, initial mode of ventilation should be continuous positive airway pressure (CPAP). However, if respiratory drive is not sufficient or CPAP fails, baby should be intubated and put on mechanical ventilation.

INITIATION OF INVASIVE VENTILATION

Intubation and Mechanical Ventilation

- Threshold for intubation may vary among neonatal units. Usually we decide to intubate a neonate once he fails on CPAP (as mentioned above).
- In a preterm neonate, decision of intubation may be taken even earlier to give benefit of early surfactant therapy. Subsequently, baby may be rapidly extubated after surfactant delivery *(INSURE: INtubation-SUrfactant administration-Rapid Extubation)*. In this regimen, as soon as infant is symptomatic, infant is intubated, surfactant instilled into trachea and infant is then extubated to CPAP within few minutes. This practice is claimed to shorten subsequent ventilation.
- In most of infants >28 weeks it may be worthwhile to give a fair trial of CPAP before considering intubation and mechanical ventilation/ INSURE, as intubation itself might destabilize them and most of them do with CPAP alone. In smaller infants (<28 weeks), benefits of INSURE may outweigh any harm incurred.

Intubation

- Select appropriate size endotracheal tube (ET) (Table 1). Tube should neither be very tightly fitting, nor having high peri-tubal leak (>20–25%). Usual guidelines are based on infants weight.
- Keep appropriate size mask, bag, oxygen tubing, reservoir, suction catheter ready before proceeding. An appropriate size mask should cover chin, mouth, and nose but not eyes. Maintain thorough aseptic precautions. If baby is too agitated, sedate him with IV midazolam (0.1 mg/kg). If intubation attempt is getting prolonged or baby has severe

Table 1: Weight and size of endotracheal tube (ET).	
Weight	Inner diameter of ET
<1 kg	2.5 mm
1–2 kg	3 mm
2–3 kg	3.5 mm
>3 kg	4 mm

desaturation, interrupt the procedure, reoxygenate with supplemental oxygen or bag and mask. Be gentle, do not panic. If needed call for help, rather than taking it to your pride.

- Do not place the ET too deep into the trachea. Always look at vocal cord guide on ET tube (dark line at the tip), and keep it at level of vocal cord. Look for B/L equal air entry, before securing it. Optimal tube position should be later reconfirmed on chest X-ray. If tube is closer to carina, pull it out. Note the cm marking at the corner of mouth. This reading will be a future guide for reintubation and tube fixation. A rough rule for length of tube from corner of mouth is: 6 + birth weight in Kg.

Tip to lip distance = 6 + birth weight in kg

- However, this formula overestimates the distance at times. Always check tube position by auscultation and on X-ray.

NEONATAL PATIENT-TRIGGERED VENTILATION

Before we move to patient-triggered ventilation (PTV) and various trigger mechanisms, we should know critical events during a mechanical breath:

A. **What initiates the breath?**
B. **What limits the breath?**
C. **What cycles the breath?**

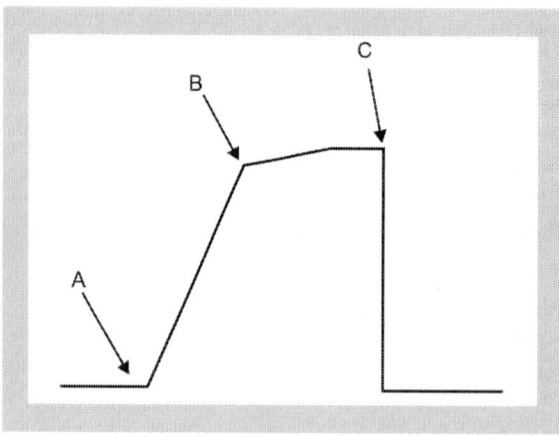

- **A:** In convention intermittent mandatory ventilation (IMV), breath is initiated once a preset time (as decided by set ventilatory rate) has elapsed. This is called time triggering. In more sophisticated ventilators, change in flow or pressure in the ventilatory circuit or realization of abdominal movements, as induced by patient's inspiratory effort is detected by ventilator and a breath is initiated. This is called patient triggering.
- **B:** In conventional ventilation 2nd point, i.e. limit is pressure, that is the breath is limited to a point when preset pressure is achieved. This is called pressure-limited ventilation. More recently, volume guarantee ventilation is being used increasingly, in which breath is limited, once preset volume is achieved.
- **C:** Third point is what cycles the breath? This can be time, in which breath is terminated, once a preset inspiratory time (Ti) is elapsed and expiration is allowed. This is called time cycling. Other mechanism is flow cycling, in which ventilator senses decelerating inspiratory flow and breath is terminated, once flow rate falls to a critical point. This is called flow cycling. This will be discussed in more detail later.

Initial assisted ventilation in 1960s was time cycled pressure limited ventilation, where ventilator delivered intermittent mechanical breath at preset interval (IMV), irrespective of infant's spontaneous effort.

As expected, there is asynchrony between ventilatory breath and patient's spontaneous breath in such type of ventilation. This asynchrony may have many untoward effects. Asynchrony may impair gas exchange as well as might lead to air trapping and pneumothorax. There is also association of asynchrony with alteration in blood pressure, cerebral blood flow, and intra-ventricular hemorrhage.

This asynchrony can be avoided if patient's spontaneous effort and the onset of mechanical inspiration could be coordinated. PTV is one of such innovation, which achieves synchronization between spontaneous and mechanical breaths. These synchronized ventilatory modes are characterized by the delivery of mechanical breaths in response to a signal derived from the patient's inspiratory effort. Synchronized intermittent mandatory ventilation (SIMV), assist/control (A/C) ventilation and pressure support ventilation (PSV) are examples of PTV.

Signal Detection: Flow Sensor

Different ventilators have different trigger signal mechanisms for detection of patient's inspiratory efforts with some advantages/disadvantages over one another.

Following is tabulated list of these methods:

Synchronized intermittent mandatory ventilation (Fig. 1): In this mode, mechanical breaths are delivered in synchrony with patient's inspiratory

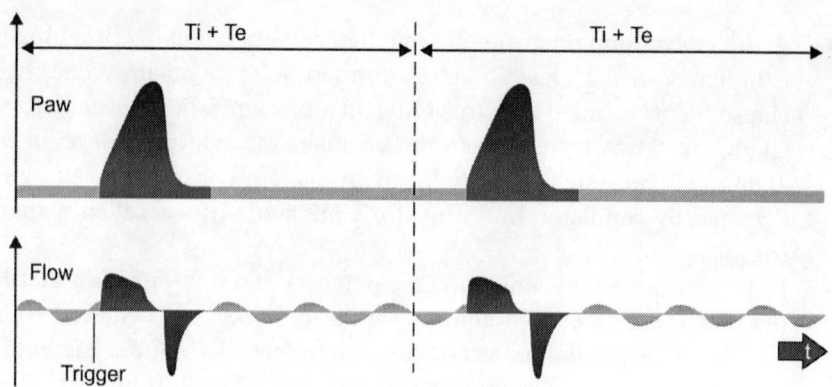

Fig. 1: Synchronized intermittent mandatory ventilation.
(Ti: inspiratory time; Te: expiratory time; Paw: peak airway pressure)

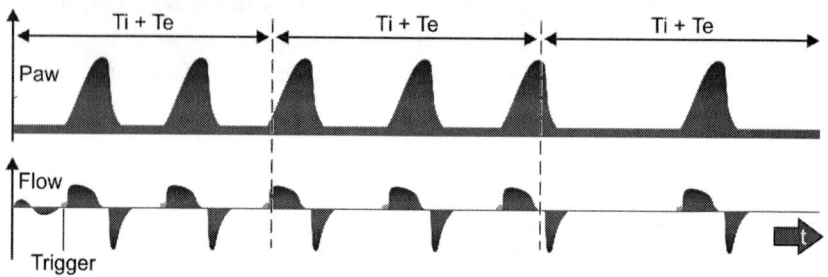

Fig. 2: Assist/control ventilation.
(Ti: inspiratory time; Te: expiratory time; Paw: peak airway pressure)

effort. In between the mandatory breath, patient can breathe spontaneously from continuous flow in the circuit. In this mode, onset of mechanical breath coincides with patient's inspiration but expiration is not synchronized as Ti is preset and might be different from patient's spontaneous Ti. As a result, patient might start expiration, while ventilator is still in inspiratory phase. This might lead to fight against ventilator during expiration. This situation can be avoided by optimizing the Ti according to patient's Ti.

Assist/control ventilation (Fig. 2): This is also time cycled pressure limited ventilation, where every breath triggered by patient is supported. In case patient does not have spontaneous effort, ventilator delivers mandatory breaths as preset rate. Here also inspiration is synchronized but possibility of expiratory asynchrony still remains there. Merit over SIMV is that all of patient's breaths are supported.

Flow cycled ventilation (Fig. 3): In this mode of ventilation, every inspiratory effort of the patient triggers the ventilator. But unlike other modes, Ti is not pre-selected. Rather Ti is decided by time constant of the lung unit, so inspiration and expiration both are synchronized. Inspiration is initiated with patient's spontaneous efforts. During decelerating phase of inspiratory flow

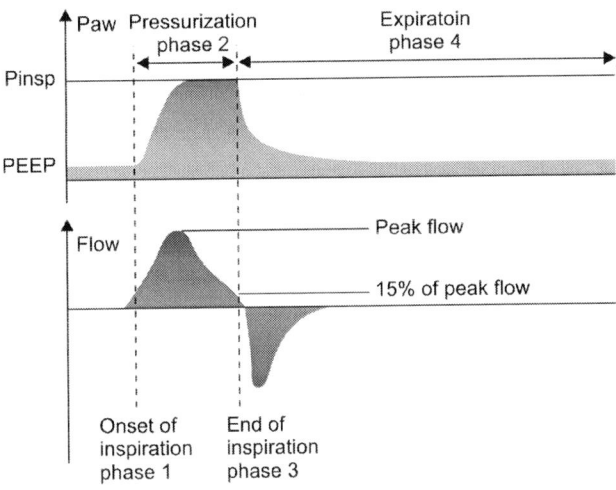

Fig. 3: Flow cycled ventilation.
(PEEP: positive end expiratory pressure)

breath is terminated when flow rate falls to certain percentage of peak flow rate, which is called termination sensitivity. Termination sensitivity usually varies from 5% to 20%.

Pressure support ventilation: It is a pressure limited ventilatory mode in which each breath is patient-triggered and supported. It provides breath-by-breath ventilatory support by means of a positive pressure wave synchronized with the inspiratory effort of the patient, both patient-initiated and patient-terminated. Thus, during a cycle of PSV, four phases are seen:
1. Recognition of the beginning of inspiration
2. Pressurization
3. Recognition of the end of inspiration
4. Expiration

If flow cycling is used instead of time cycling, inspiration is terminated at a percentage of peak flow rather than time, thus providing full synchronization between patient and ventilator. Thus, A/C ventilation can be provided either as a time cycled or flow cycled mode. Flow-cycling is also incorporated in PSV which provides synchrony during both inspiration and expiration. Flow cycled A/C and PSV on surface look the same but PSV has additional features designed to regulate inspiratory gas flow in such a way that it provides a "boost" to spontaneous breaths to help overcome the work of breathing (WOB) imposed by the narrow lumen endotracheal tube, ventilator circuit, and demand valve.

As inspiratory flow in PSV is servo controlled, patient can breathe as much, as fast and for as long as he or she wants. In that sense, it resembles spontaneous breaths and appears to be more physiologic as the patient has full control on his or her breathing.

Advantages of PSV:

- Better synchrony between patient and ventilator
- Increased patient comfort
- Reduced need for sedation
- Decrease in WOB
- Shorter duration of weaning process

Synchronized intermittent mandatory ventilation + pressure control (PC)/ pressure support ventilation: Alternative is to put baby on SIMV + PSV mode, if available. In this mode, full support is provided through set SIMV rate. For rest of spontaneous breath, a partial pressure support (PS) is added.

Selecting "Mode of ET ventilation"

- *We usually use either SIMV or PSV mode*
- Many clinicians prefer volume guarantee modes (VG—Volume guarantee; VAPS—Volume-assured pressure support; PRVC—Pressure-regulated volume control; etc.). In these modes, caregiver sets the desired tidal volume (VT) (4–6 mL/kg) and then peak inspiratory pressure (PIP) is constantly manipulated by the ventilator so as to keep the VT into target range. Whereas in pressure modes (SIMV, PSV), caregiver sets a pressure, so as to generate desired VT. In this case VT will keep changing as per changing lung compliance. If compliance improves, delivered VT will increase and vice-versa.
- Message is that we shall not get blindly carried away by any particular mode. Keep looking if your set mode and settings are suitable for baby or not. Basic fundament should be to provide adequate support to the baby so as to assist in his WOB, without taking total control of the situation.

OPTIMIZING "VENTILATORY SETTINGS"

- *Positive end expiratory pressure (PEEP)*: Set a PEEP of 4–6 cm H_2O to start with. Later adjustments can be made by looking at FRC on chest X-ray. Optimal FRC will be dome of right diaphragm at 7–9th posterior ribs. If X-ray shows hyperinflation, decrease PEEP by 1–2 and vice-versa.
- *Peak inspiratory pressure (PIP)*: Adjust the PIP so as to achieve a VT 3–5 mL. This will cause visible chest rise (but not too much of chest excursions).
- *Inspiratory time (Ti)*: Adjust the inspiratory time so that there is minimal gap between inspiratory and expiratory flow waveforms. Ti is usually kept short in hyaline membrane disease (HMD) i.e close to 0.25 sec and little longer in MAS (0.35 sec). In normal lung ventilation, Ti may be as high as 0.5 sec. It is better to look at flow waveforms for final adjustment or switch to PSV mode.
- *Rate*: Adjust the rate to provide optimal support. In severe disease set higher rate, you may require to set a rate as high as 70–80 per minute. In mild disease a rate of 30–40 might be sufficient. One way of dealing

the situation could be shifting to PSV mode and allowing all the breaths to be supported. Or in case of SIMV, we may set ventilatory rate so much that unsupported breaths are not more than 25–35% of total. Final manipulation of rate is done on looking at PCO_2 in blood gas. If there is hypocapnia, decrease the rate (and PIP, if very high); if there is hypercapnia, increase the rate. As a lung protective strategy, many clinicians will tolerate a PCO_2 as high as 55–60, as long as pH is >7.2.

- *FiO_2*: Adjust FiO_2 so as to maintain saturation 85–95%. In meconium aspiration syndrome (MAS) [± persistent pulmonary hypertension (PPHN)] target SPO_2 may be 90–95%.
- *Flow rate*: Set flow rate 6–8 L/min.
- An X-ray should be obtained within ½–1 hour of initiating ventilation, which will define the position of ET tube, FRC as well condition of lung parenchyma.
- Maintain a ventilatory chart, on which all important parameters are noted every hourly.
  Other supportive measures:
- *Investigate and treat the underlying disorders, as indicated by clinical scenario*: Sepsis, pneumonia, air leak, pulmonary hemorrhage, shock, Patent ductus arteriosus (PDA), PPHN, etc.

NEONATAL VENTILATION SETTINGS (TABLE 2)

Monitoring of a Ventilated Neonate

The aim of monitoring is simple and clear to follow in real time specific physiological values that can change rapidly and alter the patient's clinical status. Especially in the intensive care setting, in which the vast majority of patients are admitted because of a primary respiratory problem or of respiratory complications during their illness, monitoring of the cardiorespiratory system alerts the clinician to sudden untoward events, aids in diagnosis, helps manage diagnosis, facilitates prognosis, and enables assessment of therapeutic response.

On routine neonatal intensive care unit (NICU), round daily monitoring includes the following things:

- Clinical monitoring
- Noninvasive monitoring
- Invasive monitoring

Clinical Monitoring

Physical examination

- Heart rate (HR), respiratory rate (RR), WOB, SPO_2, perfusion, temperature, etc.
- Quantify WOB (Downe score or Silverman score) (Table 3)

Table 2: Suggested ventilatory strategies for common neonatal disorders.

Disease	Initial strategy	Blood gas target
RDS	• Rapid rates (> 60/min) • Moderate PEEP (4–5 cm H_2O) • Low PIP (10–20 cm H_2O) • Ti 0.3–0.4 sec • Tidal volume 4–6 mL/kg body weight	pH 7.25–7.35 PaO_2 50–70 mm Hg $PaCO_2$ 40–55 mm Hg
MAS without PPHN	• Relatively rapid rate (40–60/min) • Low to moderate PEEP (4–5 cm H_2O) • Adequate Te (0.5–0.7 sec) • If gas trapping occurs, increase Te to 0.7–1 sec and decrease PEEP	pH 7.3–7.4 PaO_2 60–80 mm Hg $PaCO_2$ 40–50 mm Hg
Apnea of prematurity	• Relatively slow rates (10–15/min) • Minimal peak pressures (7–15 cm H_2O) • PEEP 3 cm H_2O • FiO_2 usually low (<0.25)	pH 7.25–7.35 PaO_2 50–70 mm Hg $PaCO_2$ 55–65 mm Hg
Hypoxic ischemic encephalopathy	• Rates 30–45/min or slower depending upon spontaneous rate • PIP 12–20 cm H_2O • PEEP 4–6 cm H_2O • FiO_2 to maintain saturations between 92–96%	pH 7.35–7.45 PaO_2 60–90 mm Hg $PaCO_2$ 35–45 mm Hg

(MAS: meconium aspiration syndrome; PEEP: positive end expiratory pressure; PIP: peak inspiratory pressure; PPHN: persistent pulmonary hypertension; RDS: respiratory distress syndrome)

Table 3: Downe's score for assessment of severity of respiratory distress.

	Score 0	Score 1	Score 2
Cyanosis	No cyanosis	Cyanosis on FiO_2 <40%	Cyanosis on FiO_2 >40%
Respiratory rate (RR)	<60	60–80	>80
S/C retractions	No	Mild	Severe
Air entry	Normal	Diminished	Absent
Grunting	No grunting	Audible with stethoscope	Audible without stethoscope

Noninvasive Monitoring

- Pulse oximetry
- *Transcutaneous (Tc)*: Tc PO_2/Tc PCO_2
- *ET CO_2*: Capnography
- Pulmonary graphics
- ECG
- *Apnea monitor*: Chest wall movement
- Chest X-ray/Cold light for air leaks

Invasive Monitoring

- Blood gas-arterial, venous, capillary

Capillary blood gas: The capillary blood is sampled by heel stab. The method of arterialization is heel warming, usually by immersing the heel in warm water (40–45°C) for 5–10 minutes prior to heel stab, or using a warmed towel or surgical gloves (with hot water).

- There is clinically acceptable agreement between capillary and arterial *pH and* PCO_2. With regard to PO_2 → values significantly lesser than arterial blood.

Venous

- *Central venous:* In comparison with arterial blood gas, pH 0.03–0.05 units lower and the PCO_2 is 4–5 mm Hg higher, with little or no increase in serum HCO_3.
- *Peripheral venous:* In comparison with arterial blood gas, pH is 0.02–0.04 units lower than the arterial pH, HCO_3 is 1–2 mEq/L higher, and the PCO_2 is 3–8 mm Hg.

Pulse oximeter: In premature neonates, oxygen toxicity is associated with the development of retinopathy of prematurity (ROP) and bronchopulmonary dysplasia (BPD). Reducing the levels and time of oxygen exposure in this patient population will likely decrease these morbidities.

The goal of SPO_2 level targeting for premature neonates is to adequately deliver oxygen to the tissue without causing the complications of oxygen toxicity. Premature neonates' SPO_2 readings are often labile and difficult to keep within a narrow range. The care-team must aim to maintain SPO_2 levels within this range.

- For the high-risk premature neonate, the SPO_2 target range is 88–92%, with monitor alarm limits set at 85% and 94%.
- For neonates in the high risk group that are in air, the upper alarm limit can be set at 100%.

Permissive hypercapnia: Ventilator–induced lung injury remains an important cause of neonatal morbidity. Permissive hypercapnia is a ventilatory strategy that may reduce injury to the developing lung through a variety of mechanisms.

- Baby stable on ventilator. CXR: good FRC. ABG: pH: >7.2, PCO_2: 55–65 mm.
- Because it will target to correct this, that means you have to increase pressure which may lead to more tidal volume delivery and can cause volutrauma.

Pulmonary graphics: Although there is truly no substitute for clinical assessment at the bedside of a mechanically ventilated infant, real-time pulmonary graphics do provide useful information regarding the breath-to-breath performance of the ventilator and its interaction with the baby. Graphic monitoring assists the clinician at the bedside in several ways. It can be helpful in fine-tuning or adjusting ventilator parameters. One can track and determine the progress of a disease such as respiratory distress syndrome by following compliance measurements.

Pressure-volume loop: The pressure-volume loop begins at PEEP. As the pressure delivered to the lung increases, there is a concomitant increase in the volume of gas delivered to the lung. The inspiratory limb ends at PIP, and the expiratory or deflationary limb begins, whereby pressure and volume fall as the lung empties. The shape of this loop is referred to as hysteresis and describes the mechanical properties of the lung as it is filled and emptied. A loop indicating good compliance will be described as upright (compliance axis > 45°) (Figs. 4 to 7), and a loop indicating poor compliance is described as flat, or lying on its side.

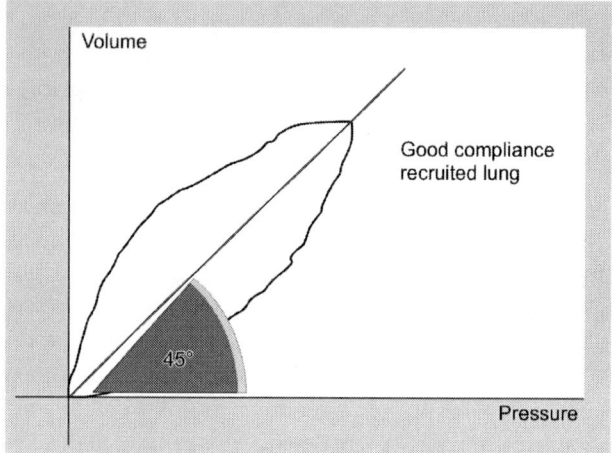

Fig. 4: Good compliance (CL) indicated by slope of pressure volume curve approximately 45°.

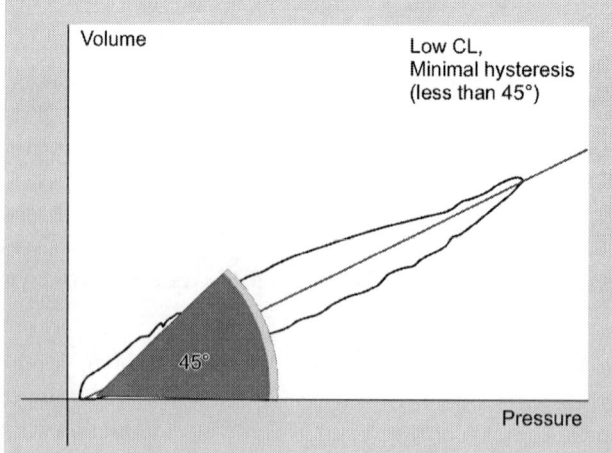

Fig. 5: Low compliance (CL) indicated by slope of Pressure volume curve less than 45°.

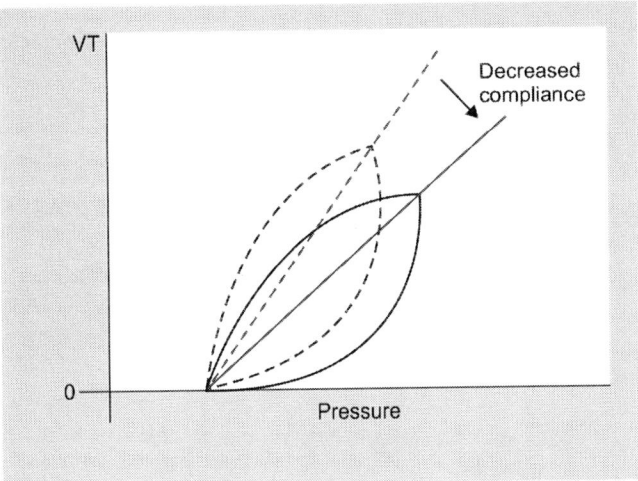

Fig. 6: Decreased compliance reduces tidal volume (VT) per unit change in pressure (from dotted curve to solid curve).
(VT: tidal volume)

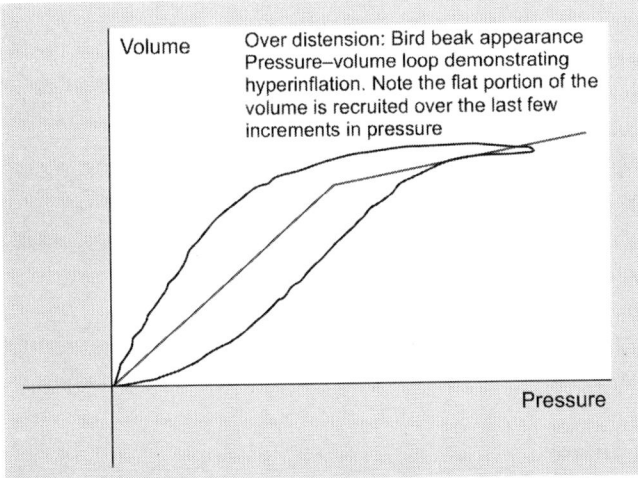

Fig. 7: Pressure volume loop showing over distension (bird beak effect).

Flow–volume loop (Fig. 8)

- The tidal flow-volume relationship describes the pattern of airflow during tidal breathing. It is characterized by the VT; peak inspiratory and expiratory airflow (which generally occurs during mid-respiratory cycle); and no evidence of flow limitation other than at end expiration or end inspiration.
- Generally, any inspiratory-expiratory volume discrepancy should be less than 10%. Airflow limitation is described as abrupt downward deviation of the flow signal toward baseline and away from its normal direction.

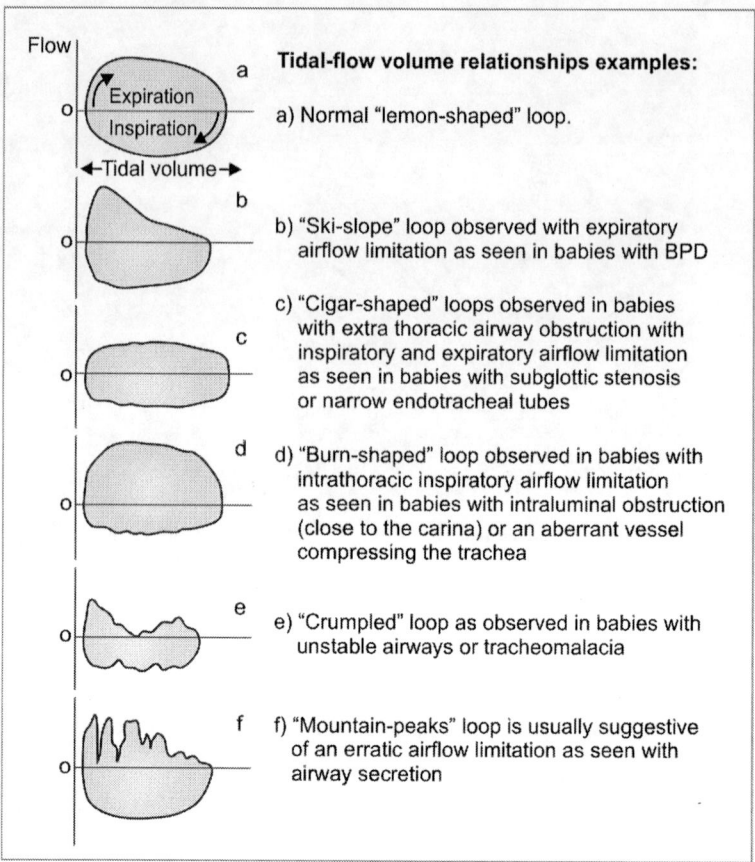

Flow

a

o Expiration
Inspiration

←Tidal volume→

Tidal-flow volume relationships examples:

a) Normal "lemon-shaped" loop.

b

b) "Ski-slope" loop observed with expiratory airflow limitation as seen in babies with BPD

c

c) "Cigar-shaped" loops observed in babies with extra thoracic airway obstruction with inspiratory and expiratory airflow limitation as seen in babies with subglottic stenosis or narrow endotracheal tubes

d

d) "Burn-shaped" loop observed in babies with intrathoracic inspiratory airflow limitation as seen in babies with intraluminal obstruction (close to the carina) or an aberrant vessel compressing the trachea

e

e) "Crumpled" loop as observed in babies with unstable airways or tracheomalacia

f

f) "Mountain-peaks" loop is usually suggestive of an erratic airflow limitation as seen with airway secretion

Fig. 8: Flow–volume loop showing various morphological changes seen in different lung conditions affecting gas flow and lung volumes.

A complete flow limitation is defined as 80% or greater reduction of the airflow signal.

KEY MESSAGES

- During conventional ventilation neonates are ventilated with continuous flow, pressure limited, and time cycled ventilators. Various triggered ventilation modes have been developed for neonates: SIMV, A/C, and more recently PSV.
- Pressure support ventilation gives the patient optimum liberty during ventilation. The patient decides over start of inspiration and start of expiration and therefore controls inspiration time, breathing frequency, and minute volume. It is not only baby friendly but also doctor friendly.
- Monitoring of a neonate on ventilation includes hourly vitals HR, RR, temperature, SPO_2, BP, perfusion (CRT), respiratory distress and synchrony with ventilator, abdominal and neurological status.

- Ventilatory parameters both *set parameters* (PIP, PEEP, inspiratory time, rate, flow rate, FiO$_2$) as well as *measured parameters* (PIP, PEEP, FiO$_2$, MAP, VT, minute ventilation (MV), compliance and resistance) should be noted periodically. Monitoring of ventilator graphics can detect abnormalities early and alert the treating intensivist.
- Intermittent arterial blood gas should be obtained while patient is on ET ventilation, frequency of which will vary according to the severity of disease and fluctuations in ventilatory settings.
  - If disease is severe and condition of baby is unstable and/or there are significant alterations in ventilatory parameters, blood gas should be repeated frequently (every 2–4 hourly).
  - Once condition stabilizes, frequency of gases can be decreased to 2–3 gases per day or even lesser. Minor manipulations in settings can be done by looking at measured parameters alone (VT and MV).
- In case of any acute deterioration systematic examination should be done in following order: *DOPE*
  - Tube displacement (D)
  - Tube obstruction (O)
  - Pneumothorax (P)
  - Equipment malfunction (E)
  - Sepsis/pulmonary hemorrhage
  - PDA, etc.

SUGGESTED READING

1. Baumer JH. International randomised controlled trial of patient triggered ventilation in neonatal respiratory distress syndrome. Arch Dis Child Fetal Neonatal Ed. 2000;82:F5-F10.
2. Beck J, Reilly M, Grasselli G, et al. Patient-ventilator interaction during neurally adjusted ventilatory assist in low birth weight infants. Pediatr Res. 2009;65:663-8.
3. Beresford MW, Shaw NJ, Manning D. Randomised controlled trial of patient triggered and conventional fast rate ventilation in neonatal respiratory distress syndrome. Arch Dis Child Fetal Neonatal Ed. 2000;82:F14.
4. Bernstein G, Mannino FL, Heldt GP, et al. Randomized multicenter trial comparing synchronized and conventional intermittent mandatory ventilation in neonates. J Pediatr. 1996;128:453-63.
5. Claure N, Bancalari E. New modes of mechanical ventilation in the preterm newborn: evidence of benefit. Arch Dis Child Fetal Neonatal Ed. 2007;92:F508.
6. Cleary JP, Bernstein G, Mannino FL, et al. Improved oxygenation during synchronized intermittent mandatory ventilation in neonates with respiratory distress syndrome: a randomized, crossover study. J Pediatr. 1995;126:407.
7. Do Boer RC, Jones A, Ward PS, et al. Long term trigger ventilation in neonatal respiratory distress syndrome. Arch Dis Child. 1993; 68: 308-11
8. Donn SM, Nicks JJ, Becker MA. Flow-synchronized ventilation of preterm infants with respiratory distress syndrome. J Perinatol. 1994;14:90-4.
9. Donn SM, Sinha SK. Minimising ventilator induced lung injury in preterm infants. Arch Dis Child Fetal Neonatal Ed. 2006;91:F226-30.

10. Dreyfuss D, Saumon G. Ventilator-induced lung injury: lessons from experimental studies. Am J Respir Crit Care Med. 1998;157:294-323.

11. Greenough A, Rossor TE, Sundaresan A, et al. Synchronized mechanical ventilation for respiratory support in newborn infants. Cochrane Database Syst Rev. 2016;9:CD000456.

12. Grover A, Field D. Volume-targeted ventilation in the neonate: time to change? Arch Dis Child Fetal Neonatal Ed. 2008;93:F7-13.

13. Guthrie SO, Lynn C, Lafleur BJ, et al. A crossover analysis of mandatory minute ventilation compared to synchronized intermittent mandatory ventilation in neonates. J Perinatol. 2005;25:643-6.

14. Klingenberg C, Wheeler KI, McCallion N, et al. Volume-targeted versus pressure-limited ventilation in neonates. Cochrane Database Syst Rev. 2017;10:CD003666.

15. Klingenberg C, Wheeler KI, Owen LS, et al. An international survey of volume-targeted neonatal ventilation. Arch Dis Child Fetal Neonatal Ed. 2011;96:F146-8.

16. Lee J, Kim HS, Sohn JA, et al. Randomized crossover study of neurally adjusted ventilatory assist in preterm infants. J Pediatr. 2012;161:808.

17. McCallion N, Davis PG, Morley CJ. Volume-targeted versus pressure-limited ventilation in the neonate. Cochrane Database Syst Rev. 2005;(3):CD003666.

18. McCallion N, Lau R, Morley CJ, et al. Neonatal volume guarantee ventilation: effects of spontaneous breathing, triggered and untriggered inflations. Arch Dis Child Fetal Neonatal Ed. 2008;93:F36-9.

19. Ramanathan R, Sardesai S. Lung protective ventilatory strategies in very low birth weight infants. J Perinatol. 2008;28 Suppl 1:S41.

20. Reyes ZC, Claure N, Tauscher MK, et al. Randomized, controlled trial comparing synchronized intermittent mandatory ventilation and synchronized intermittent mandatory ventilation plus pressure support in preterm infants. Pediatrics. 2006; 118:1409-17.

21. van Velzen, A, De Jaegere A, van der Lee J. Feasibility of weaning and direct extubation from open lung high-frequency ventilation in preterm infants. Pediatr Crit Care Med. 2009;10:71-5.

Chapter 8

High-Frequency Ventilation in Neonates

Kumar Ankur

Much progress has been made in the treatment of neonatal respiratory failure over the past few decades. However, lung injury and pulmonary morbidities secondary to mechanical ventilation remain an ongoing problem in the care of premature infants. High-frequency ventilation (HFV) is a form of mechanical ventilation that uses small tidal volumes and extremely rapid ventilator rates. Whatever the HFV system, the presumed linear relationship between ventilator rate and carbon dioxide (CO_2) elimination improves with decreasing ventilator frequency as long as the inspiratory-to-expiratory time ratio (I:E) is held constant.

PRINCIPLES OF GAS EXCHANGE

Chang described the multiple modes of gas transport that occur during HFV (Figs. 1 and 2).

- *Bulk convection*: Direct ventilation of the alveoli that are lying close to the trachea is called the bulk convection. With a decreased tidal volume [as in high-frequency oscillator (HFO)], a small fraction of the lung receives fresh gas with each inspiration, therefore allowing sufficient gas exchange to occur in that particular lung region. As long as the tidal volume remains above a certain limit, direct alveolar ventilation will contribute in some way to gas exchange during HFO.

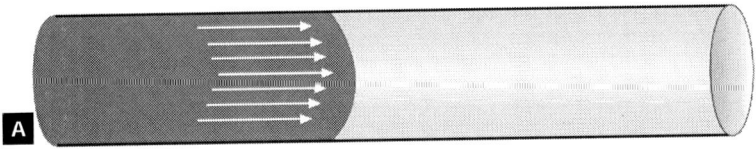

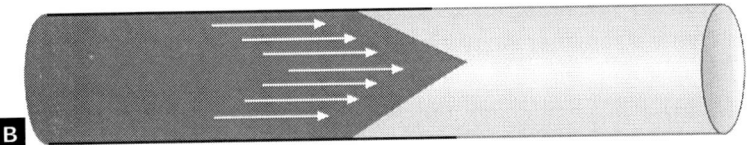

Figs. 1A and B: Taylor dispersion.

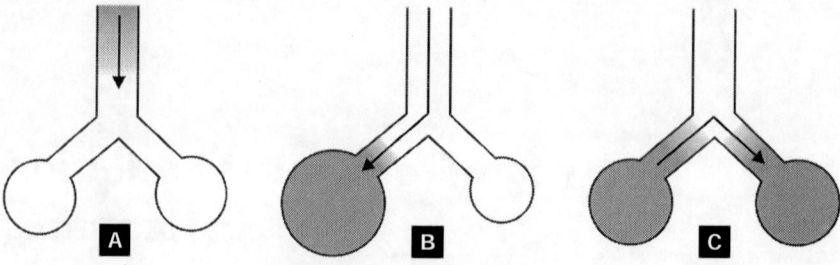

Figs. 2A to C: Pendulum shift.

- *Taylor dispersion*: Augmented diffusion occurs because of turbulent air currents that result from interaction between axial velocity and the radial concentration gradient in the airway.
- *Pendelluft effect*: The alveoli are ventilated asynchronously, as opposed to synchronously in conventional ventilation. This asynchronous ventilation occurs when small neighboring regions of the lung are different in compliance, air resistance or the time constants of their filling or emptying. This method of gas transport is termed as "pendelluft", which is defined as transient movement of respiratory gases out a certain and into neighboring alveoli either at the instant of Zero flow at the end of inspiration, or in the opposite direction at the end of expiration.
- *Asymmetric velocity profiles*: Convective gas transport is enhanced by asymmetry between inspiratory and expiratory velocity profiles that occur at branch points in the airway. The velocity profile of the inhaled gas is initially parabolic, but on exhalation is flat. After a full cycle, gas particles initially near the center of the flow are displaced to then right while those near the wall are displaced to the left.
- *Molecular diffusion*: Diffusion occurring near the alveolocapillary membrane with the random thermal oscillation of the gas molecule. This suggests that as long as the gas molecules are of a temperature that is above absolute zero, then molecular diffusion will always occur.

TYPES OF HIGH-FREQUENCY VENTILATION

Currently, there are three general types of HFV:

1. High-frequency positive pressure ventilation (HFPPV), which is produced by conventional or modified conventional mechanical ventilation (CMV) operating at rapid rates.
2. High-frequency jet ventilation (HFJV), which is produced by ventilators that deliver a high-velocity jet of gases directly into the airway.
3. High-frequency oscillatory ventilation (HFOV), which is produced by a device that moves air back and forth at the airway opening and produces minimal bulk gas flow.

HIGH-FREQUENCY OSCILLATORS

High-frequency oscillators are a type of HFV that use piston pumps or vibrating diaphragms, operating at frequencies ranging from 180 breaths/min to 2,400 breaths/min (3–40 Hz), to vibrate air in and out of the lungs. During HFOV, inspiration and expiration are both active (proximal airway pressures are negative during expiration). Oscillators produce little bulk gas delivery. A continuous flow of fresh gas rushes past the source, generating or powering the oscillations. The amplitude of the pressure oscillations within the airway determines the tiny tidal volumes that are delivered to the lungs around a constant mean airway pressure (MAP). This allows avoidance of high peak airway pressures for ventilation as well as maintenance of lung recruitment by avoidance of low end-expiratory pressures. A bias flow system supplies fresh gas (Fig. 3).

Variables on High-Frequency Oscillator

Three parameters determine oscillatory ventilation (Fig. 3): MAP around which the pressure oscillates; secondly, the oscillatory volume, which results from pressure swings and essentially determines the effectiveness of this type of ventilation; thirdly, the oscillatory frequency denotes the number of cycles per unit of time.

Oxygenation

During HFO, oxygenation is controlled by the inspired oxygen concentration and the MAP which controls lung volume. Oxygenation during HFO is independent of frequency and tidal volume, except at very low values. Two "volume or pressure strategies" can be employed during HFO; low volume/low pressure or high volume/high pressure. The former strategy is used with the aim of reducing barotraumas and the latter to maintain lung volume above its closing pressure and ensure lung recruitment. The high volume strategy

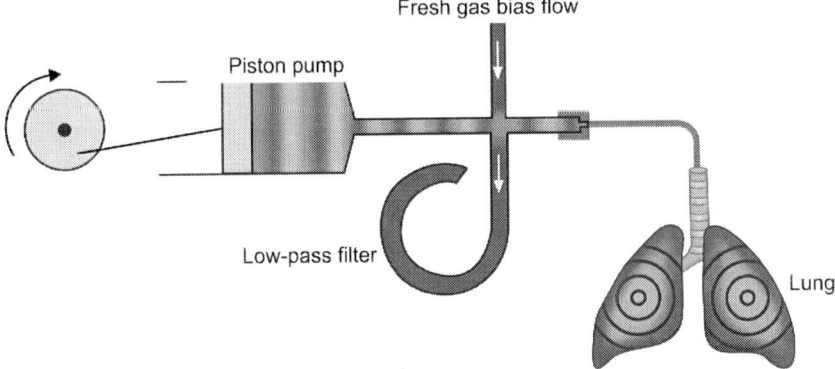

Fig. 3: Operating principle of high-frequency oscillatory ventilation.

can improve pulmonary mechanics and is associated with a reduction in inspired oxygen concentration and diminished structural injury. Increasing MAP on transfer from conventional ventilation to HFO (high volume strategy) improves oxygenation; whereas transfer to HFO at the same MAP as used on conventional ventilation had a variable effect on oxygenation. The MAP necessary to optimize oxygenation during HFO is directly correlated with disease severity. Infants with severe respiratory distress syndrome (RDS) with poor gas exchange on conventional ventilation have very low lung volumes. Not surprisingly, then, such infants require the largest changes in MAP to optimize their lung volume adherence oxygenation. Such a strategy, however, is not appropriate to the healthy lungs as this may lead to overdistention.

For any infant, there is a MAP level at which lung volume is optimum and hence so is oxygenation. Increasing MAP above that optimum level will impair oxygenation, as well reducing it below that level. The optimum MAP level will depend on the infant's disease severity and hence lung volume. The relationship between the MAP displayed on any given oscillator and the mean alveolar pressure in the infant's lung will vary with the device. In the SensorMedics at 30% inspiration the mean alveolar pressure is lower than displayed; the same is true for the Infant Star. For the Hummingbird and possibly other sine wave generators with an I/E ratio of 1:1, the displayed and actual pressures are about equal but, if using a Drager Babylog 8000, the intrapulmonary pressures will be higher than the displayed pressure. This has practical implications if a hospital has more than one type of oscillators. For example, a switch from a SensorMedics 3100A to a Drager ventilator at a display pressure of 12 cm H_2O could result in a 5–8 cm H_2O abrupt increase in distending pressure.

Ventilation

Ventilation in CMV is calculated by the product of respiratory rate (f) times tidal volume (VT). In contrast ventilation in HFV is calculated by the equation $f^a \times VT^b$ where "a" is found to be between 0.75 and 1.24 and "b" is between 1.5 and 2.2. For clinical application, the equation is simplified to $f \times VT^2$. Thus, CO_2 elimination is more strongly affected by changes in VT than in frequency. This explains why even small changes in VT would produce big effect on ventilation. Furthermore due to the characteristics of ventilator machine, the delivered tidal volume is inversely proportional to frequency. To avoid wide variations in delivered tidal volume the oscillatory rate is generally held constant during the clinical application of HFV.

Frequency

During HFO, the delivered volume might be expected to be greatest at the resonant frequency of the respiratory system. The resonant frequency of the preterm lung varies between 15 Hz and 20 Hz. The problem with the using high frequency to match the resonant frequency of the lung is that volume delivered by the commercially available oscillators decreases as frequency is increased. Thus, in clinical setting while using HFO in very preterm babies, one should use a frequency between 12 Hz and 15 Hz so as to facilitate the oxygenation as tidal volume recruitment moving in and out of the lung is less but in cases of term babies with respiratory acidosis the frequency of 10 Hz or less is optimum as the volume delivery to the lung increases.

INDICATION FOR HIGH-FREQUENCY VENTILATION

- Failure of conventional ventilation in the term infant [persistent pulmonary hypertension (PPHN) of the newborn, meconium aspiration syndrome (MAS)]
- Air-leak syndromes [pneumothorax, pulmonary interstitial emphysema (PIE)]
- Failure of conventional ventilation in the preterm infant (severe RDS, PIE, pulmonary hypoplasia) or to reduce barotraumas when conventional ventilator settings are high.

ELECTIVE HIGH-FREQUENCY OSCILLATORY VENTILATION

Some authors are of the view that starting HFV as a primary mode of respiratory support results in less pulmonary injury. A meta-analysis of 11 trials has shown HFOV had no significant effect on mortality or on short-term neurological abnormality. Although, a reduction in bronchopulmonary dysplasia (BPD) survivors at term was highlighted, the effect of HFOV was modest. The "HFOV" trials have, however, been different in the details of their study design and the results obtained. The data are limited and the results are mixed as to whether HFJV may reduce incidence of chronic lung disease (CLD). Keszler and colleagues, in a multicenter controlled trial of 130 babies who had RDS, demonstrated a decreased incidence of CLD at 36 weeks corrected gestational age, as well as a decreased need for home oxygen therapy in the HFJV-treated group.

HIGH-FREQUENCY OSCILLATORY VENTILATION AS A RESCUE MODE

High-frequency oscillatory ventilation is frequently used to "rescue" infants who have respiratory failure, due to a variety of conditions as has been mentioned above. Most of this is from nonrandomized trials or case series. For example, there are reports of infants with congenital diaphragmatic hernia and refractory hypoxemia on conventional ventilation improving when transferred to HFOV and similarly oxygenation in infants with pulmonary hypertension, but no long-term benefits have been highlighted. Oxygenation in infants with severe PIE has also been documented to improve when infants are transferred from convention ventilation to HFOV. Here have been two randomized trials of HFOV in infants with severe respiratory failure, both report only short-term outcomes. In term-born infants, HFOV was shown to be more effective rescue support than conventional ventilation, but there were no significant differences in the requirement for extracorporeal membrane oxygenation (ECMO) or duration of ventilator or oxygen dependency between the two respiratory support modes. In preterm infants, although HFOV use was associated with a significant reduction in new pulmonary air leak, intracranial hemorrhage was increased.

TRANSFER FROM CONVENTIONAL VENTILATION

- Use appropriate sized endotracheal (ET) tube: Down the length of ET tube there is attenuation of the oscillatory amplitude signal. The degree of attenuation was greatest with smaller ET tubes and lower oscillatory amplitudes with approximately 20% loss of amplitudes with smaller tubes.
- Make sure that hypotension is corrected before starting high frequency as the hypotension is exacerbated by HFO.
- Use a higher MAP (by 2 cm H_2O) than what the child was while on conventional ventilation. MAP should be increased by 1 cm every 10–15 minutes as the improvement in oxygenation because of the increased lung volume can be seen in that time only.
- The oscillatory amplitude is increased until the chest wall is seen vibrating. Vibrations to the umbilicus are considered adequate but beyond that are supposed to be excessive. However, this is a rough starting guideline and should always be correlated with blood gas examinations.
- Perform a chest X-ray soon after commencing HFO to ensure adequate lung expansion has occurred and there is no evidence of overexpansion.
- Once lung volume is established, any procedure which requires the infant to be disconnected from the oscillator should be done as infrequently and as quickly as possible so as to prevent frequent loss of volume, e.g. suctioning. It is preferable to use a closed system suctioning device.
- If the child is not improving despite increasing MAP on ventilator, then other causes should be sought before labeling as failure of HFO like anemia, PPHN, hypotension, pneumothorax, etc.

WEANING FROM HIGH FREQUENCY

It is important to maintain lung volume to optimize oxygenation, thus, as recovery from RDS begins; the inspired oxygen concentration should be turned down before altering the MAP level. Once the inspired oxygen concentration has been reduced to 30%, the MAP is the reduced in 2 cm H_2O steps at a rate dictated by the blood gases. If weaning is performed too rapidly, atelectasis will occur and it is necessary to increase the MAP level above that at which the weaning process occurred to optimize respiratory status once more. Once the MAP level has been reduced to 8 cm H_2O, there are two options for further weaning. One option is to extubate the infant directly from HFO. The second option is to change the infant to a shorter period of patient triggered ventilation (PTV) prior to extubation; such a policy is facilitated by the machines that offer a choice of oscillation, triggered and conventional ventilation. A period on PTV can be useful to confirm that the infant has adequate respiratory drive to ensure successful extubation.

ADVERSE EFFECTS OF HIGH-FREQUENCY VENTILATION

- *Gas trapping*: Leading to lung over inflation which may cause adverse cardiopulmonary function or air leak. This has not been found to be a significant problem during HFOV in premature infants in experienced centers.
- *Pulmonary interstitial emphysema*: There have been few cases of PIE developing in babies on Hummingbird ventilator. Author postulated that the unusually low MAP used might be the main cause of PIE. At low MAP and low compliance gas cannot be transported into the atelectatic alveoli. This led to an increase in the amplitude of oscillations in the peripheral airway resulting in overexpansion of the airways and hence airway injury.
- *Intraventricular hemorrhage (IVH) and periventricular leukomalacia (PVL)*: A meta-analysis of studies on the association of IVH and PVL with HFV in premature infants with RDS showed that a significant association was present only when the HIFI study was included, while analysis of the more recent studies without the HIFI study did not show any association. So possibly the current load of ventilators using the high volume strategy is not associated with increased IVH and PVL.
- *Noise pollution*: The noise produced by Infant Star 500 and SensorMedics 3100A were 53 (49-54) and 59 (56-64) dB respectively. These noise levels were lower than the recommended highest level of 85 dB by the Occupational Safety and Health Administration. However, we have to be cautious in using HFV in patients receiving aminoglycosides. These infants are recommended not to be exposed to noise levels of > 58 dB.
- *Tracheal damage*: This is a well-documented complication of HFJV in neonates, but fortunately not described in HFOV. It is essential to adequately humidify [90% relative humidity (RH)] the breathing gas otherwise severe irreversible damage to the trachea may result. Viscous secretion could obstruct bronchi and deteriorate the pulmonary situation. Excessive humidification on the other hand can lead to condensation in the paten circuit, the ET tube and the airways, completely undoing the effect of HFV.

KEY MESSAGES

- High-frequency oscillatory ventilation used with a high lung volume strategy is at least as safe as CMV with the current lot of ventilators and may even be lifesaving and used as a rescue therapy.
- Experience is an important element in the safe and efficient use of HFOV particularly in premature infants.
- The long-term risk-benefit ratio for HFV is not well documented.
- Follow-up studies should be performed to investigate the long-term survival, lung function and neurodevelopment of infants who have been treated with HFV in the neonatal period before this exciting form of ventilation is more widely accepted and used.

SUGGESTED READING

1. Calvert S. The role of high frequency oscillatory ventilation in very preterm infants. Biol Neonate. 2002;81 Suppl 1:25-7.
2. Clark RH, Gerstmann DR. Controversies in high frequency ventilation. Clin Perinatol. 1998;25(1):113-22.
3. Cools F, Askie LM, Offringa M, et al. Elective high-frequency oscillatory versus conventional ventilation in preterm infants: a systematic review and meta-analysis of individual patients' data. Lancet. 2010;375:2082.
4. Cools F, Henderson-Smart DJ, Offringa M, et al. Elective high-frequency oscillatory ventilation versus conventional ventilation for acute pulmonary dysfunction in preterm infants. Cochrane Database Syst Rev. 2009;(3):CD000104.
5. Cools F, Offringa M, Askie LM. Elective high frequency oscillatory ventilation versus conventional ventilation for acute pulmonary dysfunction in preterm infants. Cochrane Database Syst Rev. 2015;(3):CD000104.
6. Courtney SE, Asselin JM. High frequency jet and oscillatory ventilation for neoantes: which strategy and when? Respir Care Clin N Am. 2006;12(3):453-67.
7. Eichenwald EC, Stark AR. High-frequency ventilation: current status. Pediatr Rev. 1999;20:e127-33.
8. Froese AB, Kinsella JP. High-frequency oscillatory ventilation: lessons from the neonatal/pediatric experience. Crit Care Med. 2005;33(3 Suppl);S115-21.
9. Greenough A. High frequency oscillation and liquid ventilation. Paediatr Respir Rev. 2006;7 Suppl 1:S186-8.
10. Haney C, Allingham TM. Nursing care of the neonate receiving high-frequency jet ventilation. J Obstet Gynecol Neonatal Nurs. 1992;21(3):187-95.
11. HiFO Study Group. Randomized study of high-frequency oscillatory ventilation in infants with severe respiratory distress syndrome. J Pediatr. 1993; 122:609-19.
12. Keszler M, Donn SM, Bucciarelli RL, et al. Multicenter controlled trial comparing high-frequency jet ventilation and conventional mechanical ventilation in newborn infants with pulmonary interstitial emphysema. J Pediatr. 1991;119: 85-93.
13. Lampland AL, Mammel MC. The role of high-frequency ventilation in neonates: evidence-based recommendations. Clin Perinatol. 2007;34(1):129-44.
14. Rojas-Reyes MX, Orrego-Rojas PA. Rescue high-frequency jet ventilation versus conventional ventilation for severe pulmonary dysfunction in preterm infants. Cochrane Database Syst Rev. 2015;(10):CD000437.

15. Soll RF. The clinical impact of high frequency ventilation: review of the Cochrane meta-analysis. J Perinatol. 2006;26 Suppl 1:S38-42; discussion S43-5.
16. Thome UH, Carlo WA, Pohlandt F. Ventilation strategies and outcomes in randomised trials of high frequency ventilation. Arch Dis Child Fetal Neonatal Ed. 2005;90(6):F466-73.
17. Wheeler HJ, Nokes LD, Powell T. A review of high frequency oscillation ventilation in the neonate. J Med Eng Technol. 2007;31(5):367-74.
18. Wiswell TE, Graziani LJ, Kornhauser MS, et al. High-frequency jet ventilation in the early management of respiratory distress syndrome is associated with a greater risk for adverse outcomes. Pediatrics. 1996;98:1035-43.
19. Yoder BA, Siler-Khodr T, Winter VT, et al. High-frequency oscillatory ventilation: effects on lung function, mechanics, and airway cytokines in the immature baboon model for neonatal chronic lung disease. Am J Respir Crit Care Med. 2000;162:1867-76.
20. Zivanovic S, Peacock J, Alcazar-Paris M, et al. Late outcomes of a randomized trial of high-frequency oscillation in neonates. N Engl J Med. 2014;370:1121-30.

Newer Modes of Ventilation

Anil Sachdev

Newer ventilators can be set to modes other than the pressure-control and volume-control modes of older machines. The alternative modes of ventilation were developed to prevent ventilator lung injury, patient-ventilator asynchrony, promote better oxygenation and faster weaning, and be easier to use. However, evidence of their benefit is scant. Until now, we have lacked a standard nomenclature for mechanical ventilation, leading to confusion. Regardless of the mode used, the goals are to avoid lung injury, keep the patient comfortable, and wean the patient from mechanical ventilation as soon as possible. In this chapter, we review several of these alternative modes [adaptive pressure control (APC), adaptive support ventilation (ASV), proportional assist ventilation (PAV), airway pressure-release ventilation (APRV), biphasic positive airway pressure (biphasic PAP), mandatory minute ventilation (MMV), and high-frequency oscillatory ventilation (HFOV)], explaining how they work and contrasting their theoretical benefits and the actual evidence of benefit (Flowchart 1).

PRESSURE-REGULATED VOLUME CONTROL

Pressure-regulated volume control (PRVC) ventilation is an example of a dual-control ventilation mode, also known as hybrid modes of ventilation. This mode is a form of closed-loop ventilation that has combined the features of volume and pressure ventilation. First introduced on the Servo 300 ventilator, it is now available on most modern ventilators under different names, e.g. Autoflow (Drager Evita), Volume Guarantee (Datex-Ohmeda, Drager Babylog), Adaptive pressure ventilation (Hamilton Galileo), and Variable pressure control (Venturi).

This dual mode combines the benefits of decelerating flow of pressure-controlled ventilation (PCV) with the safety of a volume guarantee. In essence, the clinician sets a target tidal volume and maximal pressure level. The ventilator attempts to achieve the volume target using a pressure-control gas-delivery format at the lowest possible airway pressure. This is achieved by altering the peak flow and inspiratory time breath-to-breath in response to changing airway resistance or compliance characteristics. PRVC

Flowchart 1: Classification of modes of ventilation.

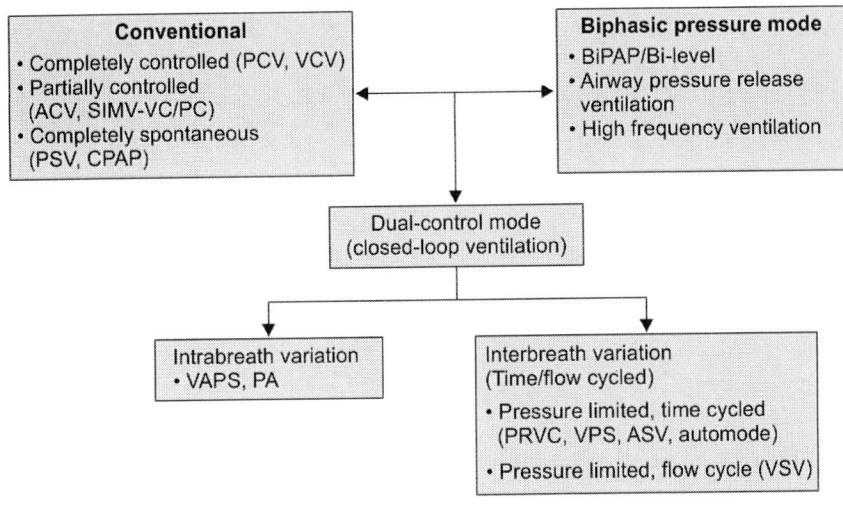

(ACV: assist control ventilation; ASV: adaptive support ventilation; BiPAP: bilevel positive airway pressure; CPAP: continuous positive airway pressure; PA: pressure augmentation; PCV: pressure control ventilation; PRVC: pressure-regulated volume control; SIMV: synchronized intermittent mandatory ventilation; VAPS: volume-assured pressure support; VCV: volume control ventilation; VPS: variable pressure support; VSV: volume support ventilation)

breaths have a variable decelerating flow pattern. The breaths are time-cycled. During PRVC, the pressure and volume are regulated. All breaths are volume targeted, with pressure adjusted to reach that volume target. PRVC often incorporates a "compliance curve" that is developed within the ventilator computer, as it gives several initial breaths at varying tidal volumes that increase incrementally up to the set value (Flowchart 2). From this information, the ventilator computes the pressure target required to deliver the desired tidal volume.

When activated, the first delivered breath is a "test breath" at some minimal pressure level (5–10 cm H_2O), along with an inspiratory "hold" maneuver, which is used to calculate patient compliance. The program in the ventilator then determines the plateau pressure required to achieve the desired tidal volume. The next few breaths may be delivered at a pressure below the calculated pressure needed to deliver the target tidal volume as a further test. This is also done anytime ventilation has been interrupted (opening the ventilator circuit, suctioning, etc.). Using this information, the calculated pressure is applied to deliver breaths (Flowchart 2).

Depending on the respiratory system compliance, the pressure associated with the tidal breath can vary over time. If the tidal volume is exceeded, the pressure limit is decreased by 1–3 cm H_2O on each breath until the target tidal volume is reached. Similarly, if the volume is low, pressure is increased

Flowchart 2: Breath-to-breath pressure adjustments to deliver target tidal volume.

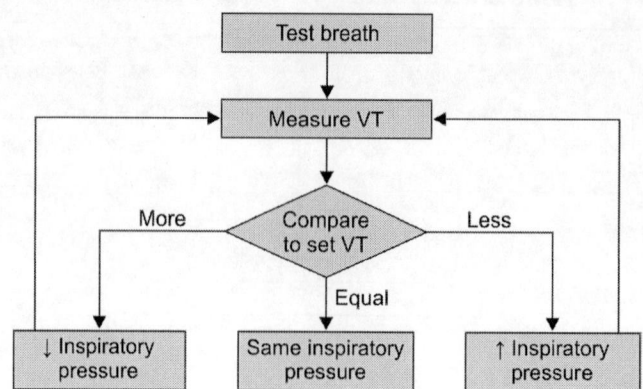

by 1–3 cm H_2O on each breath until the target volume is met. The pressure required to ensure the volume breath can be increased up to a maximum of within 5 mm Hg of the set pressure alarm limit. Thus, specific tidal volume and minute ventilation is assured, while pressure-induced lung damage is minimized. The duration of inspiration is determined by the respiratory rate and the inspiration-to-expiration (I:E) ratio or inspiratory time (i.e. this is a time-cycled mode of ventilation). In the Siemens 300 ventilator, PRVC is only active during continuous mandatory ventilation (CMV) whereas in other ventilators, this type of dual-control mode is also active in synchronized intermittent mandatory ventilation (SIMV). The proposed advantage of this mode is a constant tidal volume with automatic weaning of the pressure limit as the patient's compliance improves.

Initial Settings

Ventilatory setting will depend on type and severity of disease.
- Respiratory rate—physiological for age
  - If patient's spontaneous respiratory rate is less than set rate, then ventilator gives additional control breaths to make up difference, whereas if patient's spontaneous rate > set rate, no control breaths are provided.
- Target tidal volume—initial setting: 6–8 mL/kg predicted body weight
- Upper pressure limit—since ventilator delivers pressure of up to 5 cm H_2O below upper pressure alarm limit set to 35–40 cm H_2O to ensure "safe" pressures
- Inspired oxygen concentration—initial setting 100%
- I:E ratio—initial setting: 1:2 (inspiratory time of 33%)
- Positive end-expiratory pressure (PEEP)—initial setting: 5–10 cm H_2O
- Rise time—5% of inspiratory time usually satisfactory.

Pressure-regulated volume control is one of the recommended modes of ventilation in patients with acute lung injury (ALI)/acute respiratory distress syndrome (ARDS). During ARDS if volume control ventilation is used, higher peak inspiratory pressures (PIP) would be required to ensure delivery of set tidal volume. Conventional ventilation may lead to overdistention of the normally functioning lung while expanding collapsed parts. Thus, mechanical ventilation may exacerbate the pulmonary pathology and/or delay recovery. In two studies of patients with ARDS, it was concluded that survival is better when high ventilation pressures are avoided. In another study Sachdev et al. comparing PRVC and volume control ventilation in two groups of children with acute lung diseases concluded that significantly lower mean airway pressure was required to improve oxygenation parameters in PRVC group. A study by Guldager et al. showed the advantage of using the PRVC mode for ventilation during acute respiratory failure. In this study, PIP was lower for all patients using the PRVC mode compared to the VC mode (statistically significant difference in peak pressures of 4 cm H_2O) and alveolar ventilation was unchanged as indicated by the constant $PaCO_2$. They concluded that though this difference in peak pressure is small, it may be more relevant in situations where larger tidal volumes are contemplated. D'Angio et al. in a study comparing SIMV versus PRVC found no differences in time to extubation or pulmonary outcomes. Piotrowski et al. also found in a study comparing intermittent mandatory ventilation versus PRVC in neonates with respiratory distress syndrome that there was no decrease in duration of mechanical ventilation or incidence of bronchopulmonary dysplasia. Kallet et al. also found that during lung-protective ventilation, PRVC offered no advantage in reducing work of breathing, compared to volume-controlled ventilation with a high-flow rate, and in some patients did not allow control of tidal volume to be as precise as expected. But some other small studies have found that PRVC resulted in faster weaning.

Advantages

It "Guarantees" tidal volume with minimum risk of barotraumas and decelerating flow pattern, that provides better distribution of ventilation and oxygenation.

Disadvantages

In this mode, pressure delivery to achieve target tidal volume will dependent on the character of previous breath. If patient makes intermittently significant inspiratory effort, it can result in variable tidal volume.

To conclude, PRVC is a new dual mode of ventilation that is becoming increasingly popular as it offers advantages of both target volume ventilation with pressure control, but specific studies on whether it allows for easier, faster weaning, better patient comfort or improved outcomes, are currently conflicting and need to be explored further.

AIRWAY PRESSURE-RELEASE VENTILATION

Airway pressure-release ventilation is a mode of ventilation that was described in 1987 by Stock et al. It has gained popularity recently due to the decreased need of sedation and neuromuscular blockade while using this mode of ventilation. It has also been identified as safe mode of ventilation for ARDS and ALI. APRV has also been shown to facilitate spontaneous breathing, decrease peak airway pressures, and improve oxygenation and ventilation compared to other modes of ventilation (Table 1). It has been described as continuous positive pressure ventilation (CPAP) with intermittent, regular and brief release of pressure. The release phase results in alveolar ventilation and removal of carbon dioxide (CO_2). APRV, unlike CPAP, facilitates both oxygenation and CO_2 clearance and originally was described as an improved method of ventilatory support in the presence of ALI and inadequate CO_2 ventilation. Technically, APRV is a time-triggered, pressure-limited, time-cycled mode of mechanical ventilation.

Physiological Effects

Oxygenation is better with APRV with spontaneous breathing than with mechanical ventilation alone. This effect is at least attributable to recruitment of collapsed lung tissue and increased aeration in dependent areas of lung. Putensen et al. showed improved ventilation perfusion matching and increased systemic flow in APRV with spontaneous breathing. APRV with spontaneous breathing increased ventilation in the juxtadiaphragmatic regions, predominantly in the dependent areas. Spontaneous breathing had a significant effect on the spatial distribution of ventilation and pulmonary

Table 1: Summary of advantages and disadvantages of airway pressure-release ventilation.

Advantages	Disadvantages
• High mean arterial pressure (MAP) with low peak pressure • Maintain normal cyclic decrease in pleural pressure • Allow inverse ratio ventilation, increases oxygen delivery • Augment venous return, increases cardiac index • Reduces need for sedation/paralysis • Improves renal perfusion, increases osmolar clearance, increases urine output • Decreased basal atelectasis, may decrease dead space • Improve patient ventilatory synchrony with spontaneous respiration	• Pressure-targeted mode, variable tidal volume delivery • CO_2 elimination depends on spontaneous breaths • Increase in airway resistance hampers CO_2 elimination • Increase work of breathing with asynchrony between spontaneous and pressure release breath • Not useful in large bronchopleural fistula and raise intracranial pressure • Limited experience • Auto-PEEP is usually present, contraindicated in high expiratory resistance

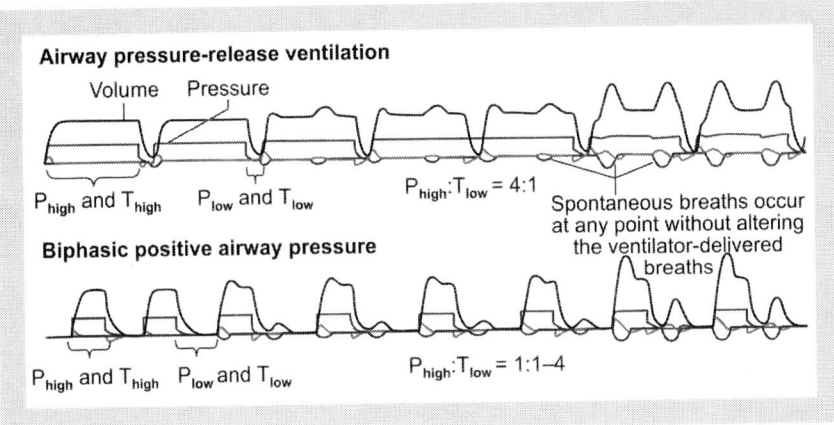

Fig. 1: Differences between airway pressure-release ventilation (APRV) and biphasic positive airway pressure modes. APRV (top) and biphasic positive airway pressure (bottom) are forms of pressure-controlled intermittent mandatory ventilation in which spontaneous breaths can occur at any point without altering the ventilator-delivered breaths. The difference is that the time spent in high pressure is greater in APRV.

perfusion. It has been shown to improve cardiac output, renal blood flow, glomerular filtration, and achieve high mean airway pressure with low peak airway pressure. APRV was associated with increases in lung compliance and oxygenation and reduction of shunting (Fig. 1).

Initial Ventilator Settings

There are four commonly used terms in APRV: (1) pressure high (P high), (2) pressure low (P low), (3) time high (T high), and (4) time low (T low) (Fig. 1).

- *P high*: It is the baseline airway pressure and is higher of the two airway pressure. Initial P high is kept same as plateau pressure measured on volume-control mode provided it is lower than 30 cm H_2O.
- *P low*: It is the airway pressure level resulting from pressure release. Other authors have described P low as the PEEP level, the release pressure, or the P2 pressure. It is usually set at 0 cm of H_2O.
- *T high*: It is the time during which P high is maintained. It is set at 3–4 seconds, then adjusted if necessary.
- *T low*: It is the time for which P low is held or pressure is released. It is probably the most difficult variable to set because it needs to be short enough to avoid derecruitment but still long enough to allow alveolar ventilation. It is usually set at 0.6–0.8 seconds.

Adjustments

- Hypoxemia: Adjust these ventilator settings to improve oxygenation
  - Increase pressure gradient (P high–P low) —increase P high by 2–5 cm H_2O.

- Airway pressure release frequency = 60/cycle time (T high + T low)—decrease frequency of pressure release (prolong T high by 0.5–1 sec) (if T low remains constant)
- Increase fraction of inspired oxygen (FiO_2).
  - Hypercapnia: Adjust these ventilator settings to relieve hypercapnia
    - Tolerate "permissive hypercapnia" (pH ≤ 7.15)
    - Reduce T high by 0.5–1 second; it may affect recruitment by lowering the Paw.

Advantages and Disadvantages

Summary of advantages and disadvantages of airway pressure-release ventilation has been shown in Table 1.

VOLUME SUPPORT VENTILATION

In volume support ventilation (VSV), patient triggers every breath. Ventilator automatically adjusts the inspiratory pressure to ensure the lowest possible inspiratory pressure to deliver the preset tidal volume. Tidal volume is used as feedback control to adjust the pressure support level. Inspiratory pressure is maintained constant during inspiration. Inspiratory flow is decelerating. Patient determines the breathing rate and the inspiratory time. If there is apnea, there is automatic backup with PRVC mode of ventilation. Inspiration stops and expiration starts when the peak flow drops to 5–15% of initial flow (Fig. 2). As the upper pressure limit is reached, the ventilator immediately

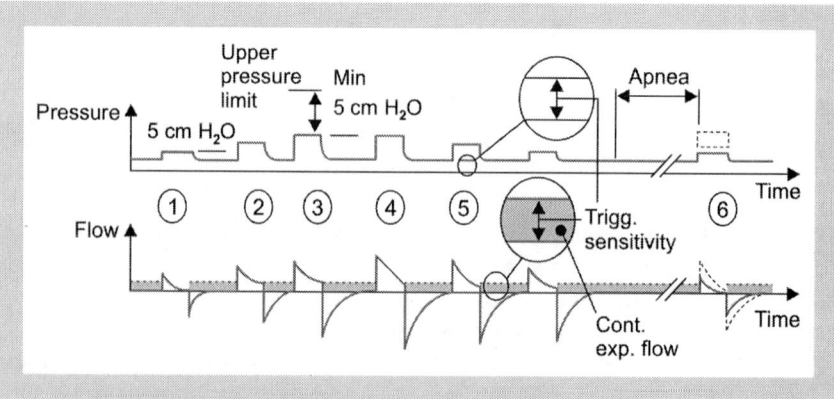

Test breath (5 cm H_2O)
1. Pressure is increased slowly until target volume is achieved
2. Maximum available pressure is 5 cm H_2O below upper pressure limit
3. VT higher than set VT delivered results in lower pressure
4. Patient can trigger breath
5. If apnea, ventilator switches to PRVC (Automode)

Fig. 2: Breath-to-breath analysis of patient in pressure time and flow time waveform with volume support ventilation.

changes to expiration and gives alarm for "high airway" pressure. If the difference between the upper pressures limit and peak airway pressure is less than 5 cm of H_2O, a "limited pressure" alarm is given. The tidal volume delivered will be less than the preset. Maximum inspiratory time is 80% of the respiratory cycle. VSV indicated in postoperative patient recovering from anesthesia, spontaneous breathing patient who requires minimum tidal volume, patients who are asynchronous with the ventilator, and as a weaning mode especially in patient with neuromuscular weakness. Volume support is a PRVC-like modification of pressure support. The difference between this and PRVC is the difference between PCV and PS—volume support is flow-cycled.

Advantages

Automatic weaning of pressure support as tidal volume matches minimum required tidal volume.

Disadvantages

Sustain spontaneous effort required, tidal volume selected may be too large or small for patient, auto-PEEP may affect proper functioning, varying mean airway pressure with each breath, sudden increase in respiratory rate and demand may result in a decrease in ventilator support.

PROPORTIONAL ASSIST VENTILATION

Patients who have normal respiratory drive but who have difficulty in sustaining adequate spontaneous ventilation are often subjected to pressure support ventilation (PSV), in which the ventilator generates a constant pressure throughout inspiration regardless of the intensity of the patient's effort (Fig. 3). In 1992, Younes and colleagues developed PAV as an alternative in which the ventilator generates pressure in proportion to the patient's effort. PAV became commercially available in Europe in 1999 and was approved in

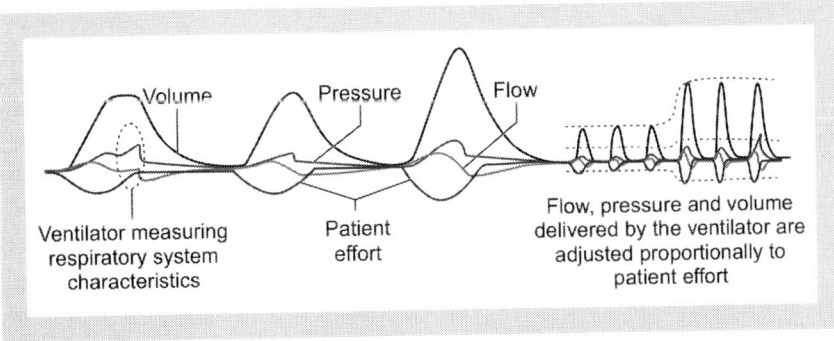

Fig. 3: Volume delivery adjusted proportionally to the patient's effort in proportional assist ventilation mode.

the United States in 2006, available on the Puritan Bennett 840 ventilator. PAV has also been used for noninvasive ventilation. Other names for PAV are proportional pressure support (Drager Medical).

Both PSV and PAV are spontaneous modes. The patient controls the timing and size of the breath. There are no preset pressures, flow, or volume goals, but safety limits on the volume and pressure delivered can be set. With PSV, the pressure applied by the ventilator rises to a preset level that is held constant until a cycling criterion is reached. The inspiratory flow and tidal volume are the result of the patient's inspiratory effort, the level of pressure applied, and the respiratory system mechanics. In contrast, during PAV, the pressure applied is a function of patient effort—the greater the inspiratory effort, the greater the increase in applied pressure. The operator sets the percentage of support to be delivered by the ventilator. The ventilator intermittently measures the compliance and resistance of the patient's respiratory system and the instantaneous patient-generated flow and volume, and on the basis of these it delivers a proportional amount of inspiratory pressure.

Initial Settings in Proportional Assist Ventilation

- Airway type (endotracheal tube, tracheostomy)
- Airway size (inner diameter)
- Percentage of work supported (assist range 5–95%)
- Tidal volume and pressure limit
- Expiratory sensitivity (normally, as inspiration ends, flow should stop; this parameter tells the ventilator at what flow to end inspiration).

Advantages

In theory, PAV should reduce the work of breathing, improve synchrony, automatically adapt to changing patient lung mechanics and effort, decrease the need for ventilator intervention and manipulation, decrease the need for sedation, and improve sleep. The probability of spontaneous breathing without assistance was significantly better in critically ill patients ventilated with PAV than with PSV. No trial has reported the effect of PAV on deaths.

VOLUME-ASSURED PRESSURE SUPPORT

Volume-assured pressure support (VAPS) is also based on closed-loop ventilation but in this mode intrabreath variation is present rather than interbreath variation. It means character of breath changes within the breath from pressure control to volume control if minimum tidal volume has not been achieved. It combines high initial flow of pressure-limited breath with a constant volume delivery of volume-limited breath within same breath. In this mode of ventilator, use both type of breaths (pressure- and volume-limited) within the same breath to achieve target minimum tidal volume. Type of breath will depends on the adequacy of the patient's effort. If patient

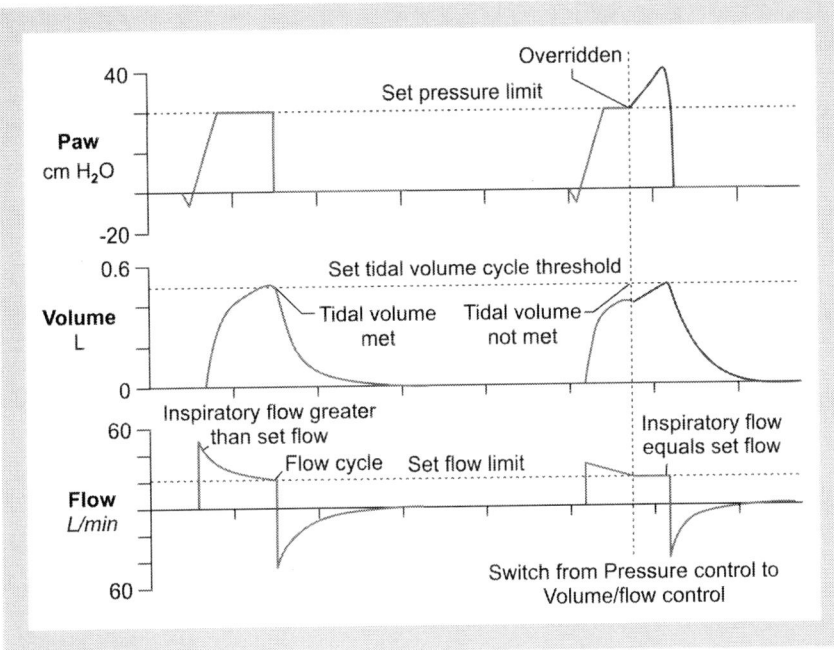

Fig. 4: Pulmonary mechanics waveforms in volume assured pressure support (VAPS) mode showing change in mode of ventilation within same breath to achieve target minimum tidal volume.

had adequate respiratory effort, then pressure supported breath will be delivered. If patient had inadequate respiratory effort, then controlled breath (flow-targeted and volume-cycled) will be delivered rather than pressure supported (Fig. 4).

Advantages

Patient will receive minimum pressure support and peak flow to achieve minimum tidal volume. Decrease work of breathing in comparisons to conventional ventilation (Table 2).

ADAPTIVE SUPPORT VENTILATION

Adaptive support ventilation is a positive pressure mode of mechanical ventilation that is closed-loop controlled. ASV evolved as a form of MMV implemented with APC. MMV is a mode that allows the operator to preset target minute ventilation, and the ventilator then supplies mandatory breaths, either volume- or pressure-controlled, if the patient's spontaneous breaths generate lower minute ventilation. ASV automatically selects the appropriate tidal volume and frequency for mandatory breaths and the appropriate tidal volume for spontaneous breaths on the basis of the respiratory system mechanics and target minute alveolar ventilation. In the

Table 2: Comparisons between different modes of ventilation.		
Pressure-regulated volume control	*Volume support ventilation*	*Volume-assured pressure support*
• Interbreath variation • Use the set tidal volume as the "target" for each breath • Normal cycling may stop inspiration below or above set tidal volume • Pressure used based on mechanics measurements	• Interbreath variation • Use the set tidal volume as the "target" for each breath • Normal cycling starts when the peak flow drops to 5–15% of initial flow • If inspiratory demand decreases, ventilator can increase up to 150% of set tidal volume in next breath by increasing inspiratory pressure up to a limit • Tidal volume/Pressure mechanics measured	• Intrabreath variation • Use the set tidal volume as a minimum • Normal cycling occurs at or above the set tidal volume • Character of breath changed within the breath from pressure control to volume control if minimum tidal volume has not been achieved • Tidal volume mechanics not measured

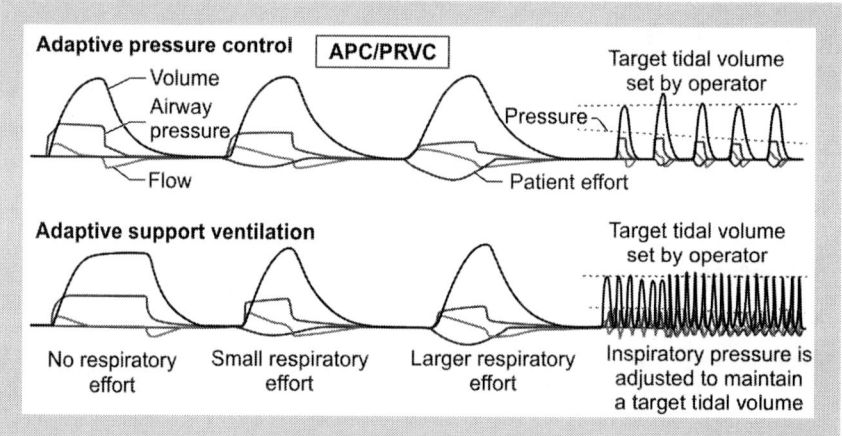

Fig. 5: Differences between PRVC (APC) and ASV mode. Adaptive support ventilation (bottom) automatically selects the appropriate tidal volume and frequency for mandatory breaths and the appropriate tidal volume for spontaneous breaths on the basis of the respiratory system mechanics and the target minute ventilation.

ASV mode, every breath is synchronized with patient effort if such an effort exists, and otherwise, full mechanical ventilation is provided to the patient. Targeted tidal volume will be given as pressure control or pressure support breaths (Fig. 5).

Advantages

It provides decelerating flow waveform to improved gas distribution with guaranteed tidal volume. It also decreases work of breathing. Automatic weaning is possible with disease reversal.

Initial Ventilatory Settings

It is first commercially available mode that automatically selects all the ventilator settings except PEEP and FiO_2.

- Gender and height (to calculate the ideal body weight)
- Percent of normal predicted minute ventilation goal. Delivers 200 mL/min/kg of minute ventilation for children. It can be set from 20% to 200%.
- FiO_2 and PEEP
- High-pressure alarm: 5 cm H_2O above PEEP to 10 cm H_2O below set Pmax.

MANDATORY MINUTE VENTILATION

Mandatory minute ventilation was first described by Hewlett et al. in 1977. MMV is the first closed-loop mode which simply means that the ventilator changes its output based on measured input variables. This mode allows the patient to breathe spontaneously with guaranteed minimum minute ventilation preset by clinician. This can be accomplished by the use of increasing levels of pressure support or by delivery of mandatory breaths (time-triggered, volume-controlled). If spontaneous breathing is used, breaths are pressure-controlled; pressure, flow or volume-triggered; pressure-limited; and flow-cycled. Essentially the patient is receiving PSV with varying pressure support level. In contrast to SIMV, MMV gives mandatory breaths only if spontaneous breathing has fallen below preselected minimum ventilation.

Advantages

Major difference with SIMV mode is that it decreases mechanical breaths and it may reduce some long-term complications associated with mechanical ventilation.

NEURALLY ADJUSTED VENTILATORY ASSIST

Neurally adjusted ventilatory assist (NAVA) is a unique mode of ventilation which is based on neural respiratory output. The act of taking a breath is controlled by the respiratory center in the brain, which decides the characteristics of each breath, timing and size. The respiratory center sends a signal along the phrenic nerve, excites the diaphragm muscle cells, leading to muscle contraction and descent of the diaphragm dome. As a result, the pressure in the airway drops, causing an inflow of air into the lungs

Flowchart 3: Neuroventilatory control sequence, from neural inspiratory signal to (mechanical) inspiration.

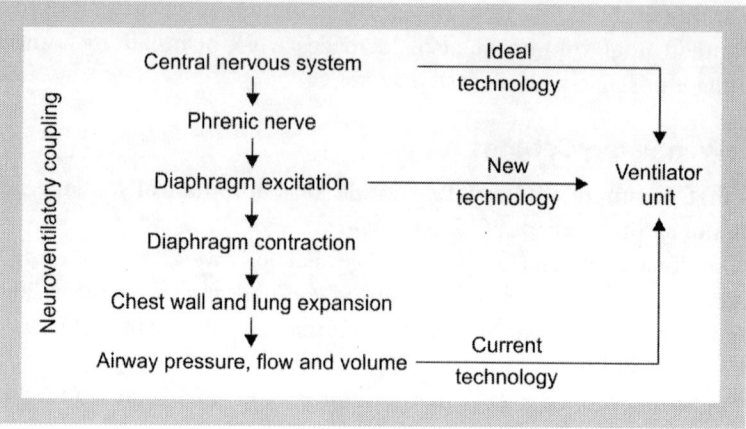

(Flowchart 3). With NAVA, the electrical activity of the diaphragm (Edi) is captured, fed to the ventilator and used to assist the patient's breathing in synchrony with and in proportion to the patient's own efforts, regardless of patient category or size. As the work of the ventilator and the diaphragm is controlled by the same signal, coupling between the diaphragm and the ventilator is synchronized simultaneously. As the work of breathing increases and the respiratory center ask the diaphragm for more effort, the neurally controlled system increases the amount of ventilator support.

AUTOMODE

This mode design to allow the ventilator to be interactive with the patient's needs by making breath-by-breath adjustments in both control and support modes. In the absence of triggering, the machine functions in a control mode. When the patient begins to make satisfactory inspiratory efforts (two consecutive triggered breaths), the ventilator switches to the support mode. All breaths are patient-triggered, pressure-limited, and flow-cycled. A switching of modes is indicated by a blinking light. Ventilator automatically shifts between controlled, supported, and spontaneous ventilation as required. When patient was shifted from time-cycled to flow-cycled ventilation, which can lead to decrease in mean airway pressure and hypoxemia.

HIGH-FREQUENCY OSCILLATORY VENTILATION

Different modes are available in high-frequency ventilation. Here we will discuss only HFOV, which is most commonly used. HFOV is a form of pressure-controlled intermittent mandatory ventilation. In contrast to conventional pressure-controlled intermittent mandatory ventilation, in which relatively small spontaneous breaths may be superimposed on relatively large

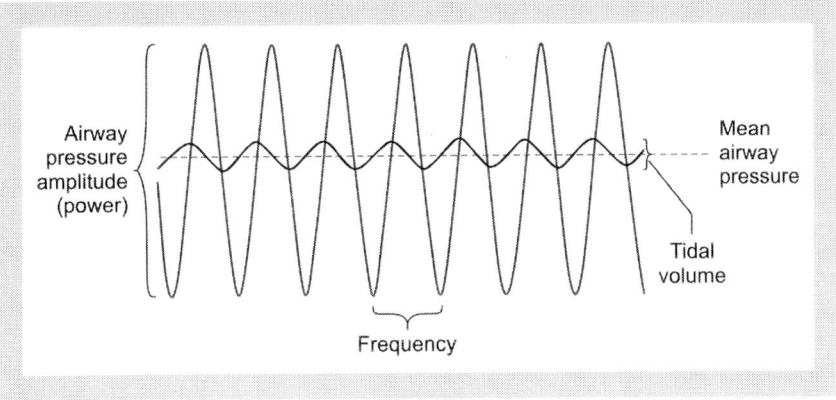

Fig. 6: High-frequency oscillatory ventilation delivers very small mandatory breaths (oscillations) at frequencies of up to 900 breaths/minute.

mandatory breaths, HFOV superimposes very small mandatory breaths (oscillations) on top of spontaneous breaths (Fig. 6). HFOV can be delivered only with a special ventilator. The ventilator delivers a constant flow (bias flow), while a valve creates resistance to maintain airway pressure, on top of which a piston pump oscillates at frequencies of 3–15 Hz. This creates a constant airway pressure with small oscillations. For appropriate amplitude settings, "chest wiggle factor" is assessed clinically.

It is an attractive mode of ventilation because of its unique ability to provide adequate gas exchange using tidal volumes below dead space volume in the setting of continuous alveolar recruitment. Theoretically, HFOV should provide the ultimate open-lung strategy of ventilation, with preservation of end-expiratory lung volume (EELV), minimization of cyclic stretch, and avoidance of parenchymal over distention at end-inspiration, amounting to ventilation on the most compliant portion of the volume-pressure curve while avoiding extremes of lung volume. Oxygenation is achieved with high mean airway pressure to achieve lung recruitment and ventilation is achieved with an oscillating piston that creates cycles of pressure above and below the mean airway pressure at a supraphysiological respiratory rates (180–900/min), resulting in small tidal volumes (1–2.5 mL/kg). Exhalation is active rather than passive process as occurs in all other conventional and high-frequency mode. In this mode control of oxygenation and ventilation are independent. The initial ventilatory settings in HFOV depend on age, type and severity of the disease (Table 3).

Adjustments

After initial ventilator settings, the oxygenation and ventilation are adjusted independently. Mean airway pressure is adjusted to achieve $SaO_2 > 90\%$ while CO_2 elimination is increased by adjusting the amplitude and decreasing frequency on machine.

	FiO$_2$	Bias flow	Ti	Hz	Paw	Power
Table 3: Initial ventilator settings in high-frequency oscillatory ventilation (HFOV).						
Neonate (not preterm)	1.0	20 L/min	33%	13–12	3–5 cm above CMV P$_{aw}$	0–2
<10 kg	1.0	20 L/min	33%	12–10		0–4
10–30 kg	1.0	20–30 L/min	33%	12–8		4
>30 kg	1.0	≥ 30 L/min	33–(50)%	6		4–6

(Hz: Hertz; Paw: mean airway pressure; Ti: inspiratory time).

Weaning:
- Decrease FiO$_2$, MAP, and amplitude
- Switch to conventional ventilation when
  - Reversal of disease process
  - Adequate gas exchange and improving oxygenation indices
  - MAP < 15 (12–18 cm H$_2$O)
  - FiO$_2$ < 0.5 (0.4–0.6).

High-frequency oscillatory ventilation should not be used in patients with shock, severe airway obstruction, intracranial hemorrhage, or refractory barotraumas. It must be used cautiously with severe acidosis, because CO$_2$ excretion may be limited. Different studies have found no differences in survival or duration of mechanical ventilation between the two groups while comparing conventional and HFOV, but few children who receive HFOV remained dependent on supplemental O$_2$ at 30 days. It has been suggested that HFOV should be employed early in the course of severe ARDS.

KEY MESSAGES

- Regardless of the mode, our goals are to avoid lung injury, keep the patient comfortable, and wean the patient from mechanical ventilation as soon as possible.
- Conventional modes are passive and operator-dependent, but newer modes are adaptively interactive, goal-oriented and patient-centered.
- Further clinical trials are needed to make a recommendation for various modes of ventilation according to disease and patient status.

SUGGESTED READING

1. Amato MB, Barbas CS, Bonassa J, et al. Volume-assured pressure support ventilation (VAPSV). A new approach for reducing muscle workload during acute respiratory failure. Chest. 1992;102(4):1225-34.
2. Balke B, Ware RW. Basic principles of ventilator machinery. In: Tobin MJ (Ed). Principles and Practice of Mechanical Ventilation, 2nd edition. Philadelphia: McGraw-Hill; 2006. pp. 77-8.
3. Bengtsson JA, Edberg, KE. Neurally adjusted ventilatory assist in children: an observational study. Pediatr Criti Care Med. 2010;11:253-7.

4. Chatburn RL. Classification of ventilator modes: update and proposal for implementation. Respir Care. 2007;52:301-23.
5. Clark RH, Gerstmann DL, Null DM Jr, et al. Prospective randomized comparison of high-frequency oscillatory and conventional ventilation in respiratory distress syndrome. Pediatrics. 1992;89:5-12.
6. East TD, Bohm SH, Wallace CJ, et al. A successful computerized protocol for clinical management of pressure control inverse ratio ventilation in ARDS patients. Chest. l992;101:697-710.
7. Ferguson ND, Cook DJ, Guyatt GH, et al. High-frequency oscillation in early acute respiratory distress syndrome. N Engl J Med. 2013;368:795-805.
8. Hasan A. The conventional modes of mechanical ventilation. In: Hasan A (Ed). Understanding Mechanical Ventilation: A Practical Handbook, 2nd edition. Philadelphia: Springer; 2010. pp. 72-109.
9. Marcy TW, Marini JJ. Inverse ratio ventilation in ARDS. Rationale and implementation. Chest. 1991;100:494-504.
10. Sachdev A, Chugh K, Gupta D, et al. Comparison of two ventilation modes and their clinical implications in sick children. Indian J Crit Care Med. 2005;9:205-10.
11. Schultz TR, Costarino AT, Durning SM, et al. Airway pressure release ventilation in pediatrics. Pediatr Crit Care Med. 2001;2:243-6.
12. Younes M, Puddy A, Roberts D, et al. Proportional assist ventilation. Results of an initial clinical trial. Am Rev Respir Dis. 1992;145:121-9.
13. Young D, Lamb SE, Shah S, et al. High-frequency oscillation for acute respiratory distress syndrome. N Engl J Med. 2013;368(9):806-13.

Noninvasive Ventilation

Shipra Gulati, Rajiv Uttam

Noninvasive ventilation (NIV) refers to the application of ventilatory support using techniques that do not require an invasive endotracheal airway. Multiple forms of NIV are available for use in children:

- Continuous positive airway pressure (CPAP)
- Bilevel positive airway pressure (BiPAP)
- Intermittent positive pressure breathing (IPPB)
- Humidified high-flow nasal cannula (HHFNC)
- Bilevel nasal CPAP.

Use of NIV in pediatric patients is increasing in the emergency department, critical care unit, and prehospital environment. Noninvasive positive pressure ventilation refers to the delivery of a pressurized gas to the airway via a nasal or full face mask. The earliest NIV devices were actually external negative pressure ventilators, including the body ventilator and iron lung. Negative pressure ventilators were widely used during the polio epidemics of the 1930s and 1960s, but these ventilators were problematic they were large and bulky, and they made access to patients difficult. Alternative forms of respiratory support emerged during the 1970s and 1980s along with increased interest in noninvasive positive pressure ventilation.

PATHOPHYSIOLOGY AND MECHANISM OF ACTION

Noninvasive positive pressure devices deliver pressurized gas to the airway via a mask or nasal prongs. This results in an increase in mean airway pressure, which recruits atelectatic alveoli, improves gas exchange, and reduces work of breathing (Box 1). In pediatric patients, NIV decreases work of breathing by unloading the diaphragm and accessory muscles and reducing inspiratory energy expenditure. NIV may also help stabilize the highly pliable chest wall in young infants, reducing retractions. NIV provides positive end-expiratory pressure (PEEP) which helps open collapsed alveoli, increasing functional residual capacity and improving oxygenation. NIV may also reverse hypoventilation by increasing tidal volume and minute ventilation in children with hypercapnic respiratory failure. In children with

Box 1: Noninvasive ventilation (NIV): mechanisms of action.
- Decreases work of breathing
- Increases functional residual capacity
- Recruits collapsed alveoli
- Improves respiratory gas exchange
- Reverses hypoventilation
- Maintains upper airway patency
- May increase or decrease cardiac output depending on underlying disease

occlusive apnea, noninvasive positive pressure may help reduce the number of occlusive events by maintaining upper airway patency. NIV may have negative physiologic effects, most of which are shared by invasive mechanical ventilation. Positive airway pressure increases intrathoracic pressure, which may decrease venous return and cardiac output in patients with poor cardiac function. In patients with normal cardiac function, NIV may actually improve cardiac output by decreasing left ventricular afterload.

ADVANTAGES OF NONINVASIVE VENTILATION

Noninvasive ventilation has several significant advantages over endotracheal intubation. NIV devices leave the upper airway intact, decreasing the risk of airway trauma and preserving the natural defense mechanisms of the upper airways. Additionally, patients receiving NIV do not require paralytics, and the need for sedation is greatly reduced. Older children can communicate with their health care providers while receiving NIV. NIV is also less expensive than mechanical ventilation, and studies have shown that it decreases length of hospital stay and associated cost.

NONINVASIVE VENTILATION TECHNIQUES AND EQUIPMENT

Continuous Positive Airway Pressure

Continuous positive airway pressure (CPAP) delivers a constant level of pressure support to the airways during inspiration and expiration. This constant pressure typically ranges from 5 cm H_2O to 10 cm H_2O and is delivered without regard to the respiratory cycle. CPAP can be delivered through several different external interfaces, including oronasal masks, nose masks, nasopharyngeal prongs, single-nasal prongs, and short binasal prongs. Oronasal masks (full face masks) are commonly used in older children and adults, but these masks are not generally used in neonates and young infants due to the difficulty in maintaining an adequate fit and seal. Short binasal prongs deliver equal pressure to both nostrils and have less resistance than the single-nasal prongs. Nasal CPAP has been used extensively in premature neonates, infants with bronchiolitis and lower airway obstruction (also refer to chapter 5 for details).

Bilevel Positive Airway Pressure

Bilevel positive airway pressure devices provide two levels of positive airway pressure during the respiratory cycle. A higher level of pressure is provided during inspiration [inspiratory positive airway pressure (IPAP)], and a lower level of pressure is provided during expiration [expiratory positive airway pressure (EPAP)]. The available IPAP range is 2–25 cm H_2O, with typical settings of 10–16 cm H_2O. The available EPAP range is 2–20 cm H_2O, with typical settings of 5–10 cm H_2O. BiPAP can be delivered with a set respiratory rate or a backup rate. Additionally, the cycle may be fixed as a function of time, or it may be triggered by the patient's inspiratory flow. As with CPAP, BiPAP may be provided by a machine specifically designed for this form of NIV or by a traditional ventilator set to appropriate bilevel pressure support settings. The level of pressure support in BiPAP is equivalent to the difference between the inspiratory and expiratory pressures (IPAP minus EPAP). Supplemental oxygen may be provided through the ventilatory tubing or directly through the mask. Many of the new BiPAP devices also have oxygen blenders.

Humidified High-Flow Nasal Cannula

High-flow nasal cannula devices deliver warmed humidified gas to the airways. Because the gas is nearly 100% humidified, nasal mucosal irritation is greatly reduced. This permits improved tolerance of high gas flow up to 8 L/min in infants and 40 L/min in older children. 2–3 mL/kg flow may be set. With HHFNC, many units are ventilating less and less infants with bronchiolitis and even with pneumonia. It helps in CO_2 wash out by flow dynamics as well as improved ventilation of open alveoli maintained open after the initial opening pressure as well as improves oxygenation by CPAP effect by generating positive mean airway pressure.

Please refer to chapter 6 for details.

Nasal Intermittent Positive Pressure Ventilation

A relatively new form of NIV for infants that provides periodic increases in positive pressure above a baseline fixed pressure. Nasal intermittent positive pressure ventilation (NIPPV) can be delivered via a nasal mask or nasal prongs connected to a ventilator, or it can be delivered by a free-standing device specifically designed for this form of NIV. Whereas the traditional infant nasal CPAP device contains a single flowmeter, the NIPPV device has a second flowmeter that periodically adds additional flow to the system. These periods of increased flow are known as "*sighs*" and can be delivered at a preset rate. The periodic increases in positive airway pressure may help offload the diaphragm and accessory muscles, decreasing the infant's work of breathing. The device essentially provides two levels of CPAP, but unlike BiPAP, the infant cannot trigger the device to cycle between the high and low CPAP settings. These cycles are controlled by settings on the machine.

Improved oxygenation can be achieved by increasing the amount of time on the high CPAP setting. Improved ventilation can be achieved by increasing the number of cycles between the high and low CPAP settings (see chapter 5).

APPLICATIONS OF NONINVASIVE VENTILATION

In Chronic Diseases

- Obstructive airway disease
- Obstructive sleep apnea (OSA)
  - Adenotonsillar hypertrophy
  - Craniofacial malformations as in Down syndrome or Pierre Robin syndrome
  - Neurological abnormalities as in cerebral palsy
- Restrictive airway disease
  - Poliomyelitis
  - Neuromuscular diseases as Duchenne muscular dystrophy
  - Central hypoventilation syndrome.

In Acute Diseases

- Respiratory distress syndrome
  - Hyaline membrane disease in newborns
- Apnea of prematurity
- Lower airway obstruction
  - Asthma
  - Bronchiolitis
- Upper airway obstruction
- Acute respiratory distress syndrome (ARDS) in pediatrics
- Pneumonia
- Postextubation respiratory failure
- Weaning from ventilator
- Immunocompromised patients.

CONTRAINDICATIONS TO NONINVASIVE VENTILATION

- Apnea
- Impaired mental status
- Inability to protect the airway
- Excessive oral secretions
- Uncooperative or agitated patient
- Poor mask fit
- Hemodynamic instability
- Shock
- Upper gastrointestinal bleeding
- Recent gastric, esophageal, or upper airway surgery
- Inadequate staff to appropriately monitor patient.

SIGNS OF EFFECTIVE RESPONSE TO NONINVASIVE VENTILATION

- Decreased respiratory rate
- Decreased retractions and accessory muscle use
- Reduced airway occlusion events
- Improved oxygenation on pulse oximetry and blood gases
- Improved lung volumes on chest radiographs.

REASONS TO DISCONTINUE NONINVASIVE VENTILATION

- Progressive respiratory distress
- Persistent tachypnea
- Persistent hypoxia despite supplemental oxygen
- Hemodynamic instability
- Vomiting
- Excessive secretions
- Increasing anxiety or agitation
- Increasing lethargy or worsening mental status.

ACUTE NONINVASIVE VENTILATION: MONITORING

- Pulse oximetry
- Noninvasive blood pressure (NIBP)
- Peripheral venous access
- Arterial blood gas/capillary gases
- Electrocardiogram (ECG)
- Arterial lines.

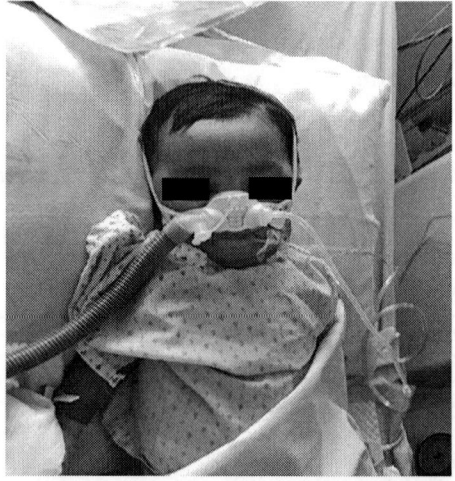

Fig. 1: A 9-month-old girl with spinal muscular dystrophy with severe necrotizing pneumonia was extubated onto BiPAP and discharged on BiPAP (smallest nasal mask NASAL PIXI).

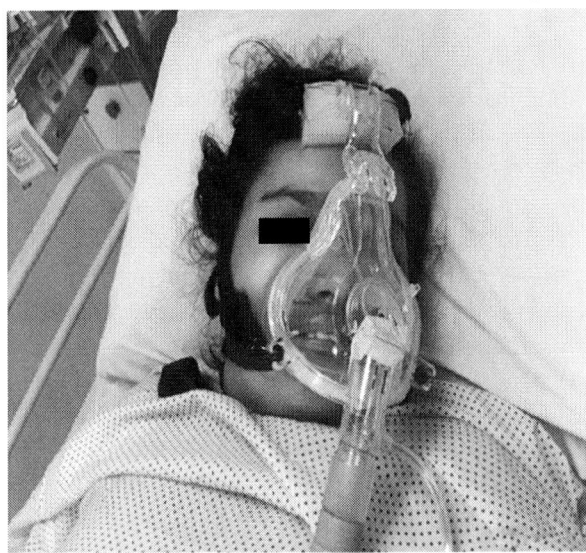

Fig. 2: An 11-year-old girl with fulminant staphylococcal infection including bilateral pneumonia with empyema with pyomyositis with multiple abscesses (BiPAP use prevented intubation and respiratory distress settled).

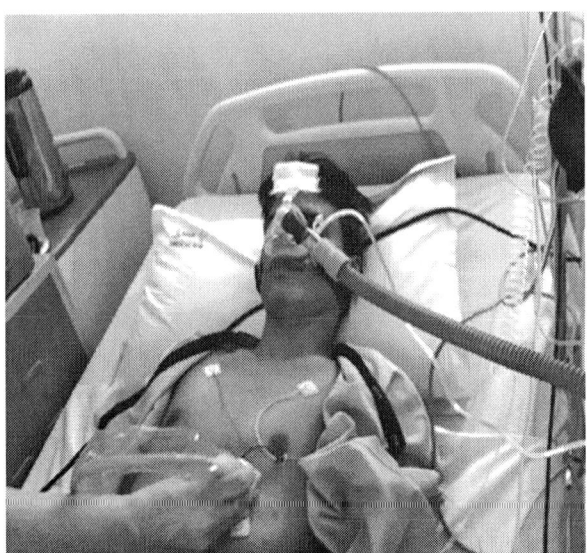

Fig. 3: A 15-year-old boy with pulmonary embolism came in respiratory distress (nasal mask used for BiPAP).

Authors have used NIV in around 50 children with almost 90% success rate (Figs. 1 to 3). NIV has decreased the rates of intubation and ventilator-associated pneumonia (VAP) in many pediatric intensive care units (PICUs); at the same time, it has decreased the emotional stress and financial burden.

KEY MESSAGES

- Noninvasive ventilation has gained popularity in last two decades even in younger children as initial modality before considering invasive mechanical ventilation. It has also been used postextubation for trial before reintubation is considered.
- Noninvasive ventilation keeps upper airway intact, decreasing the risk of airway trauma and preserving the natural defense mechanisms of the upper airways. Additionally, patients receiving NIV do not require paralytics, and the need for sedation is greatly reduced.
- Noninvasive ventilation can be used in chronic diseases such as OSA, craniofacial malformations as in Down syndrome or Pierre Robin syndrome and neurological abnormalities as in cerebral palsy, neuromuscular diseases as in Duchenne muscular dystrophy and central hypoventilation syndrome.
- Contraindications to NIV are apnea, impaired mental status, inability to protect the airway, excessive oral secretions, poor mask fit and hemodynamic instability.
- Reasons to discontinue NIV are progressive respiratory distress, persistent tachypnea, persistent hypoxia despite supplemental oxygen, etc.
- A facility for invasive ventilation must be kept available and ready whenever a patient is placed on NIV.

SUGGESTED READING

1. Abadesso C, Nunes P, Silvestre C, et al. Non-invasive ventilation in acute respiratory failure in children. Pediatr Rep. 2012;4(2):e16.
2. Basnet S, Mander G, Andoh J, et al. Safety, efficacy, and tolerability of early initiation of noninvasive positive pressure ventilation in pediatric patients admitted with status asthmaticus: a pilot study. Pediatr Crit Care Med. 2012;13(4):393-8.
3. Baudin F, Pouyau R, Cour-Andlauer F, et al. Neurally adjusted ventilator assist (NAVA) reduces asynchrony during non-invasive ventilation for severe bronchiolitis. Pediatr Pulmonol. 2015;50(12):1320-7.
4. Bernet V, Hug MI, Frey B. Predictive factors for the success of noninvasive mask ventilation in infants and children with acute respiratory failure. Pediatr Crit Care Med. 2005;6(6):660-4.
5. Chan J, Edman JC, Koltai PJ. Obstructive sleep apnea in children. Am Fam Physician. 2004;69(5):1147-55.
6. Cummings JJ, Polin RA; Committee on Fetus and Newborn, American Academy of Pediatrics. Noninvasive respiratory support. Pediatrics. 2016;137(1).
7. DiBlasi R, Courtney SE. Noninvasive respiratory support. In: Goldsmith JP, Karotkin EH, Keszler M, Suresh GK (Eds). Assisted Ventilation of the Neonate, 6th edition. Philadelphia, Pennsylvania: Elsevier; 2003. pp. 162-79.
8. Essouri S, Chevret L, Durand P, et al. Noninvasive positive pressure ventilation: five years of experience in a pediatric intensive care unit. Pediatr Crit Care Med. 2006;7(4):329-34.

9. Flight WG, Shaw J, Johnson S, et al. Long-term non-invasive ventilation in cystic fibrosis: experience over two decades. J Cyst Fibros. 2012;11(3):187-92.
10. Gupta P, Kuperstock JE, Hashmi S, et al. Efficacy and predictors of success of noninvasive ventilation for prevention of extubation failure in critically ill children with heart disease. Pediatr Cardiol. 2013;34(4):964-77.
11. Levitt MA. A prospective, randomized trial of BiPAP in severe acute congestive heart failure. J Emerg Med. 2001;21:363-9.
12. Loh LE, Chan YH, Chan I. Noninvasive ventilation in children: a review. J Pediatr. 2007;83(2 Suppl):S91-9.
13. Pediatric Acute Lung Injury Consensus Conference Group. Pediatric acute respiratory distress syndrome: consensus recommendations from the Pediatric Acute Lung Injury Consensus Conference. Pediatr Crit Care Med. 2015;16(5): 428-39.
14. Piastra M, Antonelli M, Caresta E, et al. Noninvasive ventilation in childhood acute neuromuscular respiratory failure: a pilot study. Respiration. 2006;73(6):791-8.
15. Ruza F. Noninvasive ventilation in pediatric acute respiratory failure: a challenge in pediatric intensive care units. Pediatr Crit Care Med. 2010;11:750-1.
16. Schibler A, Franklin D. Respiratory support for children in the emergency department. J Paediatr Child Health. 2016;52(2):192-6.
17. Stein H, Beck J, Dunn M. Non-invasive ventilation with neurally adjusted ventilator assist in newborns. Semin Fetal Neonatal Med. 2016;21(3):154-61.
18. Teague GW, Thompson-Batt D. Noninvasive mechanical ventilation of the infant and children. In: Walsh BK (Ed). Neonatal and Pediatric Respiratory Care, 4th edition. St. Louis, Missouri: Elsevier; 2015. pp. 287-99.

Respiratory Monitoring on Ventilator

Chandrashekhar Singha, Abhijit Singh, Navneet Kumar, Praveen Khilnani

Monitoring of the respiratory indices has the potential for predicting catastrophes and providing an opportunity for the timely institution of lifesaving measures. Along with physical examination which remains clinically relevant, noninvasive monitoring (pulse oximetry and end-tidal CO_2) and invasive monitoring [arterial blood gas (ABG) and derived indices] are important and routinely done in most pediatric intensive care units (PICUs). The appropriate integration and interpretation of all data are essential for efficient, high-quality, cost-effective, pediatric critical care.

PHYSICAL EXAMINATION

Initial assessment begins by observing the child's position (will assume a most comfortable posture like "sniffing position" during upper airway obstruction or splinting of the chest in patients of pneumonia), respiratory pattern and body habitus (shape of the chest wall). The respiratory pattern will provide information about respiratory rate (tachypnea: an early sign of distress) which varies with age (Table 1), increased work of breathing which can be assessed by the presence grunting, flaring of alae nasi, suprasternal, intercostal and subcostal retractions, use of accessory muscles of respiration and paradoxical breathing.

Evaluation of cyanosis, clubbing, friction rub, breath sounds (wheezes and crackles) through the tracheobronchial tree are reliable and reproducible.

Table 1: Normal respiratory rate.	
Age	*Respiratory rate*
Infant (birth–1 year)	30–60
Toddler (1–3 years)	24–40
Preschooler (3–6 years)	22–34
School-age (6–12 years)	18–30
Adolescent (12–18 years)	12–16

RADIOGRAPHY

A very commonly ordered investigation in PICU which has diagnostic, therapeutic and prognostic value is X-ray chest.

MONITORING VENTILATOR GRAPHICS

In this day and age, gentle ventilation is preferred and patient ventilator asynchrony is to be avoided. These are lung protective strategies which can be monitored very well by continuous graphic monitoring on the ventilator display panel. Many adverse effects can be picked up early and corrective measures can be taken. Bronchospasm, tube obstruction, circuit leak, lung overdistention, water logging in circuit, worsening lung compliance are some of the common conditions those can be detected by ventilator graphics. Please refere to chapter 13 on ventilator graphics for details.

NONINVASIVE MONITORING

Transcutaneous Oxygen and Carbon Dioxide Monitoring

Transcutaneous measurements reflect both gas exchange and skin perfusion. In this technique, a probe composed of heater, an electrode, and a thermistor is applied to the patient's skin. The skin is warmed and softened to improve diffusion and permeability. This also causes capillaries to dilate, resulting in better approximation of arterial oxygen values.

Limitations

Several disadvantages limit the use of transcutaneous monitoring to the newborn population. Skin thickness increases with age, making transcutaneous measurements less predictable. Frequent electrode site changes are required to prevent local burns. Relatively frequent calibration and comparison with ABGs are necessary.

Pulse Oximetry

Pulse oximetry is an important noninvasive monitoring technique that allows continuous evaluation of arterial oxygen saturation *and now widely accepted as the fifth vital sign.* The two basic requirements of commercially available pulse oximeters are the presence of a pulsatile tissue bed (arterial vessel) and the spectrophotometric analysis (governed by Beer-Lambert law) of oxygenated hemoglobin (Hb) and nonoxygenated Hb. Oxygenated Hb primarily absorbs infrared (940-nm) light, whereas nonoxygenated Hb primarily absorbs red (660-nm) light. A microprocessor in the pulse oximeter determines the relative proportions of red and infrared light to calculate the percentage of oxygenated versus nonoxygenated Hb in the tissue bed. In addition to the digital readout of O_2 saturation and pulse rate, most pulse oximeters display a plethysmographic waveform which can help clinicians to distinguish an artifactual signal from the true signal.

Factors that Affect the Performance of Pulse Oximetry

- *Poor cardiac output/low perfusion states*: Low perfusion states, such as low cardiac output, vasoconstriction and hypothermia may impair peripheral perfusion and made it difficult for the pulse oximeter sensor to distinguish true signal from background.
- *Motion artifact*: Excessive motion of the photosensor causes intermittent contact with the skin and mechanically modulates the path length of the transmitted light and the amplitude and intensity of the received light, producing spurious saturation values.
- *Optical interference from environment*: Falsely low and high SpO_2 readings occur with fluorescent and xenon arc surgical lamps, bilirubin lights, infrared heating lamps, and direct sunlight.
- *Dyshemoglobinemias*: Carboxy hemoglobin, methemoglobin, fetal Hb—since pulse oximeters use only two wavelengths of light and, thus, it can distinguish only two substances, Hb and HbO_2. When carboxyhemoglobin (COHb) and methemoglobin (MetHb) are also present, four wavelengths are required to determine the "fractional SaO_2", i.e. $(HbO_2 \times 100)/(Hb + HbO_2 + COHb + MetHb)$ and this can be measured by CO-oximetry. In the presence of elevated COHb levels, oximetry consistently overestimates the true SaO_2 by the amount of COHb present since it has got same absorption spectrum as of HbO_2. Elevated MetHb levels also may cause inaccurate oximetry readings. Anemia does not appear to affect the accuracy of pulse oximetry even in nonhypoxemic patients with acute anemia; pulse oximetry was accurate in measuring O_2 saturation. Severe hyperbilirubinemia (mean bilirubin, 30.6 mg/dL) does not affect the accuracy of pulse oximetry.
- *Dyes and pigments*: Intravenous dyes such as methylene blue, indocyanine green, and indigo carmine can cause falsely low SpO_2 readings. Nail polish, if blue, green or black, causes inaccurate SpO_2 readings, whereas acrylic nails do not interfere with pulse oximetry readings.

It is important to remember that pulse oximeters assess oxygen saturation only and thereby oxygenation status and give no indication of the level of CO_2 and thereby ventilation status. For this reason, they have a limited benefit in patients developing respiratory failure due to CO_2 retention.

The pulse oximeter may be used in a variety of situations that require monitoring of oxygen status and may be used either continuously or intermittently. It is not a substitute for an ABG, but can give clinicians an early warning of decreasing arterial oxyhemoglobin saturation prior to the patient exhibiting clinical signs of hypoxia. The pulse oximeter is a useful tool but the patient must be treated—not the numbers. As with all monitoring equipment, the reading should be interpreted in association with the patient's clinical condition.

Masimo Pulse Oximetry—A New Promising Way of Measuring SpO$_2$

What makes Masimo pulse oximetry different from conventional pulse oximetry?

Conventional pulse oximetry assumes that arterial blood is the only blood moving (pulsating) in the measurement site. During patient motion, the venous blood also moves, which causes conventional pulse oximetry to under-read because it cannot distinguish between the arterial and venous blood. Masimo signal technology identifies the venous blood signal, isolates it, and cancels the noise and extracts the arterial signal, and then reports the true arterial oxygen saturation and pulse rate.

Following setbacks of conventional pulse oximetry for inaccurate monitoring or signal dropout during the reading are rectified by Masimo technology:

- Patient motion or movement
- Low perfusion (low signal amplitude)
- Intense ambient light (lighting or sunlight)
- Electrosurgical instrument interference.

Capnography (End-Tidal CO$_2$ Monitoring)

Capnography is a noninvasive monitoring tool that measures CO$_2$ concentration in exhaled gas, displayed continuously as a waveform through the respiratory cycle. Typically, this measurement is made using infrared light absorption based on the concept that CO$_2$ strongly absorbs infrared light with a wavelength of 4,280 μm.

The capnogram (Fig. 1) is divided into four distinct phases:

1. Phase I (A-B) is the beginning of exhalation. It represents most of the anatomical dead space. CO$_2$ is almost zero.
2. Phase II (B-C) is where the alveolar gas begins to mix with the dead space gas and the CO$_2$ begins to rapidly rise.
3. Phase III (C-D) represents the alveolar gas, usually has a slight increase in the slope as "slow" alveoli empty. The "slow" alveoli have a lower V/Q ratio and therefore have higher CO$_2$ concentrations. In addition, diffusion of CO$_2$ into the alveoli is greater during expiration. *This is more pronounced in infants.* End-tidal CO$_2$ is measured at the maximal point of phase III (D).
4. Phase IV (D-E) is the inspirational phase.

Note that the presence of the alveolar plateau confirms that the measurement is end-tidal. Without a capnography you cannot be sure that a measured CO$_2$ value is really end-tidal.

A normal value for end-tidal CO$_2$ is approximately 38–40 mm Hg. Under normal conditions, the end-tidal CO$_2$ is usually slightly less than

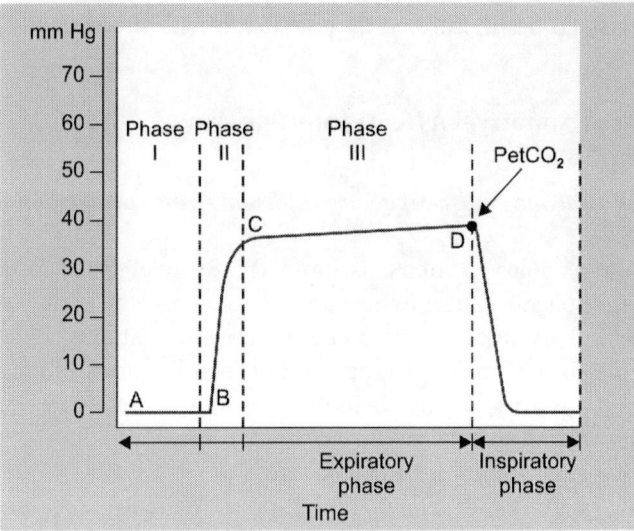

Fig. 1: Normal capnogram.

the $PaCO_2$, with a normal difference of 2–5 mm Hg. Note that this gradient may be considerably higher in situations where there is an increase in dead space. Sampling of exhaled CO_2 can be at the patient-ventilator interface (mainstream), diverted to a monitor (sidestream), or an intermediate connection. Sidestream can be used in intubated or nonintubated patients thus have wider applications but it is less accurate at higher respiratory rates.

Indications for Capnography

Indications for capnography are:
- Confirm and verify tracheal intubation placement
- Evaluate ventilator settings and circuit integrity
- Assess cardiopulmonary status and changes in pulmonary blood flow
- Assess airway management and changes in airway resistance
- Monitor effectiveness of cardiopulmonary resuscitation (CPR)
- Monitor ventilatory status of the respiratory impaired patient
- Monitor ventilation of a nonintubated patient during sedation/analgesia
- Monitor the effectiveness of ventilator weaning process, and response to change in ventilator settings (i.e. respiratory rate, flow and/or volume)
- Reduce the number and/or frequency of ABG drawings
- Aids in the treatment of neurological patients and the possibility of increasing intracranial pressures.

Other Uses

- Metabolic
  - Assess energy expenditure

- Cardiovascular
  - Monitor trend in cardiac output
  - Can use as an indirect Fick method, but actual numbers are hard to quantify
  - Measure of effectiveness in CPR
  - Diagnosis of pulmonary embolism by measuring measure gradient.

A separate chapter is included in this book on Capnography.

INVASIVE MONITORING

Arterial Blood Gas Monitoring

Evaluation of ABG provides information on the uptake of oxygen and disposal of CO_2 by the lung. In diseased lungs, indexes of oxygenation have been developed that use the data obtained from a blood gas to better define the efficiency of gas exchange and the causes of hypoxemia.

Let's elaborate now, how to determine oxygenation, and then evaluate the acid-base status systematically.

Oxygen Homeostasis

The most important interpretation in ABG is to look for the adequacy of oxygenation status. The normal partial pressure of O_2 in the arterial blood PaO_2 is 80–100 mm of Hg on breathing at atmospheric oxygen (which contains 21% of oxygen = FiO_2 21%). When the fraction of the inspired O_2 (FiO_2) concentration increases, the arterial PaO_2 increases by five times (PaO_2 = $FiO_2 \times 5$). When PaO_2 falls below 80 mm of Hg, *hypoxemia* results which can be classified as either mild PaO_2 of 60–80 mm Hg, moderate PaO_2 of 50–60 mm Hg or severe $PaO_2 <$ than 50 mm Hg. This arterial inspired oxygen concentration ratio (PaO_2/FiO_2) is the easiest index to calculate and it also is the basis for the definition of acute lung injury/acute respiratory distress syndrome (ARDS).

The alveolar-arterial (A-a) O_2 gradient, $PAO_2 - PaO_2$ helps to differentiate hypoxemia caused by hypoventilation from diffusion abnormalities, ventilation/perfusion mismatch, or shunt. Unlike oxygen (for which alveolar concentrations are higher than arterial concentrations), CO_2 freely diffuses across the lung such that the arterial and alveolar concentrations are identical. As a patient hypoventilates, CO_2 will accumulate in the body (more CO_2 is produced through metabolism than can be eliminated) and thus in the blood (where we measure it as $PaCO_2$). The CO_2 displaces the oxygen in the alveolus. It does require PAO_2, which is difficult to measure. A normal A-a gradient is 10–20 mm Hg, with the normal gradient increasing within this range as the patient ages. An increased A-a gradient identifies decreased O_2 in the arterial blood compared to the O_2 in the alveolus. This suggests a process that interferes with gas transfer, or in general terms, suggests ventilation-perfusion mismatch. A normal A-a gradient in the face of hypoxemia suggests the hypoxemia is due to hypoventilation and not due to underlying lung disorders.

$$\text{A-a gradient} = \{(FiO_2)(760 - 47) - (1.25)(PaCO_2)\} - PaO_2$$

Where does 1.25 come from?

This is a fudge factor which is derived from the respiratory quotient (RQ). The formula actually requires that the $PACO_2$ be divided by the RQ, which is defined as the ratio of CO_2 produced to O_2 consumed (and which depends on diet and metabolism). We estimate the RQ to be 0.8, and the reciprocal of 0.8 is 1.25.

Stepwise Approach to Diagnosing Acid-Base Disorders

Interpreting an ABG is a crucial skill for physicians, nurses, respiratory therapists, and other health care personnel. ABG interpretation is especially important in critically ill patients. The following six-step process helps ensure a complete interpretation of every ABG.

Normal values of ABG:
- pH: 7.35–7.45
- PCO_2: 35–45
- HCO_3: 22–26
- PaO_2: 90–99.

Six-step approach:

Step 1: Assess the internal consistency of the values using the Henderson-Hasselbalch equation:

$$[H^+] = 24\,(PaCO_2)/[HCO_3^-]$$

Step 2: Is there alkalemia or acidemia present?
- pH <7.35 acidemia
- pH >7.45 alkalemia

This is usually the primary disorder. *Remember:* an acidosis or alkalosis may be present even if the pH is in the normal range (7.35–7.45). You will need to check the $PaCO_2$, HCO_3^- and anion gap.

Step 3: Is the disturbance respiratory or metabolic? What is the relationship between the direction of change in the pH and the direction of change in the $PaCO_2$? In primary respiratory disorders, the pH and $PaCO_2$ change in *opposite* directions; in metabolic disorders, the pH and $PaCO_2$ change in the same direction (Table 2).

Step 4: Is there appropriate compensation for the primary disturbance? Usually, compensation does not return the pH to normal (7.35–7.45) (Table 3).

If the observed compensation is not the expected compensation, it is likely that more than one acid-base disorder is present.

Step 5: Calculate the anion gap (if a metabolic acidosis exists):

$$\text{AG} = [Na^+] - ([Cl^-] + [HCO_3^-]) - 12 \pm 2$$

Table 2: Changes in pH and $PaCO_2$.			
Acidosis	Respiratory	pH ↓	$PaCO_2$ ↑
Acidosis	Metabolic	pH ↓	$PaCO_2$ ↓
Alkalosis	Respiratory	pH ↑	$PaCO_2$ ↓
Alkalosis	Metabolic	pH ↑	$PaCO_2$ ↑

Table 3: Expected compensation and correction factor for acid-base disorders.		
Disorder	Expected compensation	Correction factor
Metabolic acidosis	$PaCO_2 = (1.5 \times [HCO_3^-]) + 8$	± 2
Acute respiratory acidosis	Increase in $[HCO_3^-] = \Delta PaCO_2/10$	± 3
Chronic respiratory acidosis (3–5 days)	Increase in $[HCO_3^-] = 3.5 (\Delta PaCO_2/10)$	
Metabolic alkalosis	Increase in $PaCO_2 = 40 + 0.6 (\Delta HCO_3^-)$	
Acute respiratory alkalosis	Decrease in $[HCO_3^-] = 2 (\Delta PaCO_2/10)$	
Chronic respiratory alkalosis	Decrease in $[HCO_3^-] = 5 (\Delta PaCO_2/10)$ to 7 $(\Delta PaCO_2/10)$	

- A normal anion gap is approximately 12 meq/L.
- In patients with hypoalbuminemia, the normal anion gap is lower than 12 meq/L; the "normal" anion gap in patients with hypoalbuminemia is about 2.5 meq/L lower for each 1 g/dL decrease in the plasma albumin concentration (e.g. a patient with a plasma albumin of 2.0 g/dL would be approximately 7 meq/L).
- If the anion gap is elevated, consider calculating the osmolal gap (OSM) in compatible clinical situations.
  - Elevation in AG is not explained by an obvious case [diabetic ketoacidosis (DKA), lactic acidosis, renal failure]
  - Toxic ingestion is suspected.
- OSM gap = Measured OSM – (2[Na^+] – glucose/18 – BUN/2.8
  - The OSM gap should be <10

Step 6: If an increased anion gap is present, assess the relationship between the increase in the anion gap and the decrease in $[HCO_3^-]$. Assess the ratio of the change in the anion gap (ΔAG) to the change in $[HCO3^-]$ ($\Delta[HCO_3^-]$): $\Delta AG/\Delta[HCO_3^-]$

This ratio should be between 1.0 and 2.0 if an uncomplicated anion gap metabolic acidosis is present. If this ratio falls outside of this range, then another metabolic disorder is present:

- If $\Delta AG/\Delta[HCO_3^-]$ <1.0, then a concurrent nonanion gap metabolic acidosis is likely to be present.
- If $\Delta AG/\Delta[HCO_3^-]$ >2.0, then a concurrent metabolic alkalosis is likely to be present.

It is important to remember what the expected "normal" anion gap for your patient should be, by adjusting for hypoalbuminemia (see *Step 5*, above).

KEY MESSAGES

- Respiratory monitoring is an essential tool in the care of critically ill pediatric patients.
- With the physical examination, radiographic studies, blood gas analysis, pulse oximetry, capnography and respiratory mechanics—the deleterious effect of respiratory distress in the pediatric population can be greatly ameliorated.
- All such tools should be used carefully, with their limitations in mind, and in the light of other findings.

SUGGESTED READING

1. Coss-Bu JA, Walding DL, David YB, et al. Dead space ventilation in critically ill children with lung injury. Chest. 2003;123:2050-6.
2. Donoso A, Arriagada D, Contreras D, et al. Respiratory monitoring of pediatric patients in the intensive care unit. Bol Med Hosp Infant Mex. 2016;73(3):149-65.
3. Khemani RG, Patel NR, Bart RD 3rd, et al. Comparison of the pulse oximetric saturation/fraction of inspired oxygen ratio and the PaO_2/fraction of inspired oxygen ratio in children. Chest. 2009;135:662-8.
4. Lobete C, Medina A, Rey C, et al. Correlation of oxygen saturation as measured by pulse oximetry/fraction of inspired oxygen ratio with PaO_2/fraction of inspired oxygen ratio in a heterogeneous simple of critically ill children. J Crit Care. 2013;28:538.e1-7.
5. Mayordomo-Colunga J, Pons M, López Y, et al. Predicting non-invasive ventilation failure in children from the SpO_2/FiO_2 (SF) ratio. Intensive Care Med. 2013;39:1095-103.
6. McSwain SD, Hamel DS, Smith PB, et al. End-tidal and arterial carbon dioxide measurements correlate across all levels of physiologic dead space. Respir Care. 2010;55:288-93.
7. Trachsel D, McCrindle BW, Nakagawa S, et al. Oxygenation index predicts outcome in children with acute hypoxemic respiratory failure. Am J Respir Crit Care Med. 2005;172:206-11.

Capnography and Capnometry

Madhumati Otiv

Capnography is the graphical form, while capnometry is the number that is displayed at the end of expiratory phase of a capnography.

- Noninvasive measurement of the partial pressure of carbon dioxide (CO_2) in exhaled breath expressed as the CO_2 concentration over time.
- The relationship of CO_2 concentration to time is graphically represented by the CO_2 waveform, or capnogram.
- Changes in the shape of the capnogram.
- Changes in end-tidal CO_2 ($EtCO_2$), the maximum CO_2 concentration at the end of each tidal breath, can be used to assess disease severity and response to treatment.
- Capnography is also the most reliable indicator that an endotracheal tube (ETT) is placed in the trachea after intubation.

Oxygenation and ventilation are distinct physiologic functions that must be assessed:

- *Pulse oximetry*: Instant feedback about *oxygenation*.
- *Capnography*: Instant information about *ventilation* (Fig. 1).

BASIC PRINCIPLE OF CAPNOGRAPHY

- Carbon dioxide monitors measure gas concentration, or partial pressure, using one of two configurations.

Mainstream or Sidestream

- *Mainstream* devices measure respiratory gas (in this case CO_2) directly from the airway, with the sensor located on the airway adapter at the hub of the ETT.
- *Sidestream* devices measure respiratory gas via nasal or nasal-oral cannula by aspirating a small sample from the exhaled breath through the cannula tubing to a sensor located inside the monitor.

Note: Mainstream systems are configured for intubated patients. Sidestream systems are configured for both intubated and nonintubated patients.

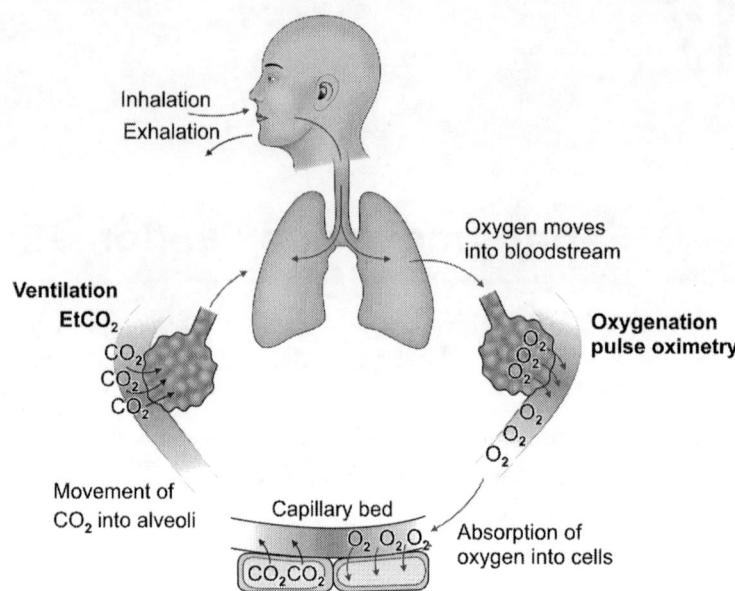

Fig. 1: Carbon dioxide: Generation by body metabolism, its transport, and elimination via lung.

Sidestream Systems

- Sidestream systems are configured to use high-flow rates (around 150 cc/min) or low-flow rates (around 50 cc/min).
- Flow rates vary according to the amount of CO_2 needed in the breath sample to obtain an accurate reading.
- Low-flow systems have a lower occlusion rate (from moisture or patient secretions) and are accurate in patients with low tidal volumes (e.g. neonates, infants, and adult patients with hypoventilation and low tidal volume breathing).
- Low-flow systems are also resistant to dilution from supplemental oxygen.
- High-flow systems sampling at ≥100 cc/min have been shown to be inaccurate in neonates, infants, young children, and in hypoventilating adult patients.

PHYSICS BEHIND CO_2 MEASUREMENT

- Capnography uses infrared (IR) radiation to make measurements.
- Molecules of CO_2 absorb IR radiation at a very specific wavelength (4.26 μm), with the amount of radiation absorbed having a nearly exponential relation to the CO_2 concentration present in the breath sample.
- Detecting these changes in IR radiation levels, using appropriate photodetectors sensitive in this spectral region, allows for the calculation of the CO_2 concentration in the gas sample.

TYPES OF EtCO$_2$ MONITORS

- CO$_2$ monitors are either quantitative or qualitative.
- Quantitative devices measure the precise EtCO$_2$ either as a number (capnometry) or a number and a waveform (capnography).
- Qualitative devices report the range in which the EtCO$_2$ falls (e.g. 0–10 mm Hg or >35 mm Hg) as opposed to a precise value (e.g. 38 mm Hg).

QUALITATIVE CAPNOMETERS

- The most commonly used qualitative capnometric device is the colorimetric EtCO$_2$ detector.
- This device consists of a piece of specially treated litmus paper that changes color when exposed to CO$_2$.
  - Purple—<3 mm Hg
  - Tan—3–15 mm Hg
  - Yellow—>15 mm Hg of EtCO$_2$
- Used is for verification of ETT placement. Exhalation of CO$_2$ from an ETT placed in the trachea will change the color of the litmus paper from purple to yellow. Improperly placed ETT in the esophagus will show no change in the color of the litmus paper, which will remain purple.
  Note:
- In patients with low perfusion states, studies using quantitative modalities (i.e. capnography) for determining tracheal location of the ETT have shown 100% sensitivity
- Studies using qualitative (i.e. colorimetric) EtCO$_2$ methods have shown variable sensitivity, because the exhaled CO$_2$ concentration can fall below the detection threshold.

CAPNOGRAM (CO$_2$ WAVEFORM)

The capnogram consists of four phases (Fig. 2):

1. *Phase I (dead space ventilation, A-B)*: Beginning of exhalation.
2. *Phase II (ascending phase, B-C)*: Rapid rise in CO$_2$ concentration in the breath stream as the CO$_2$ from the alveoli reaches the upper airway.
3. *Phase III (alveolar plateau, C-D)*: It represents the CO$_2$ concentration reaching a uniform level in the entire breath stream from alveolus to nose. Point D, occurring at the end of the alveolar plateau, represents the maximum CO$_2$ concentration at the end of the tidal breath and is appropriately named the end-tidal CO$_2$. This is the number that appears on the monitor display.
4. *Phase VI (D-E)*: It represents the inspiratory cycle.
   - Patients with normal lung function have characteristic rectangular capnograms and narrow gradients between their alveolar CO$_2$ (i.e. EtCO$_2$) and arterial CO$_2$ concentration (PaCO$_2$) of 0–5 mm Hg.

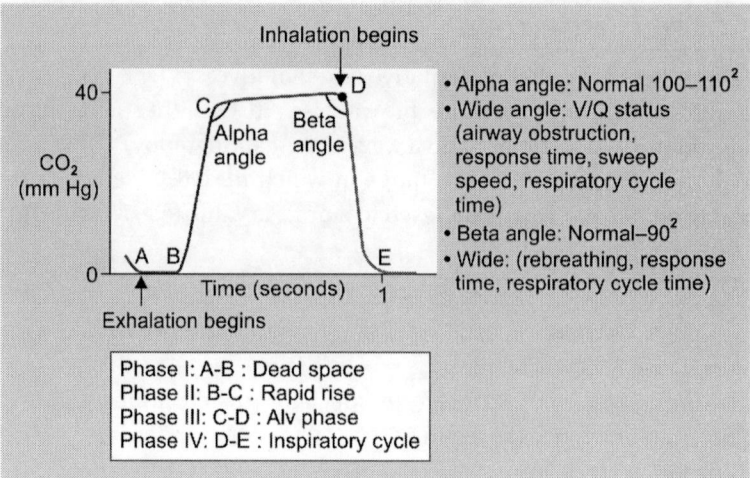

Fig. 2: Normal capnograph.

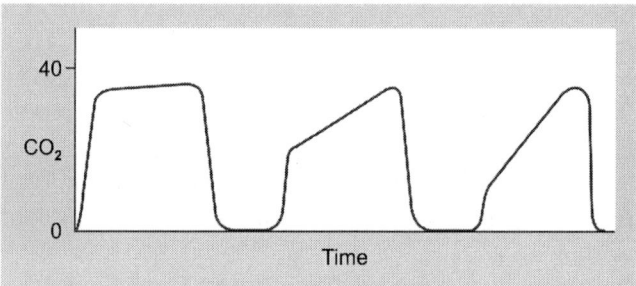

Fig. 3: Upslant in capnograph.

- Gas in the physiologic dead space accounts for this normal gradient.
- *Upslant in Capnograph (Fig. 3):* Slanting and prolongation of expiratory upstroke indicative of obstruction to gas flow caused by a partially obstructed tracheal tube or obstruction in the patient's airways (chronic obstructive lung disease or bronchospasm).
- *Low EtCO$_2$ (Fig. 4):* Low EtCO$_2$ with good alveolar plateau may be the result of hyperventilation or an increase in dead space ventilation.
- *High EtCO$_2$ (Fig. 5):* Elevated EtCO$_2$ with good alveolar plateau may be caused by hypoventilation.
- *Sudden rise of EtCO$_2$ (Fig. 6):* Sudden increase in CO$_2$: hyperthermia, glucose, hyperalimentation, CO$_2$ in peritoneal cavity, shivering, seizures, catecholamines, HCO$_3$ administration, release of tourniquet.
- *Exponential fall in EtCO$_2$ (Fig. 7):* Sudden hypotension, circulatory arrest, pulmonary embolism.
- *Paradoxical fall (Fig. 8):* Small air embolus.
- *Air leak in tubings (Fig. 9):* Leak in sampling line during ventilation.

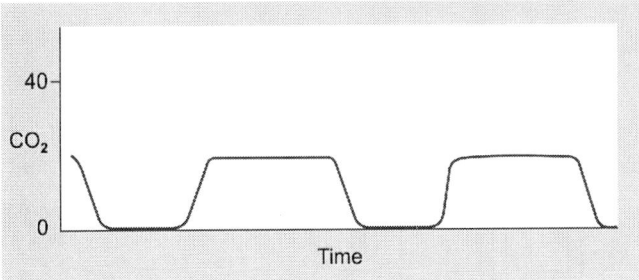

Fig. 4: Graphical representation of low EtCO$_2$.

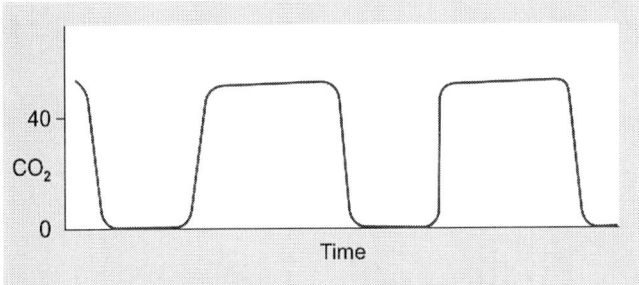

Fig. 5: Graphical representation of high EtCO$_2$.

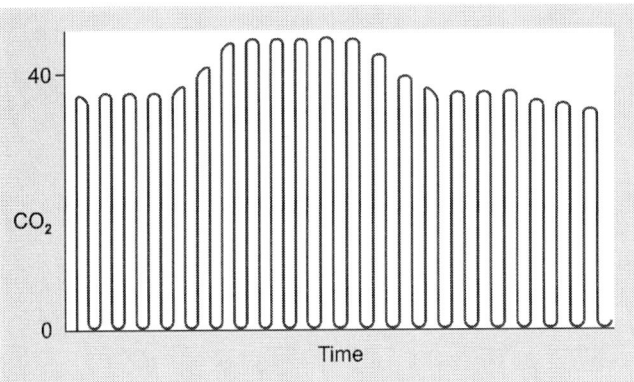

Fig. 6: Graphical representation of sudden rise of EtCO$_2$.

- *Spontaneous efforts (Fig. 10)*: Spontaneous efforts.
- *Curare effect (Fig. 11)*: Suggests that the paralytic effect has gone, and patient spontaneously breathing.
- *Improving graph (Fig. 12)*: Return of spontaneous circulation (ROSC).
- *Obstructive lung disease (Fig. 13)*: Impaired expiratory flow, and demonstrate a more rounded ascending phase and an upward slope in the alveolar plateau.

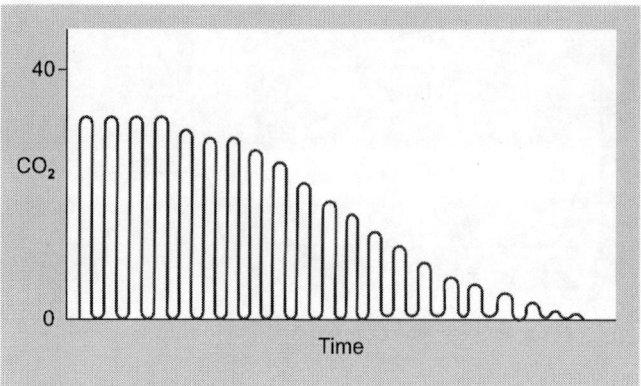

Fig. 7: Graphical representation of exponential fall in EtCO$_2$.

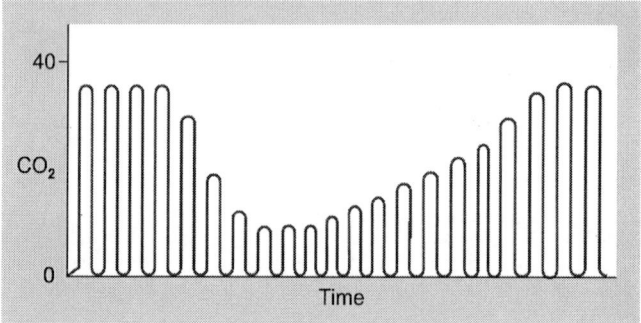

Fig. 8: Graphical representation of paradoxical fall.

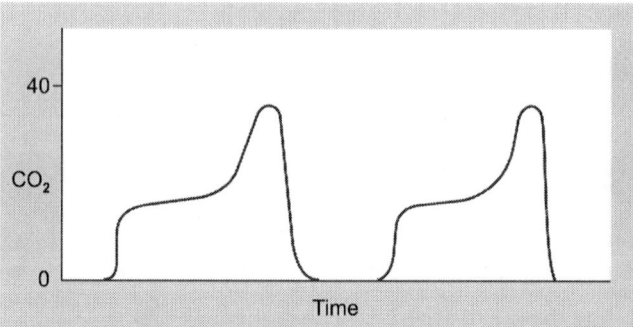

Fig. 9: Graphical representation of air leak in tubings.

- *Downslanting graph (Fig. 14)*: Expired sample contaminated by fresh gas.
- *Smooth curved waves (Fig. 15)*: Very low sampling rate with a sidestream, may result in low peak and baseline elevation.

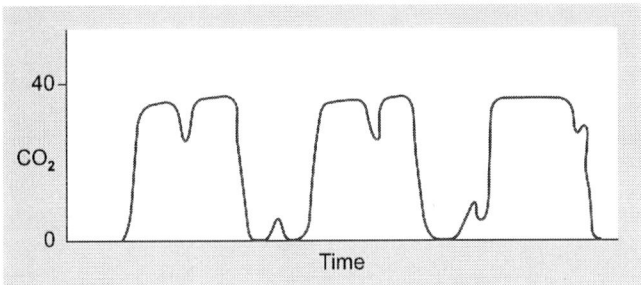

Fig. 10: Graphical representation of spontaneous efforts.

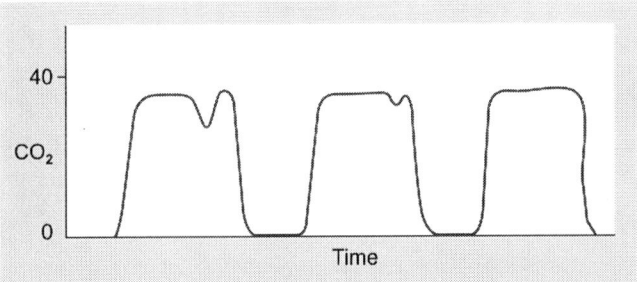

Fig. 11: Graphical representation of curare effect.

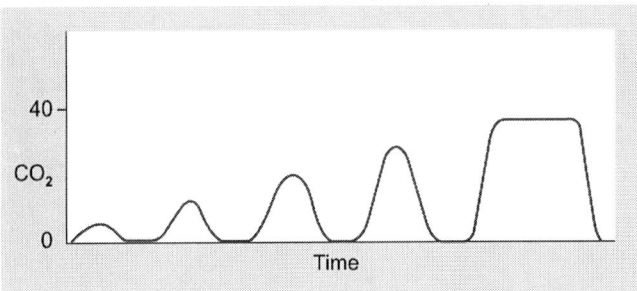

Fig. 12: Graphical representation of improving graph.

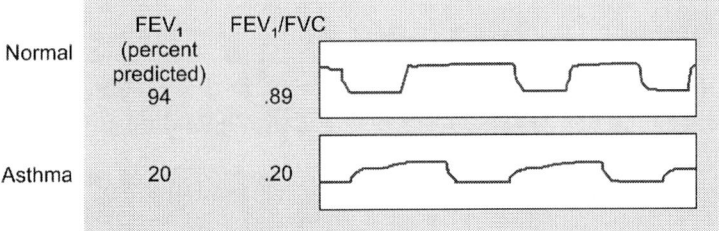

Fig. 13: Graphical representation of obstructive lung disease.

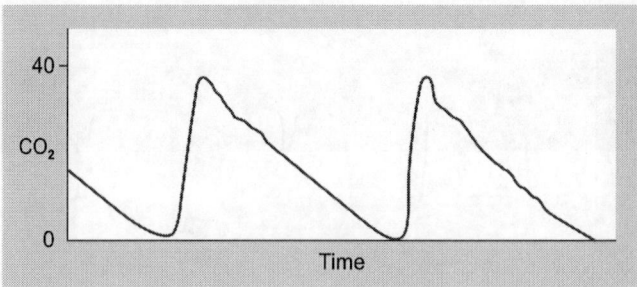

Fig. 14: Downslanting graph.

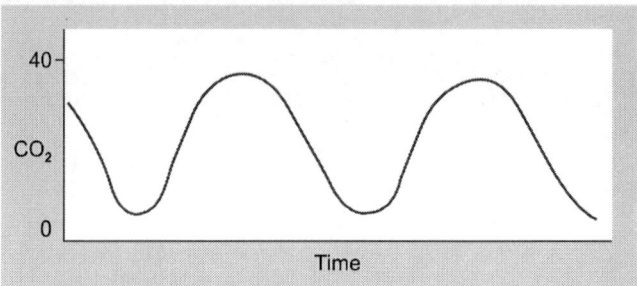

Fig. 15: Graphical representation of smooth curved waves.

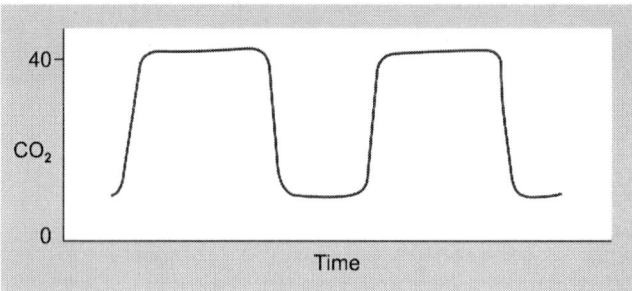

Fig. 16: Graphical representation of elevated baseline.

- *Elevated baseline (Fig. 16):* Baseline elevated due to exhausted absorbent/incompetent expiratory valve.
- *Managing graphs (Fig. 17).*

WIDENING EtCO$_2$-PaCO$_2$ GRADIENT

- In patients with abnormal lung function and ventilation-perfusion mismatch, the EtCO$_2$-PaCO$_2$ gradient widens depending on the severity of the lung disease
- Dead space calculation (%) = (PaCO$_2$ – EtCO$_2$/PaCO$_2$) × 100
  (This formula tells about, of all the CO$_2$ generated how much is not exhaled gives some idea about dead space ventilation)

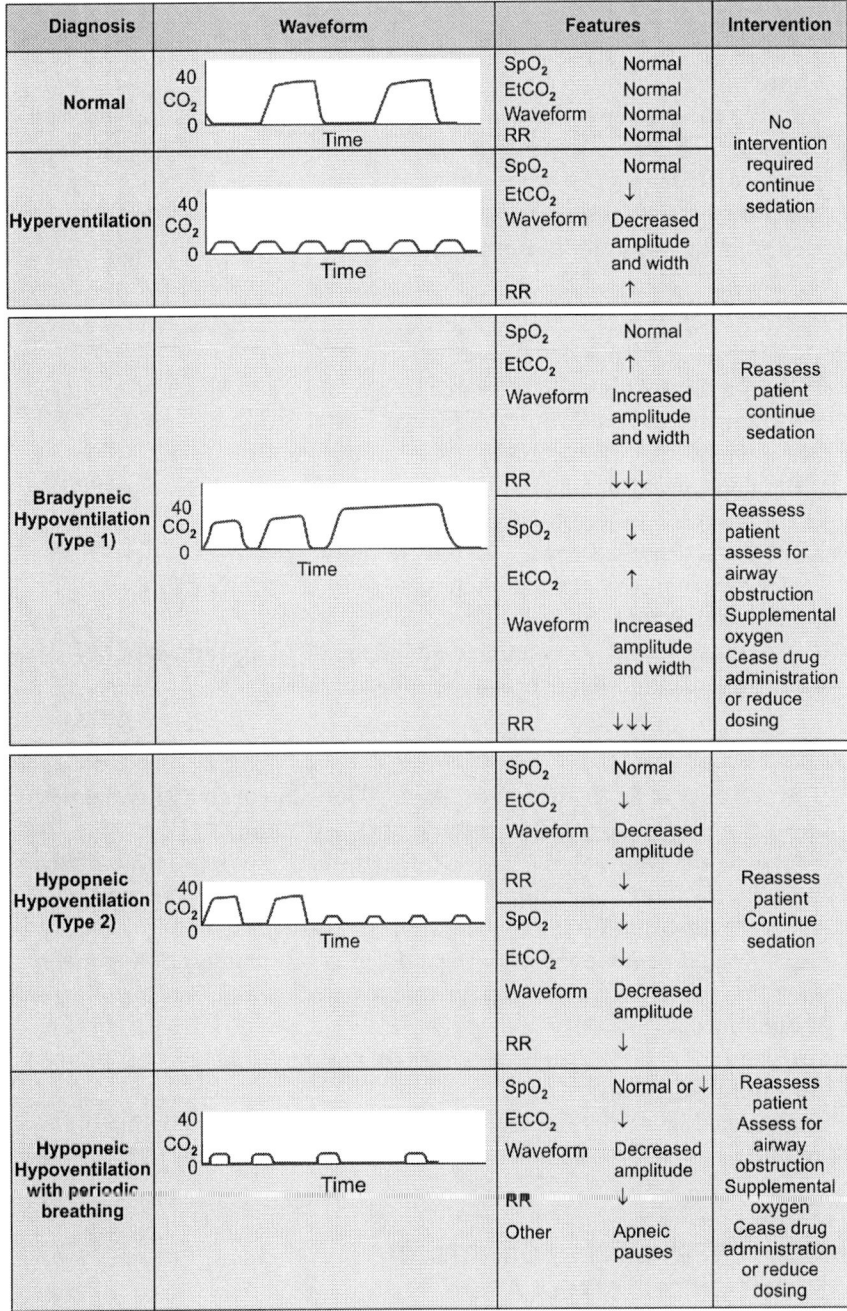

Diagnosis	Waveform	Features		Intervention
Normal		SpO$_2$	Normal	No intervention required continue sedation
		EtCO$_2$	Normal	
		Waveform	Normal	
		RR	Normal	
Hyperventilation		SpO$_2$	Normal	
		EtCO$_2$	↓	
		Waveform	Decreased amplitude and width	
		RR	↑	
Bradypneic Hypoventilation (Type 1)		SpO$_2$	Normal	Reassess patient continue sedation
		EtCO$_2$	↑	
		Waveform	Increased amplitude and width	
		RR	↓↓↓	
		SpO$_2$	↓	Reassess patient assess for airway obstruction Supplemental oxygen Cease drug administration or reduce dosing
		EtCO$_2$	↑	
		Waveform	Increased amplitude and width	
		RR	↓↓↓	
Hypopneic Hypoventilation (Type 2)		SpO$_2$	Normal	Reassess patient Continue sedation
		EtCO$_2$	↓	
		Waveform	Decreased amplitude	
		RR	↓	
		SpO$_2$	↓	
		EtCO$_2$	↓	
		Waveform	Decreased amplitude	
		RR	↓	
Hypopneic Hypoventilation with periodic breathing		SpO$_2$	Normal or ↓	Reassess patient Assess for airway obstruction Supplemental oxygen Cease drug administration or reduce dosing
		EtCO$_2$	↓	
		Waveform	Decreased amplitude	
		RR	↓	
		Other	Apneic pauses	

Fig. 17: Various abnormal ventilation patterns seen on capnography: Recognition and management.

- The EtCO$_2$ in patients with lung disease is only useful for assessing trends in ventilatory status over time; isolated EtCO$_2$ values may or may not correlate with the PaCO$_2$.

CLINICAL APPLICATIONS

- Verification of ETT placement
- Continuous monitoring of tube location during transport
- Gauging effectiveness of resuscitation and prognosis during cardiac arrest
- Titrating $EtCO_2$ levels in patients with suspected increases in intracranial pressure (ICP)
- Determining prognosis in trauma
- Determining adequacy of ventilation.

FLAT LINE WAVEFORM

- Unrecognized misplaced intubation
- Following intubation, the presence of a waveform with all four phases indicates the ETT is through the vocal cords. A normal waveform can occur when the tube has been placed in the right mainstem bronchus. A flat line waveform generally indicates esophageal placement, but can occur in several other situations, including:
  - Prolonged cardiac arrest with diffuse cellular death
  - Tracheal placement with inadequate pulmonary blood flow
  - ETT obstruction
  - Complete airway obstruction distal to the ETT (e.g. foreign body)
  - Technical malfunction of the monitor or tubing.

EFFICACY OF CAPNOMETRY

- The accuracy of $EtCO_2$ to confirm tracheal location of an ETT varies with the technology used and the condition of the patient.
- For patients who are not in cardiac arrest, studies of qualitative colorimetric $EtCO_2$ and quantitative capnography have demonstrated 100% sensitivity and 100% specificity for tracheal placement
- In contrast if capnography not used, fogging or condensation alone, of the tube, perceived as being in the trachea, occurs in 83% of esophageal intubations
- Also, chest wall movement perceived as being in trachea, can be produced by esophageal tubes
- Anesthesiologists, under ideal operating room conditions, using breath sounds as the sole means of verification, incorrectly identify ETT location in 16% of cases.

EFFECTIVENESS OF CPR FOR RETURN OF SPONTANEOUS CIRCULATION

- During cardiac arrest, when alveolar ventilation and metabolism are essentially constant, $EtCO_2$ reflects pulmonary blood flow. Therefore, $EtCO_2$ can be used as a gauge of the effectiveness of cardiac compressions.
- As effective cardiopulmonary resuscitation (CPR) leads to a higher cardiac output, $EtCO_2$ will rise, reflecting the increase in perfusion.

- The measurement of $EtCO_2$ varies directly with the cardiac output produced by chest compression and has been described in both electrical muscle stimulation (EMS) and ICU patients.
- Both of these prospective, observational studies found an $EtCO_2$ level <3 mm Hg immediately after cardiac arrest, with a higher level generated during cardiac compressions and a mean peak >7.5 mm Hg just before ROSC.
- This peak in $EtCO_2$ level is the earliest sign of ROSC and may occur before return of a palpable pulse or blood pressure.
- Early in cardiac arrest, and when the patient is receiving effective CPR, complete failure of CO_2 exchange is unlikely, and the clinician should assume an esophageal intubation exists if a waveform is absent.
- In patients with prolonged cardiac arrest and an absent waveform, the clinician should assume an esophageal intubation exists or use an alternative objective method for tube verification, such as an aspiration method.
- Physical examination criteria, such as repeat laryngoscopy and auscultation of the lungs and epigastrium, may be used, but the clinician must be aware of their limitations in discriminating between esophageal and tracheal intubation.
- $EtCO_2$ levels of $\leq$ 10 mm Hg measured 20 minutes after the initiation of advanced cardiac life support accurately predicted death in adult patients with cardiac arrest.
- The prognostic value of measuring $EtCO_2$ has been demonstrated in animal and human studies.
- During cardiac arrest, $EtCO_2$ is the earliest indicator of the ROSC.
- When the heart restarts, the dramatic increase in cardiac output, and resulting increase in perfusion, leads to a rapid increase in $EtCO_2$ as the CO_2 that has accumulated during cardiac arrest is effectively transported to the lungs and exhaled. This process manifests as a sudden rise in $EtCO_2$.
- American Heart Association (AHA) guidelines for cardiac resuscitation emphasize the importance of continuing chest compressions without interruption until a perfusing rhythm is re-established.
- Interruptions in chest compressions are followed by sustained periods of reduced blood flow, which only gradually return to preinterruption levels.
- Capnographic waveform monitoring virtually eliminates the need to stop chest compressions to check for pulses..

INCREASED ICP AND TRAUMA PROGNOSIS

- End-tidal CO_2 monitoring can help clinicians avoid inadvertent hyperventilation of patients with head injury and suspected increased ICP.
- It may also help determine the prognosis of trauma victims.

- Arterial CO_2 tension affects blood flow to the brain. High CO_2 levels result in cerebral vasodilation, while low CO_2 levels result in cerebral vasoconstriction. Sustained hypoventilation (defined as $PaCO_2$ levels ≥ 50 mm Hg) results in increased cerebral blood flow and increased ICP, which can harm head-injured patients.
- Sustained hyperventilation (defined as $PaCO_2$ ≤ 30 mm Hg) is also detrimental and is associated with worse neurologic outcome in severely brain-injured patients.
- Consequently, ventilation rates to achieve eucapnia are recommended by the Brain Trauma Foundation.

USE OF CONTINUOUS EtCO$_2$ MONITORING IN TRAUMA PATIENTS

- A prospective observational study found a lower incidence of inadvertent hyperventilation among intubated patients with severe head injury who underwent continuous $EtCO_2$ monitoring compared with those without $EtCO_2$ monitoring (5.6% vs 13.4%; OR 2.64; 95% CI 1.12–6.20).
- In a controlled study of intubated blunt trauma victims, patients assigned to capnography-guided ventilation during transport were significantly more likely to arrive at the emergency department appropriately ventilated, based on $PaCO_2$ levels obtained by arterial blood gas.
- In a prospective observational study of blunt trauma patients requiring prehospital intubation, $EtCO_2$ values obtained 20 minutes after intubation distinguished the great majority of survivors from nonsurvivors. Median $EtCO_2$ among survivors was 30.8 mm Hg and among nonsurvivors 26.3 mm Hg (95% CI of difference between medians 3 mm Hg and 6.75 mm Hg).

CLINICAL APPLICATIONS IN SPONTANEOUSLY BREATHING PATIENTS

In spontaneously breathing nonintubated patients, capnography can be used for:
- Performing rapid assessment of critically ill or seizing patients
- Determining response to treatment in acute respiratory distress
- Determining adequacy of ventilation in obtunded or unconscious patients, or in patients undergoing procedural sedation
- Detecting metabolic acidosis in diabetic patients and in children with gastroenteritis.

KEY MESSAGES

- End-tidal CO_2 is an important monitoring tool used for monitoring a mechanically ventilated patient to detect hypoventilation, ETT disconnection, and misplacement.

- Its effective use can minimize blood drawn for frequent blood gases for measurement of $PaCO_2$.
- It is also helpful in detecting sudden cardiovascular events such as embolism, cardiac arrest, severe shock and hypotension as well as during resuscitation as a tool to detect ROSC.

SUGGESTED READING

1. Block FE Jr, McDonald JS. Sidestream versus mainstream carbon dioxide analyzers. J Clin Monit. 1992;8(2):139-41.
2. Cheifetz IM, Myers TR. Respiratory therapies in the critical care setting. Should every mechanically ventilated patient be monitored with capnography from intubation to extubation? Respir Care. 2007;52(4):423-38.
3. Ghamra ZW, Arroliga AC. Volumetric capnography in acute respiratory distress syndrome: is the era of day-to-day monitoring finally here? Respir Care. 2005;50(4):457-8.
4. Hess D, Branson RD. Noninvasive respiratory monitoring equipment. Branson RD, Hess DR, Chatburn RL (Eds). Respiratory Care Equipment. Philadelphia: Lippincott; 1994. pp. 184-216.
5. Hess D. Capnometry. In: Tobin MJ (Ed). Principles and Practice of Intensive Care Monitoring. New York: McGraw-Hill; 1998. pp. 377-400.
6. Jacobus C. Noninvasive monitoring in neonatal and pediatric care. In: Walsh BK, Czervinske MP, DiBlasi RM (Eds). Perinatal and Pediatric Respiratory Care, 3rd Edition. St. Louis: Elsevier; 2009. pp. 137-46.
7. Levine RL, Wayne MA, Miller CC. End-tidal carbon dioxide and outcome of out-of-hospital cardiac arrest. N Engl J Med. 1997;337(5):301-6.
8. Shibutani K, Muraoka M, Shirasaki S, et al. Do changes in end-tidal PCO2 quantitatively reflect changes in cardiac output? Anesth Analg. 1994;79(5):829-33.
9. Silvestri S, Ralls GA, Krauss B, et al. The effectiveness of out-of-hospital use of continuous end-tidal carbon dioxide monitoring on the rate of unrecognized misplaced intubation within a regional emergency medical services system. Ann Emerg Med. 2005;45(5):497-503.
10. Singh S, Allen WD Jr., Venkataraman ST, et al. Utility of a novel quantitative handheld microstream capnometer during transport of critically ill children. Am J Emerg Med. 2006;24(3):302-7.
11. Thompson JE, Jaffe MB. Capnographic waveforms in the mechanically ventilated patient. Respir Care. 2005;50(1):100-8.
12. Walsh BK, Crotwell DN, Restrepo RD. Capnography/capnometry during mechanical ventilation: 2011. Respir Care. 2011;56(4):503-9.

Ventilator Graphics

Rachna Sharma, Ankur Ohri

Until late 1990s to early 21st century the assessment of the appropriateness of invasive ventilation was determined subjectively by noting color, observing chest excursions, listening to breath sounds, and objectively by intermittent assessment of gas exchange and radiography. Real-time pulmonary graphics are the graphical display of measured and derived values captured during the process of mechanical ventilation. These visual representations of the interaction between the mechanical ventilator and the baby receiving support for respiratory failure are critical in understanding both the support used and its effectiveness. Although ventilator waveforms and respiratory mechanics measurements are provided by all modern ventilators, this information is not yet commonly incorporated into the everyday intensive care practice. This chapter aims at simplifying ventilator graphics and projects its use as a bedside tool for better assessment.

Six steps for rapid interpretation of ventilator graphics (identify and interpret):

1. Identify the type of breath—volume and pressure
2. Identify reason for raised peak airway pressure and to differentiate low compliance from increased airway resistance
3. Interpret pressure-volume (PV) loop
4. Identify display images in common modes of ventilation
5. Interpret expiratory waveform and flow-volume (FV) loop
6. Identify signs of asynchrony.

PRINCIPLE

With the development of sensor technology, real-time pulmonary graphics were brought to intensive care units, where a microprocessor-based technology is integrated to the intended function of the ventilator. The sensor technologies fall into one of two categories: (1) thermal or (2) differential pressure type. The sensor detects either flow or pressure and converts the signal to a clinically useful analog value. For example, the flow signal can be integrated to obtain a volume measurement. The sensor also is used to detect patient effort to facilitate or "trigger" synchrony between the patient's own effort and the delivery of a mechanical breath by the ventilator. The information is presented in real-time and is a continuous display.

ADVANTAGES

Graphic monitoring assists the clinician at the bedside in several ways.
- It can be helpful in fine-tuning or adjusting ventilator parameters.
- Its monitoring may help to determine the patient's response to pharmacologic agents such as surfactant, diuretics, or bronchodilators.
- The clinician also has the ability to trend monitored events over a prolonged period of time.

DISADVANTAGES

- The understanding of graphic monitoring may at times be considered complex.
- There are many clinical situations that may be identified at the bedside and each patient is different and provides unique learning experiences.

CLASSIFICATION OF VENTILATOR GRAPHICS

Ventilator graphics are broadly classified as scalars and loops.
- Scalars (also called as waveforms) are real-time displays of control variable (volume measured in mL, pressure measured in cm H_2O, or flow measured in L/minute or L/second) plotted on vertical Y-axis in relation to time measured in seconds and plotted on horizontal X-axis.
- Loops are the tracings of one control variable against another (e.g. volume plotted against pressure or of flow against volume).

SCALARS/WAVEFORMS

Basically six shapes (waveforms) are produced with scalars in mechanical ventilation (Fig. 1).
1. Rectangular: often called as square wave or constant waveform
2. Ascending ramp: also called as accelerating ramp
3. Descending ramp: also called a decelerating ramp
4. Sinusoidal: also called the sine wave
5. Exponential rising
6. Exponential decaying.

Pressure waveforms usually are rectangular or rising exponential (similar to an ascending ramp) type (Fig. 2). Flow waveforms can take various forms—rectangular, ramp (ascending or descending), sinusoidal, and decaying exponential types. Many clinicians refer to ramp waveforms (and sometimes exponential waveforms) as either "accelerating" or "decelerating" flow patterns.

In theory, a relatively slow rise to the peak inspiratory flow—as is provided within the ascending ramp and sinusoidal waveforms—provides more time

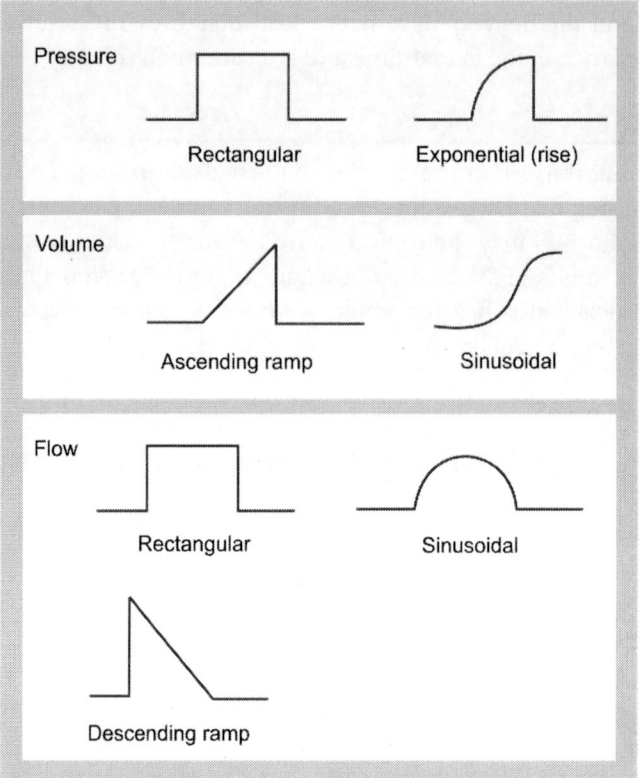

Fig. 1: Graphical representation of scalars/waveforms for pressure, volume and flow.

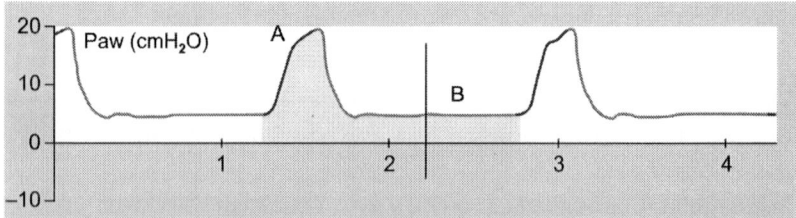

Fig. 2: Graphical representation of pressure waveform.

for gas distribution within the lungs, and thereby improves oxygenation. But slow flows in these can be uncomfortable for the patient and may cause air hunger. The constant flow waveform and the descending ramp flow waveform (the latter delivers high initial flows) are superior at preventing "flow starvation".

Pressure Waveform

The pressure waveform has upward (inspiration) and downward (expiration) scalars. Positive end-expiratory pressure (PEEP) is the baseline pressure level. If PEEP is used, the waveform will begin and end at this value and not reach zero. The uppermost point of the waveform represents peak inspiratory pressure (PIP), whereas the area under the curve is the mean airway pressure. The inspiratory time can be measured from the point of upward deflection until PIP is reached; expiratory time begins at PIP and lasts until the next positive deflection. The shape of the curve represents the breath type, e.g. volume (triangular) or pressure (square) (Fig. 2).

Oxygenation is a function of mean airway pressure (Fig. 3).

Thus, increasing the area under the curve will improve oxygenation. This can be accomplished by increases in:

- Peak inspiratory pressure
- Positive end-expiratory pressure
- Inspiratory time
- Rate.
  - Mean airway pressure (MAP) increased by increasing PIP
  - MAP increased by increasing PEEP
  - MAP increased by increasing inspiratory time
  - MAP increased by increasing rate

Flow Waveform (Fig. 4)

The flow waveform has two separate components. Anything above the zero baseline represents positive flow, or in other words, gas flow into the patient (inspiration). Inspiratory flow has two components: (1) accelerating flow (at the start of inspiration) and (2) decelerating flow (velocity slows as the lung approaches capacity). The highest point of the positive point of the waveform

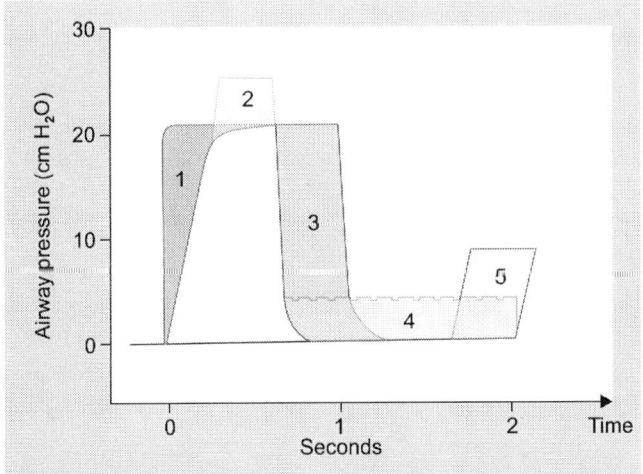

Fig 3: Graph showing factors affecting mean airway pressure (and oxygenation). 1. Inspiratory time, 2. Peak inspiratory pressure, 3. Expiratory time, 4. Positive end expiratory pressure, and 5. Pause time.

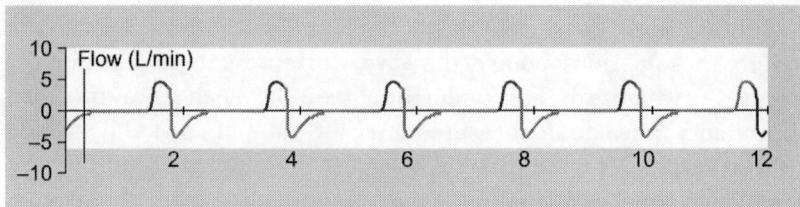

Fig. 4: Graphical representation of flow waveform.

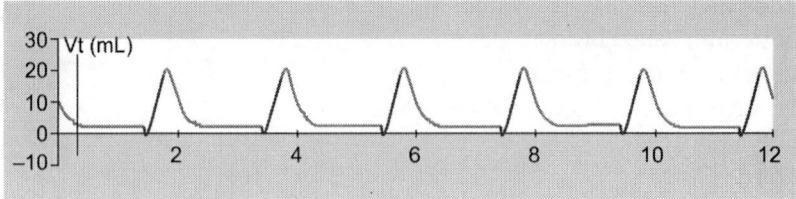

Fig. 5: Graphical representation of volume waveform.

is peak inspiratory flow. Anything below the zero baseline represents negative flow, or gas flow from the patient (expiration). The expiratory flow waveform similarly has two components: (1) accelerating flow (at the start of expiration) and (2) decelerating flow [velocity slows as the lung empties to functional residual capacity (FRC)]. The lowest negative point of the waveform is peak expiratory flow.

Volume Waveform (Fig. 5)

The volume waveform is similar in appearance to the pressure waveform, except that it starts and ends on the baseline. The shape of the pressure waveform demonstrates how volume is delivered to the baby. During pressure-targeted ventilation, peak volume delivery occurs early in inspiration, then decreases. This is in contrast to volume-targeted ventilation, which creates a "shark's fin" pressure waveform, whereby peak volume delivery occurs at the end of inspiration.

Identifying the Type of Breath

In pressure control mode [for example, pressure control mode, pressure-regulated volume control mode or synchronized intermittent mandatory ventilation pressure control (SIMV-PC) mode], pressure is an independent, or controlled, variable (Fig. 6). The set pressure will be delivered and maintained constant throughout inspiration, independent of what resistive or elastic forces of the respiratory system might be. Even though pressure is constant, the delivered tidal volume will vary as a function of compliance and resistance, and the flow will also vary exponentially with time. The volume

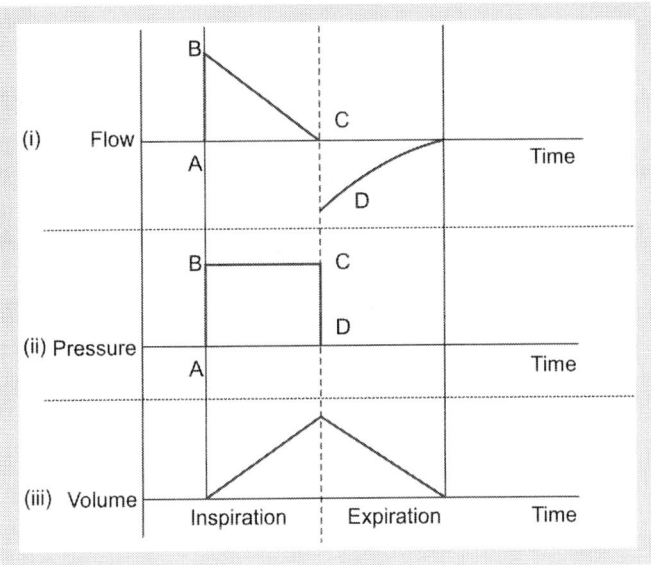

Fig. 6: Scalar changes (flow, pressure, volume) during pressure-controlled ventilation.

becomes a function of compliance, so that a decrease in compliance means less volume will be delivered for the same pressure. The events during an ideal breath in pressure control mode are the following (Fig. 6):

- *In flow-time scalar (Fig. 6, i):*
  - The beginning of inspiration (can be flow triggered in assisted control or time triggered in control mode)
  - Inspiratory flow rapidly rises to a peak, corresponding to operator set PIP.
  - Thereafter, flow rate rapidly declines as the patient's lung fill with air (the descending ramp waveform has been applied) at the same preset inspiratory pressure in pressure control mode and commencement of exhalation starts as per set inspiratory time in control mode or as per percentage of peak flow in pressure support mode.
  - Exhalation is passive, and so there is an exponential decay in the inspiratory flow down to the baseline as the lung progressively empties.
- *In pressure-time scalar (Fig. 6, ii):*
  - The beginning of inspiration. The presence of a negative deflection here would mean that the breath is patient-triggered. Its absence means that the ventilator is responsible for triggering the breath.
  - The pressure immediately rises to operator set PIP.
  - The PIP is reached and remains same till the set inspiratory time in control mode. As pressure is preset, pressure-time diagrams show either no changes, or changes which are hard to detect, as a

consequence of changes in resistance and compliance of the entire system.
- At the end of preset inspiratory time, pressure drops to zero.

All pressure modes are associated with a "descending ramp" flow pattern during inspiration. This descending flow pattern represents the speed of the gas, which is initially very high but gradually lowers as the chest fills. This characteristic flow pattern is considered more physiologic than that associated with volume-based ventilation and may contribute to better gas distribution as well.

In the volume-controlled mode, each machine breath is usually delivered with the same predetermined inspiratory flow-time profile to reach a targeted volume. Because the area under a flow-time curve defines volume, the tidal volume remains fixed and pressure becomes the dependent variable. The inspiratory pressure-time waveform varies linearly with time and will change depending on the compliance and resistance of the system. Thereby monitoring and restricting pressure becomes important in volume control mode. During volume-targeted ventilation, the most commonly used flow waveform is the square flow waveform (constant flow waveform). The events during a constant flow breath are the following (Figs. 7A and B):

- *In flow-time scalar (Fig. 7A):* Inspiration is displayed as a positive deflection and expiration as a negative deflection.
  - The beginning of inspiration.
  - Inspiratory flow rapidly rises to peak.
  - Thereafter, flow is sustained at a constant level (the square waveform has been applied) until the entire preset tidal volume has been delivered, in a given time.

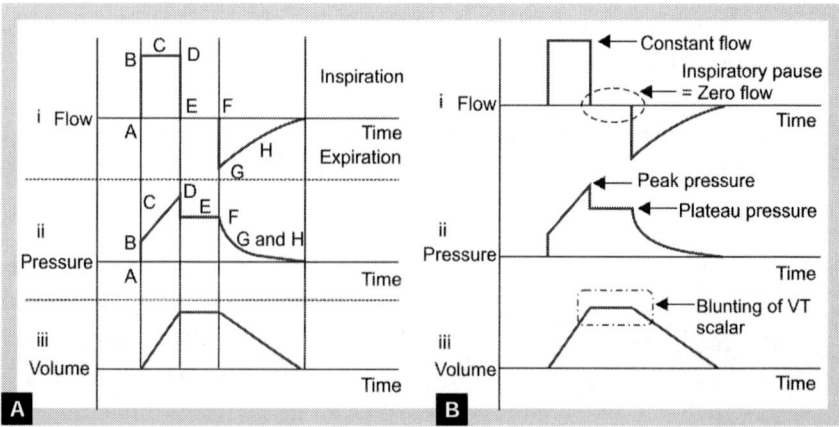

Figs. 7A and B: Scalar changes (flow, pressure, volume) during volume-controlled ventilation. (A) Describes events with markings; (B) Describes same event highlighting constant flow and inspiratory pause in flow-time scalar and corresponding plateau pressure-time scalar.

- The flow then declines sharply to zero
- During the end-inspiratory pause, the breath is briefly held within the lungs for the duration of the applied pause, helps us to measure plateau pressure.
- Commencement of exhalation.
- The peak expiratory flow is rapidly reached.
- Exhalation is passive, and so there is an exponential decay in the inspiratory flow down to the baseline as the lung empties itself.

- *In pressure-time scalar (Fig. 7A):*
  - Beginning of inspiration—presence of a negative deflection would mean that the breath is patient-triggered. Its absence means that the ventilator is responsible for triggering the breath.
  - The initial rise in airway pressure is on account of the resistance offered by the ETT and ventilator circuit. This pressure is called the flow resistive pressure or the transairway pressure (Pta).
  - As the lung begins to distend, pressure is required to overcome its resistive and elastic components. The pressure it takes to overcome elastic forces is the peak alveolar pressure (Palv).
  - When a constant flow is applied—the square waveform—there is a gradual but uniform rate of rise in the airway opening pressure until the entire tidal volume has been delivered. The PIP is reached here at point D, which strongly reflects both airway resistance and alveolar pressure.
  - The pressure settles down, when inspiratory pause is applied.
  - *End-inspiratory pause*: This represents the plateau pressure, which reflects the pressure applied to small airways and alveoli and if high is considered to be mostly responsible for stretch injury of alveoli; in pathogenesis of ventilator-induced lung injury.
  - Exhalation.

Plateau Pressure

At the end of inspiration, inspiratory hold is applied or exhalation port is occluded creating inspiratory pause, during this inspiratory pause the airway pressure falls to a plateau as the air diffuses out to the periphery of the trachea-bronchial tree. The pressure within the airway during this period of no airflow is called the pause pressure which is more popularly referred to as the plateau pressure, Pplat. The plateau pressure is a reflection of the static compliance [static compliance = corrected tidal volume/(plateau pressure – PEEP)], and so, any condition that might stiffen the lung will increase the plateau pressure.

Dynamic compliance reflects the airway resistance (nonelastic resistance) and the elastic properties of the lung and chest wall (elastic resistance). It can be calculated by dividing the volume by the pressure (i.e. PIP) measured when airflow is present. Since airflow is present, airway resistance becomes a factor in the measurement of dynamic compliance. Dynamic compliance = corrected tidal volume/(PIP – PEEP).

To differentiate low compliance from increased airway resistance, interpretation of pressure-time scalar in volume control mode with inspiratory pause is needed (Fig. 8)

In general, conditions causing changes in plateau pressure and static compliance invoke similar changes in PIP and dynamic compliance. For example, atelectasis causes an increase of plateau and PIPs (Fig. 8, iii). Since the plateau and PIPs are increased, the calculated static and dynamic compliance measurements are decreased.

In conditions where the airflow resistance is increased (e.g. bronchospasm), the PIP is increased while the plateau pressure stays unchanged (Fig. 8, ii). Since the PIP is increased, the dynamic compliance is decreased while static compliance stays the same because there is no change in the plateau pressure.

Graphics in Other Common Modes of Ventilation

Pressure Support Ventilation

Pressure support ventilation (PSV) is used to lower the work of spontaneous breathing and augment a patient's spontaneous tidal volume. PSV applies

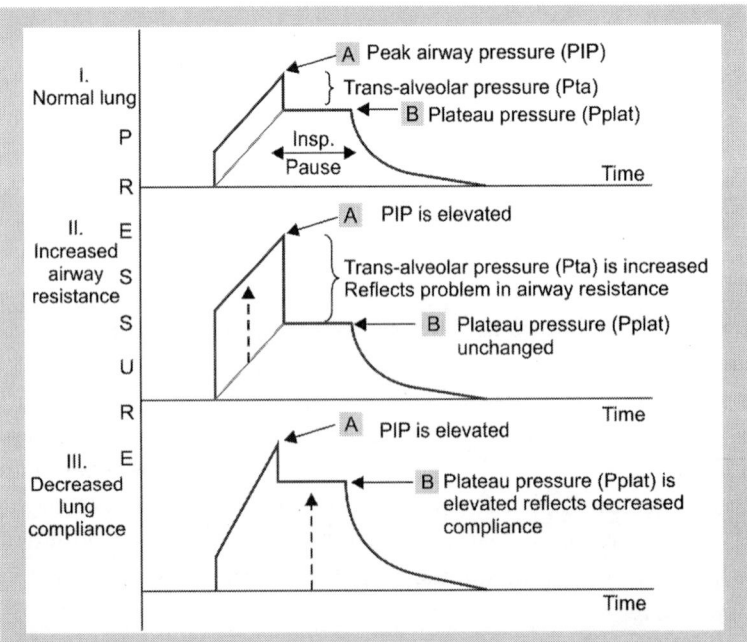

Fig. 8: Pressure-time scalar in constant flow with inspiratory pause (i) normal lung, (ii) increased airway resistance, and (iii) decreased lung compliance.

a preset pressure plateau to the patient's airway for the duration of a spontaneous breath (Fig. 9). A pressure-supported breath is therefore patient-triggered, pressure-limited, and flow-cycled. It is pressure-limited because the maximum airway pressure cannot exceed the preset pressure support level. It is flow-cycled because a pressure-supported breath cycles to expiration when the flow reaches a minimal level.

Synchronized Intermittent Mandatory Ventilation

Synchronized intermittent mandatory ventilation is a ventilator mode where mandatory breaths are delivered intermittently with volume-controlled or pressure-controlled ventilation. Between the mandatory breaths, the patient is allowed to spontaneously breathe. The ventilator delivers the mandatory breaths in synchrony with the patient's inspiratory effort (Fig. 10, breath 4). If no inspiratory effort is detected; the ventilator delivers a mandatory breath at the scheduled time. This is usually achieved by use of an assist window (Fig. 10). This window opens at intervals determined by the SIMV rate, and remains open for a specific period of time. If a patient effort detected while this window is open, a mandatory breath is delivered. If no patient effort is detected in the time that window is open, the ventilator delivers a mandatory breath.

Also in Figure 10, the second breath (A) has higher peak inspiratory flow, as patients demand may be high as compared to third breath where his peak

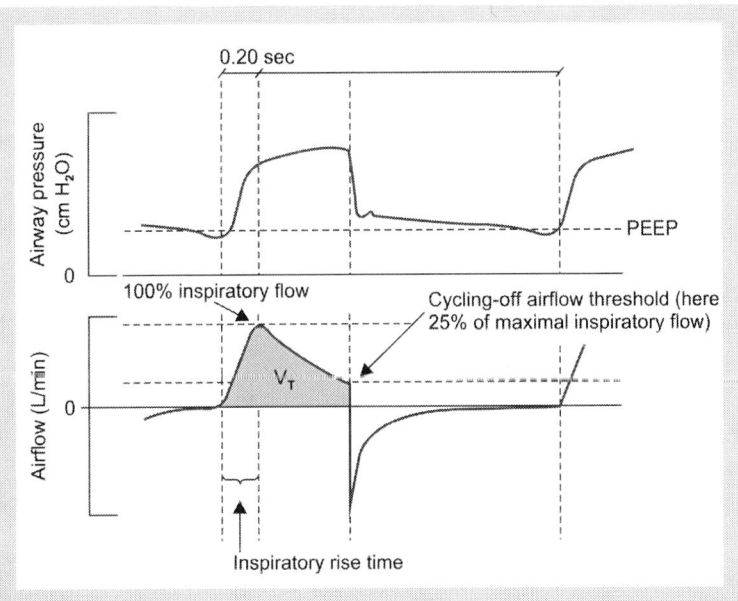

Fig. 9: Pressure- and flow-time scalars—descending flow pattern and highlighting flow-cycled mode as cycling criteria is operator set.

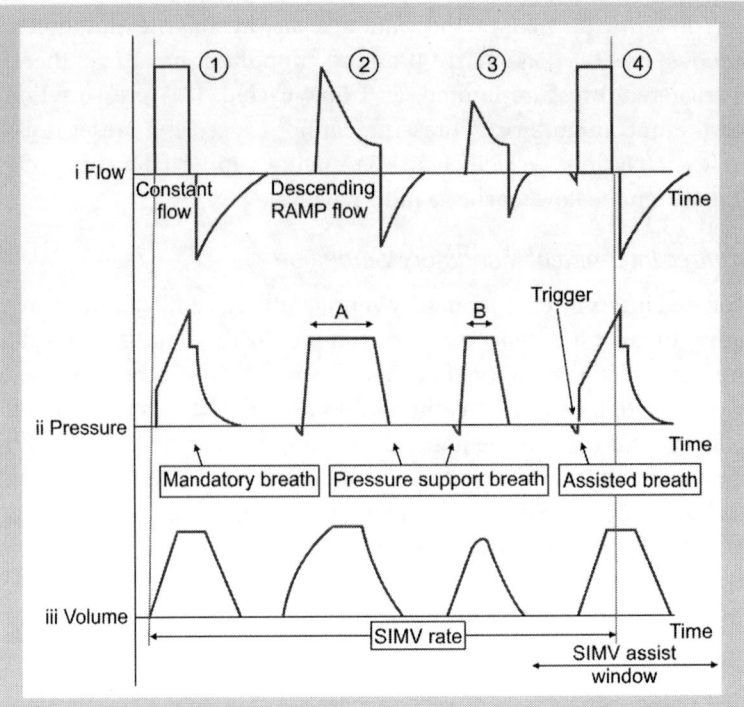

Fig. 10: Synchronized intermittent mandatory ventilation (SIMV)(volume control) + PS mode.

flow is low, as his demand may be low. Else in breath 3 the volume may also be low due to increased airway resistance; highlighting variable flow and volume delivery in PSV mode.

Airway Pressure-Release Ventilation

Airway pressure-release ventilation (APRV) mode uses longer inflation periods (T high, 3–5 sec) and short deflation periods (T low, 0.2–0.8 sec), high pressure level, which is typically set at 20–30 cm H_2O. This high pressure along with fraction of inspired oxygen (FiO_2) determines oxygenation. Ventilation is determined by the frequency with which the pressure releases to the lower pressure, the difference between the high pressure (P high) and the low pressure (P low), and the magnitude of spontaneous breathing. The low pressure setting is usually 0–5 cm H_2O. Spontaneous breathing can occur at the high pressure and low pressure settings, although the time at low pressure is usually too short to allow spontaneous breathing (Fig. 11, i). Various time ratios for high-to-low airway pressure have been used with APRV, ranging from 1:1 to 9:1. To sustain optimal recruitment, the greater part of the total time cycle (80–95%) should occur at the high airway pressure.

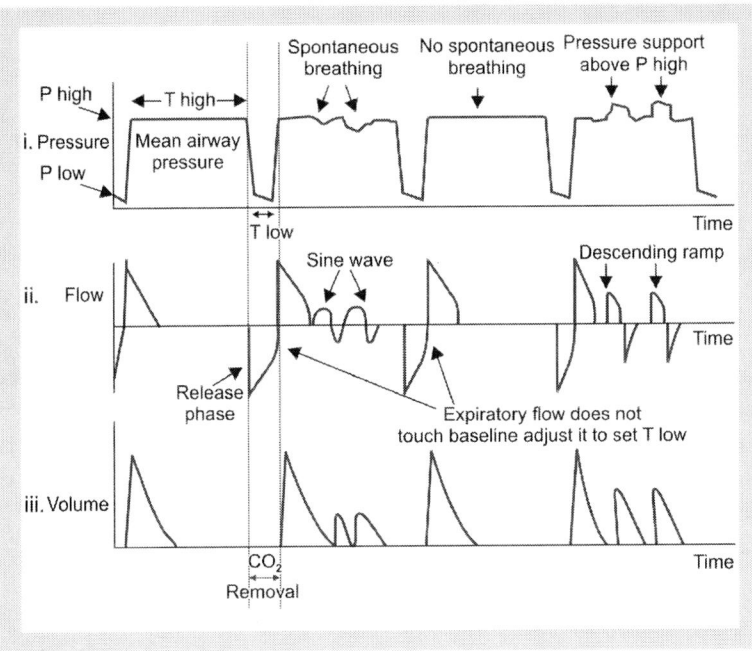

Fig. 11: Scalar graphics in airway pressure-release ventilation (APRV).

To minimize derecruitment, the time spent at low airway pressure (P low) should be brief. As when the time at low airway pressure is short, exhalation is incomplete and alveolar recruitment due to auto-PEEP results. Creating auto-PEEP is, by design, required with the usual approach to APRV in which P low is set to 0 cm H_2O. With this approach, the time at low airway pressure is set such that the expiratory flow reaches 50–75% of the peak expiratory flow. Some ventilators allow the addition of PSV to the spontaneous breaths during APRV. Spontaneous breathing during the high airway pressure phase of APRV has the potential to generate negative pleural pressures, which may add to the alveolar stretch applied from the ventilator. When PSV is triggered during the P high phase, the higher baseline lung volume distends further as the sum of P high, PSV, and pleural pressure which overall raises transpulmonary pressure. Furthermore, the imposition of PSV to APRV may reduce the benefit of spontaneous breathing by altering sinusoidal spontaneous breaths to decelerating assisted mechanical breaths as flow and pressure development may be uncoupled from patient effort.

LOOPS

Pulmonary mechanics can also be assessed when changes in pressure versus volume or flow versus volume are graphed over time and these are called loops.

Pressure-Volume Loop

Pressure-volume loop displays the relationship of pressure to volume (Fig. 12). Pressure is displayed along the horizontal axis and volume is displayed on the vertical axis. Inspiration is represented by the up-sweep from the baseline (PEEP) terminating at PIP. Expiration is the down-sweep from PIP back to baseline. The shape of this loop is referred to as hysteresis. A line drawn from each endpoint represents pulmonary compliance. The bottom of the loop will be at the set PEEP level. It will be at 0 if there is no PEEP set (Fig. 13).

Static PV loop: The static PV loop is obtained as a result of the supersyringe method. Volume graphed against pressure yields the compliance curve. Thus, the PV loop shows how compliance develops as volume increases. The lower inflection point (LIP) and the upper inflection point (UIP) can be taken from the static PV loop (Fig. 14). In the lower section (A) the pressure per volume increase rises particularly rapidly. It continues in a straight line (B) with gradual slope once a lung-opening pressure (LIP) has been exceeded.

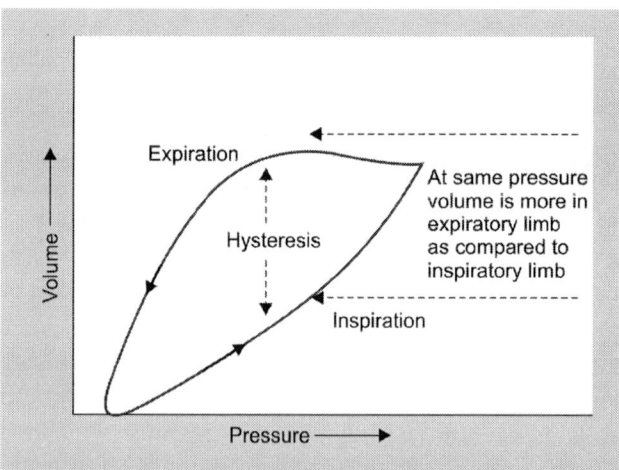

Fig. 12: Pressure-volume loop.

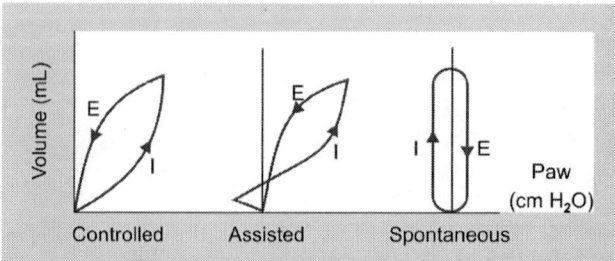

Fig. 13: Spontaneous breaths go clockwise and positive pressure breaths go counterclockwise.

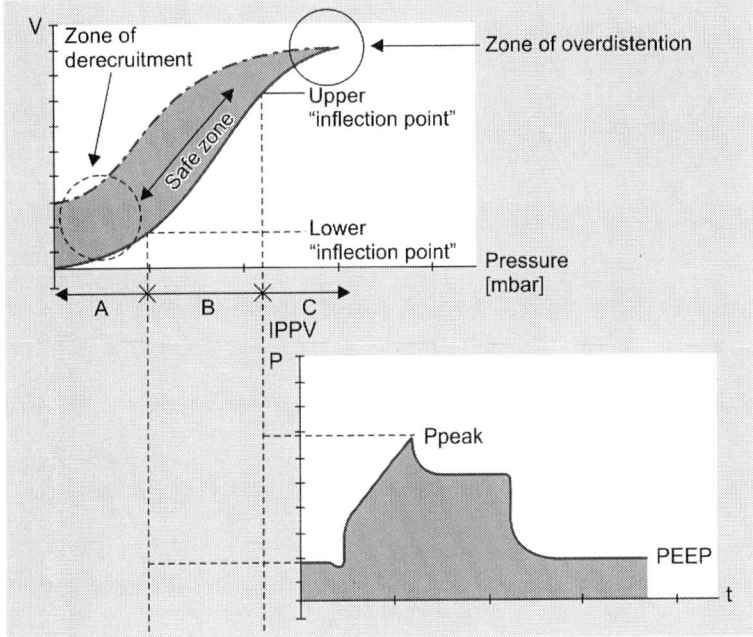

Fig. 14: Pressure-volume (PV) loop is shown in comparison to pressure-time (PT) scalar in volume control ventilation.

If the lung reaches the limits of its compliance, the rise in pressure per volume increase becomes bigger again (UIP) (C). The LIP is thought to represent the pressure at which a large number of alveoli are recruited and PEEP is used to overcome LIP. However, recruitment is likely to occur along the entire inflation in PV loop. An UIP on the pressure-volume curve is thought to indicate overdistention. However, the UIP might represent the end of recruitment rather than the point of overdistention.

Dynamic pressure-volume loop (Fig. 15): The expiration waveform is same in both and inspiratory waveform is different. In pressure control ventilation (Fig. 15, i), it is a box like shape as here the pressure in breathing system is kept at a constant level in inspiration. In volume control ventilation (Fig. 15, ii), flow is constant, allowing pressure to change as per dynamics of system.

Pressure-volume loop in volume-targeted ventilation: Figure 16 shows a PV loop during a mandatory breath.

As compliance is determined by change in volume per unit change in pressure (DV/DP), the PV loop is essentially a "compliance loop", and it provides useful information on the characteristics of a patient's compliance (Fig. 17B). A slope is drawn from the beginning point dividing the inspiratory limb and the expiratory limb. A shift of the slope toward the pressure axis indicates a decrease in compliance. A shift of the slope toward the volume axis indicates an increase in compliance.

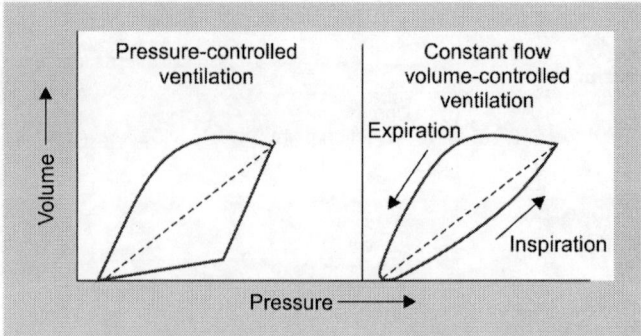

Fig. 15: Dynamic pressure-volume loop.

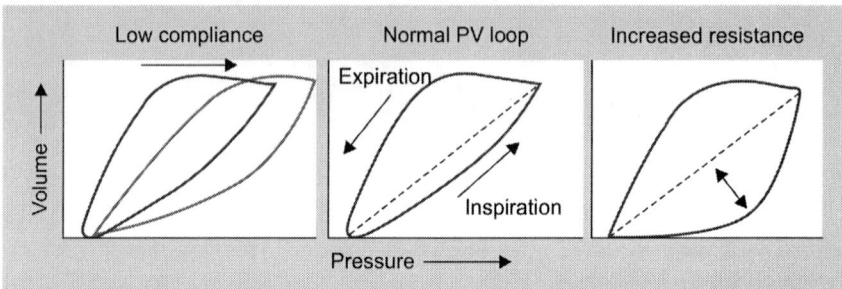

Fig. 16: Pressure-volume (PV) loop on volume-targeted ventilation.

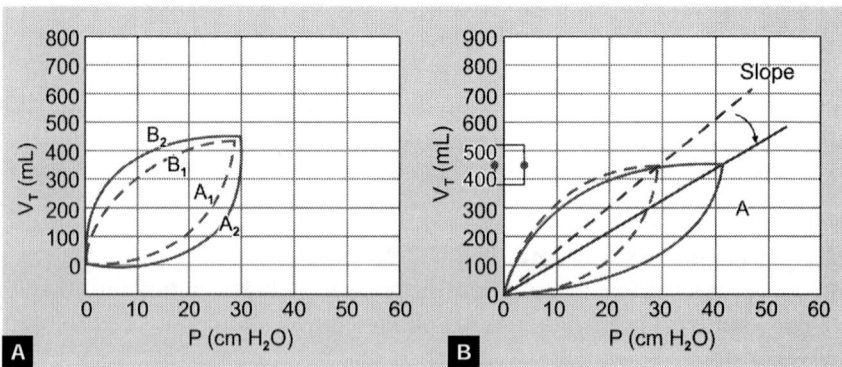

Figs. 17A and B: Pressure-volume (PV) loop in volume-targeted ventilation. (A) Increased bowing of PV loop from dotted to solid lines suggests an increase in airflow resistance. Bowing of inspiratory limb (from A1 to A2) may be caused by excessive inspiratory flow. Bowing of the expiratory limb (from B1 to B2) may be caused by an increase in expiratory flow resistance such as bronchospasm.

An increased bowing of the PV loop suggests an overall increase in air flow resistance (Fig. 17A). Increase in air flow resistance may be caused by excessive inspiratory flow or increased expiratory flow resistance.

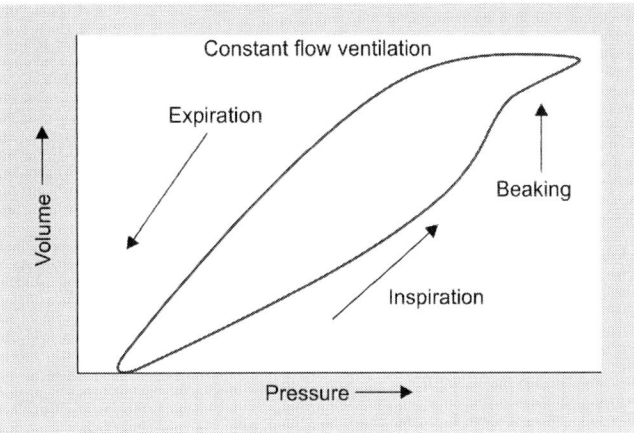

Fig. 18: Pressure-volume loop showing overdistention.

Beaking of PV loop: When overdistended, the lung is again noncompliant and less accommodative of tidal volumes. As it fills up, it increasingly stiffens, there is less volume change for a given applied pressure toward the end of the breath, than there is at the beginning of the breath. The flattening of the terminal part of the inspiratory curve gives a characteristic beaked shape to the PV loop (Fig. 18).

Pressure-volume loop during pressure-targeted ventilation: The pressure is controlled at the preset value. With the deterioration in lung compliance or increased resistance, the tidal volume falls and the loop tilts downward and to the right (Fig. 19).

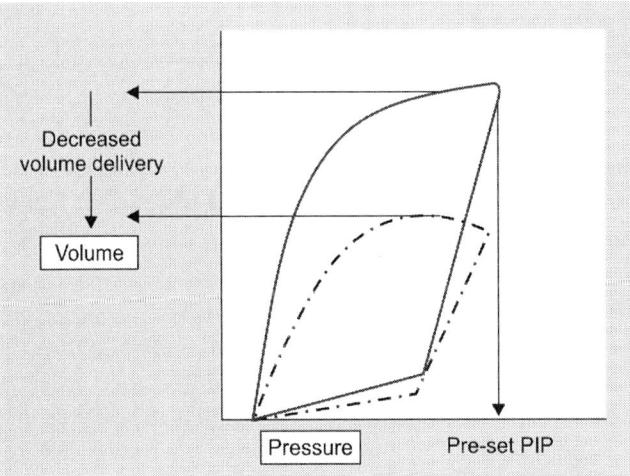

Fig. 19: Pressure-volume (PV) loop during pressure-targeted ventilation. Solid line shows normal PV loop on pressure-targeted ventilation and dotted line shows shifting of loop down and right as compliance/resistance worsens.

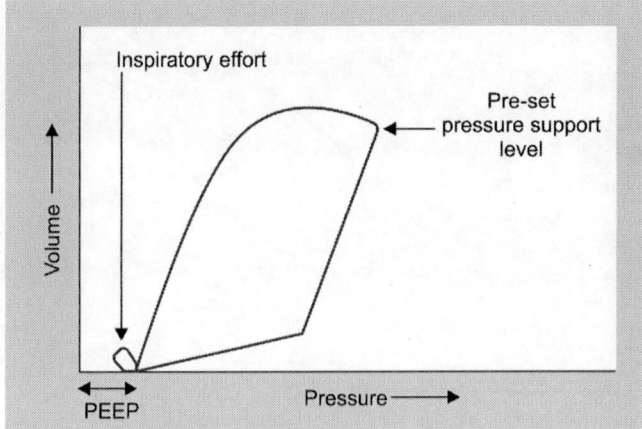

Fig. 20: Pressure-volume loop in pressure support mode of ventilation.

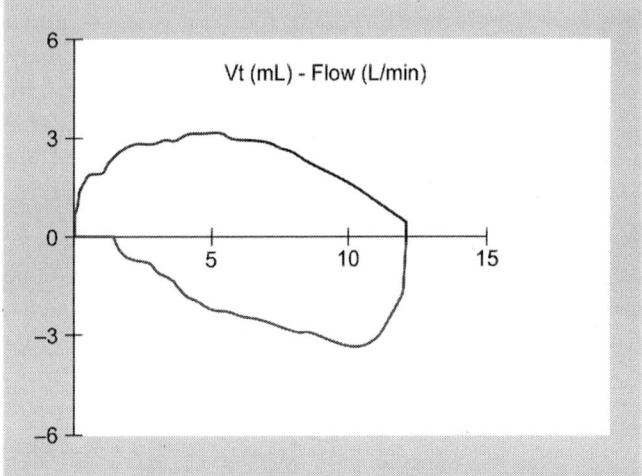

Fig. 21: A normal flow-volume loop.

Pressure-volume loop on pressure support mode of ventilation: As all breaths are patient-triggered, in PV loop we see a small trigger tail. The larger the trigger tail, the greater the patient effort, therefore greater work (Fig. 20).

Flow-Volume Loop

The FV loop displays the relationship between volume and flow. Volume is plotted on the horizontal axis and flow is plotted on the vertical axis. The breath starts at the zero axis and moves upward and to the right on inspiration, terminating at the delivered inspiratory volume and downward, to the left, back to zero on expiration (Fig. 21).

The FV loop changes shape when either inspiratory resistance (flattened inspiratory limb) or expiratory resistance (flattened expiratory limb) is

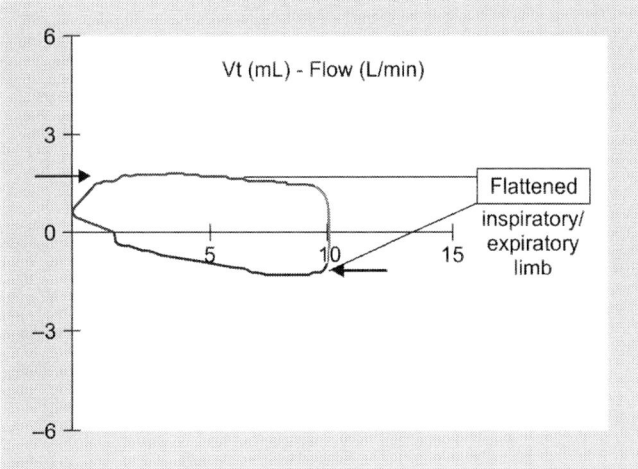

Fig. 22: Flow-volume showing inspiratory and expiratory resistance.

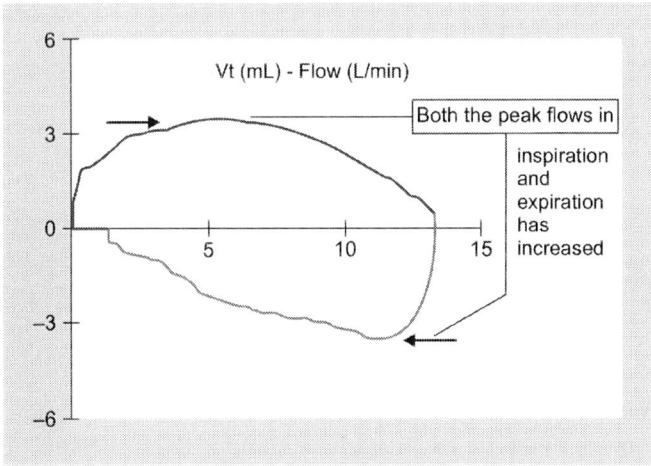

Fig. 23: Flow-volume showing improvement after a dose of bronchodilator.

increased (Fig. 22). The response to bronchodilators can also be assessed from observing the improvement in peak inspiratory/expiratory flow in the FV loop (Fig. 23).

TROUBLESHOOTING BY SCALARS AND LOOPS

Leaks

Leaks may be suspected by looking at the volume waveform (volume-time scalar), whereby the expiratory portion also fails to reach the baseline (see Fig. 7). The FV and PV loops can also suggest the same when expiratory limb fails to reach the origin (Figs. 24 to 26).

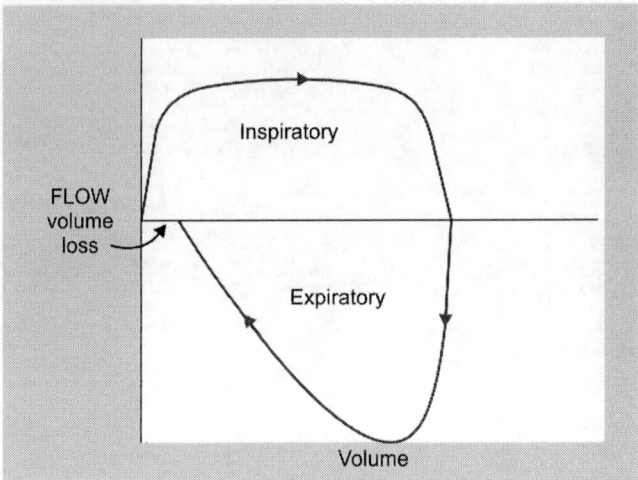

Fig. 24: Flow-volume loop showing loss of expiratory volume as it does not return to the origin.

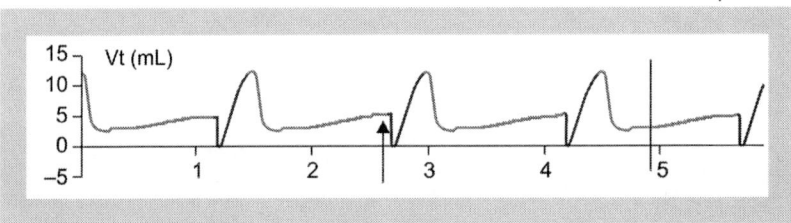

Fig. 25: Volume-time scalar showing that expiratory flow does not completely return to baseline before the next breath.

Auto-PEEP

In the presence of increased expiratory airflow resistance, the time available (expiratory time) to empty the inspired volume may not be sufficient. The next inspiration may start before the completion of the expiration leading to air trapping. Thus, the respiratory system is unable to return to its normal relaxation volume at the end of expiration, leading to higher FRC and thus, air trapping. This condition of air trapping is otherwise called dynamic hyperinflation (DHI). The DHI results in positive alveolar pressure at the end of expiration, referred to as auto-PEEP, occult PEEP or intrinsic PEEP. Sometimes DHI and auto-PEEP can occur in the absence of airflow limitation in mechanically intubated patients. The causes are usually due to rapid respiratory rate, high tidal volumes, inspiratory time more than expiratory time, small bore endotracheal and ventilatory tubes (Figs. 27 to 29).

Turbulence

It can be noted in both FV and PV loops (Fig. 30).

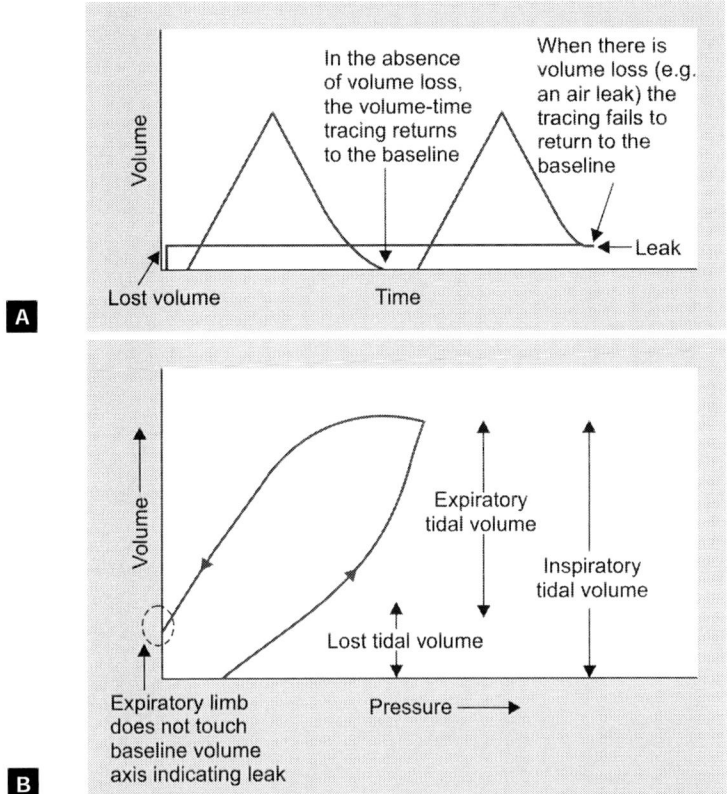

Figs. 26A and B: Graphic representation of leak around endotracheal tube. (A) Volume-time scalar; (B) Pressure-volume loop showing large endotracheal tube leak where the expiratory portion fails to reach the origin

Turbulence can also be detected in all the scalars and is most commonly due to secretions in the tube (Fig. 31).

IDENTIFY SIGNS OF ASYNCHRONY

Asynchrony is the disharmony or "tug of war" between the two interacting systems (ventilator and neural respiratory drive of the patient). This leads to deleterious effects: patient discomfort, increased work of breathing (WOB), increased sedation requirement and weaning failure. Asynchrony should be identified and understood well so necessary interventions can be done to optimize patient ventilator interaction.

Asynchrony can occur in various phases of the breath cycle:
- *Trigger asynchrony*: Improper interaction at initiation of breath.
- *Flow asynchrony*: Imbalance between ventilator flow delivery and patient demand during inspiration.
- *Cycling asynchrony*: Improper breath termination.

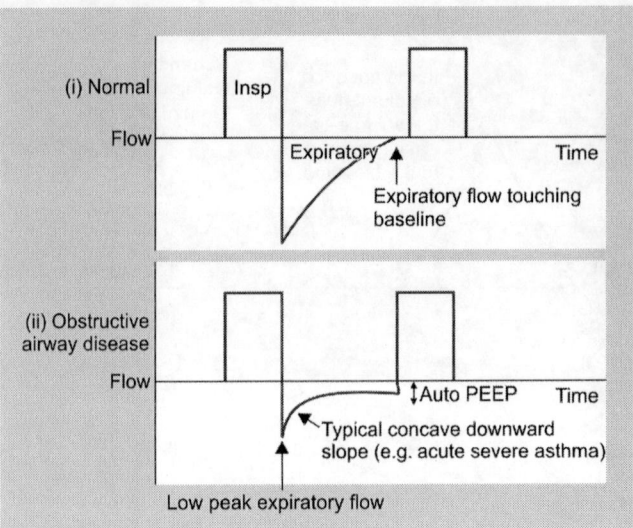

Fig. 27: Graphical representation of auto-positive end-expiratory pressure (PEEP) in flow-time scalar showing low peak expiratory flow, scooping in the expiratory waveform and the start of inspiration before the expiratory waveform touches the baseline causing air trapping (auto-PEEP).

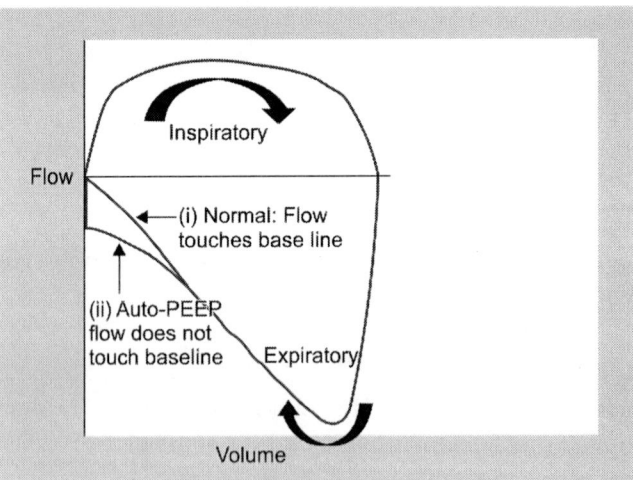

Fig. 28: Flow-volume loop—expiratory flow does not return to the baseline.

Trigger Asynchrony

This can be of three types:
1. Ineffective trigger
2. Double trigger
3. Autotrigger.

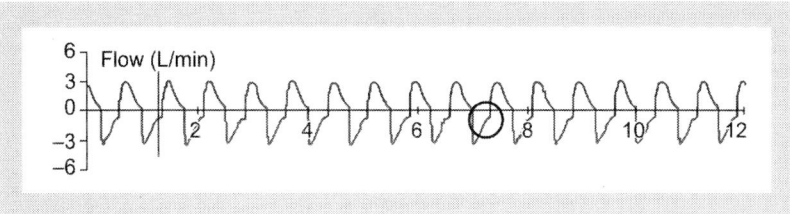

Fig. 29: Flow waveform showing air trappings. The decelerating expiratory limb fails to reach the baseline before the next breath begins (circled), preventing complete emptying of the lung.

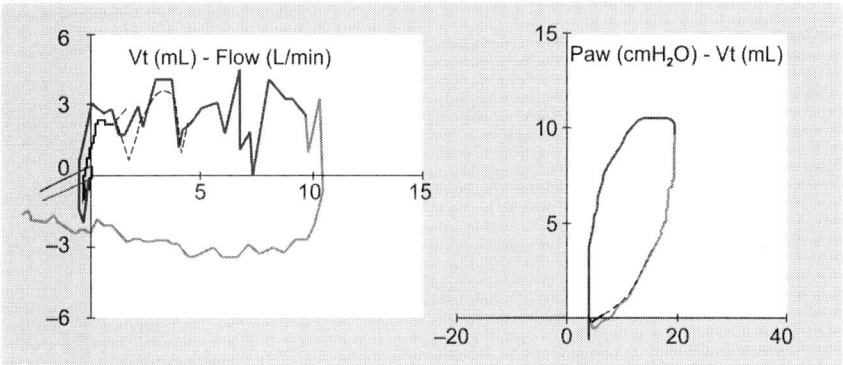

Fig. 30: The "noisy", irregular appearance to the loops in turbulence.

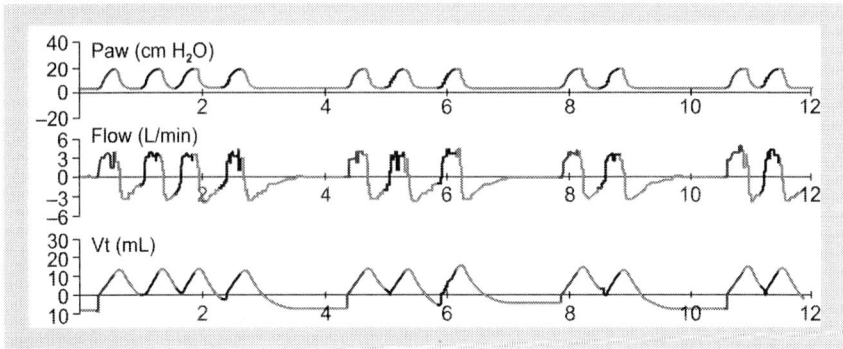

Fig. 31: Irregular waveforms indicating turbulence.

Ineffective Triggering

It is the most common type of trigger asynchrony. This occurs when patient produces respiratory muscular effort which is however not sufficient to initiate mechanical breath. This leads to wasted patient WOB and may result in respiratory fatigue (Fig. 32).

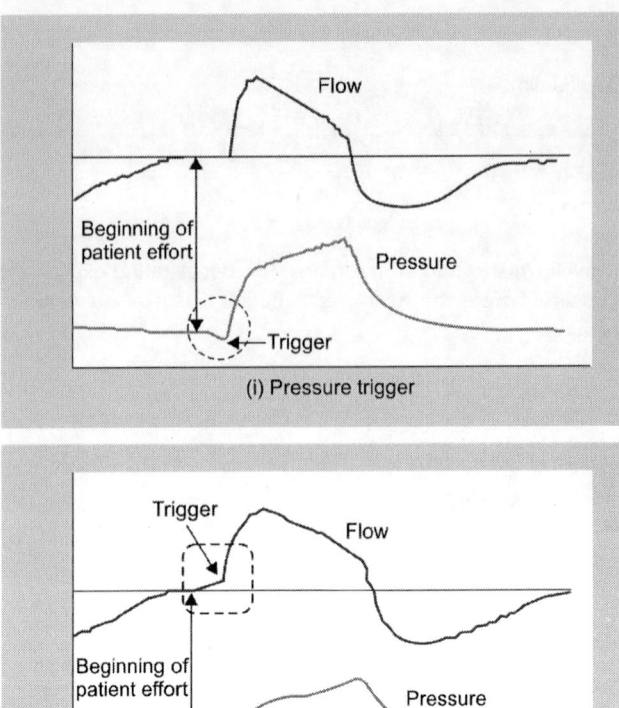

Fig. 32: Graphical representation of pressure and flow trigger.

Factors responsible for ineffective triggering are:

- Ventilator-related:
  - *Insensitive trigger*: Patient effort is unable to reach the set trigger threshold (pressure or flow). This can be corrected by reducing the threshold as appropriate.
  - *Inspiratory delay time*: Total time delay from the initial patient effort until the pressure waveform returns to baseline. Although flow triggering is assumed to be more advantageous than pressure triggering in this aspect, recent advances in pressure transducers have resulted in comparable results.
  - *Resistance of artificial airway*: Larger pressure drop occurs across a narrower ET or constricted airway which requires higher patient effort to overcome.
- Patient-related:
  - Inability to overcome effects auto-PEEP.
  - Oversedation—decreased respiratory drive.
  - Respiratory muscle weakness.

Double Triggering

Double triggering (also called breath stacking) occurs when a patient's inspiratory effort is strong and continues throughout the preset ventilator inspiratory time and remains present thereafter. This patient's inspiratory effort toward end of tidal volume delivery triggers another breath. Thus, tidal volume is again delivered before complete exhalation of the previous breath. Thus, the patient receives, in effect, a double tidal volume, and is at risk of lung overinflation. Double triggering can be caused by aggressive patient efforts in conjunction with small VT and short inspiratory times. During PSV with a high flow termination criterion, double triggering is also possible (Fig. 33).

Autotriggering

Autotriggering occurs when the ventilator delivers an assisted breath that was not initiated by the patient. Autotriggering may also be due to expiratory leak, water or noise in circuit, cardiac oscillations or inappropriately sensitive

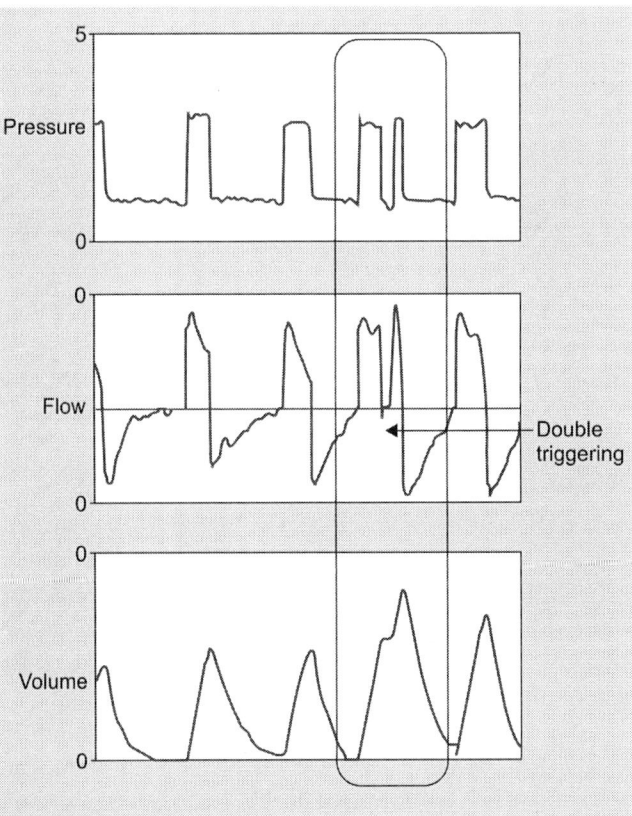

Fig. 33: An example of double trigger in pressure support ventilation.

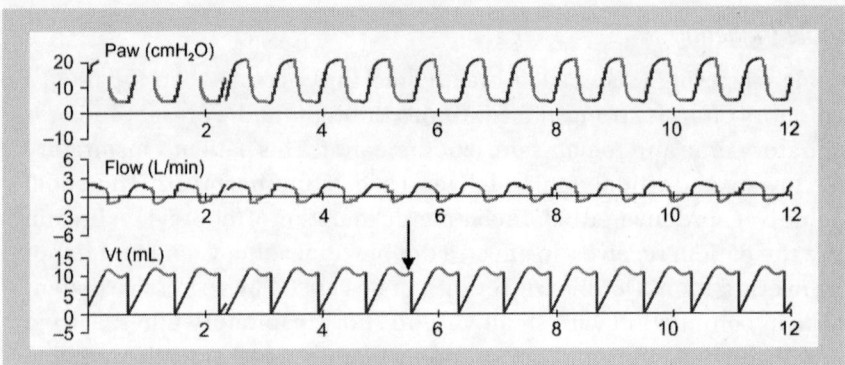

Fig. 34: Ventilatory graphics representing autocycling. In autocycling, the rhythmic breaths come without a pause as well as the large leak.

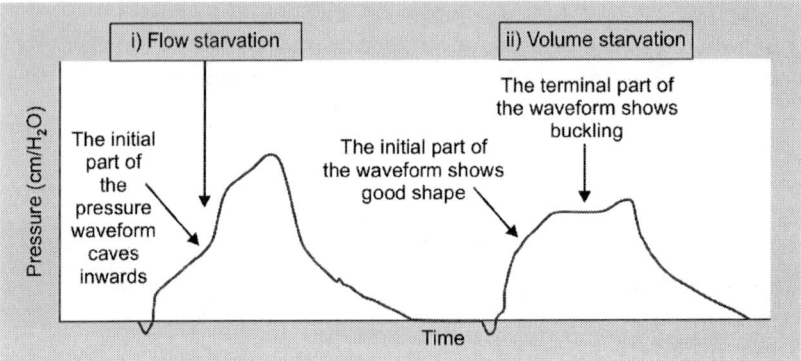

Fig. 35: Pressure-time scalar showing flow and volume starvation.

triggering thresholds. It needs to be corrected by adjustment of trigger sensitivity on the ventilator.

The pulmonary waveforms (all three forms) also indicate autocycling (Fig. 34).

Flow Asynchrony

This occurs when the ventilator flow does not match the patient flow (either too fast or slow or inadequate). This type of asynchrony is also common and may occur with either flow- or pressure-targeted ventilation. Ideally the amount of work done by the patient should be just enough to trigger ventilator. However, in reality, respiratory muscles continue to contract even after ventilator is triggered. Hence it is important to synchronize ventilator flow delivery with the patient to limit WOB and avoid respiratory muscle fatigue. Flow asynchrony can be identified on the pressure-time scalar which reveals a dip (scooped out appearance) during assisted inspiration (Fig. 35). This occurs when the ventilator flow is below the patient's desired flow,

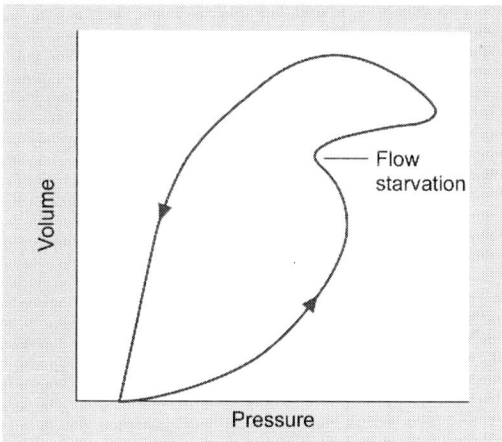

Fig. 36: Pressure-volume loop showing flow starvation.

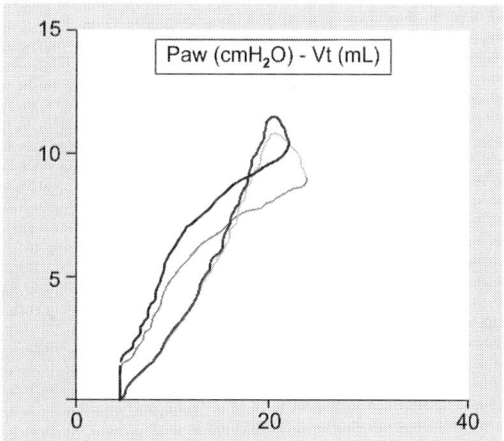

Fig. 37: Figure-of-eight appearance indicating air hunger. Severe flow limitation may appear as a "figure-of-eight" on the PV loop.

and the patient "pulls down" the pressure-time waveform and can also be visualized in PV loop (Figs. 36 and 37).

Cycling Phase Asynchrony

Cycling is the termination of inspiration by ventilator and switch to expiration. When there is a mismatch between the timing of ventilator and patient with respect to termination of inspiration it leads to cycling asynchrony. This is of two types: (1) delayed cycling and (2) premature cycling.

Delayed Cycling

When ventilator continues its inspiratory flow although patient has begun expiratory effort. This leads to a pressure spike at end of ventilator-assisted

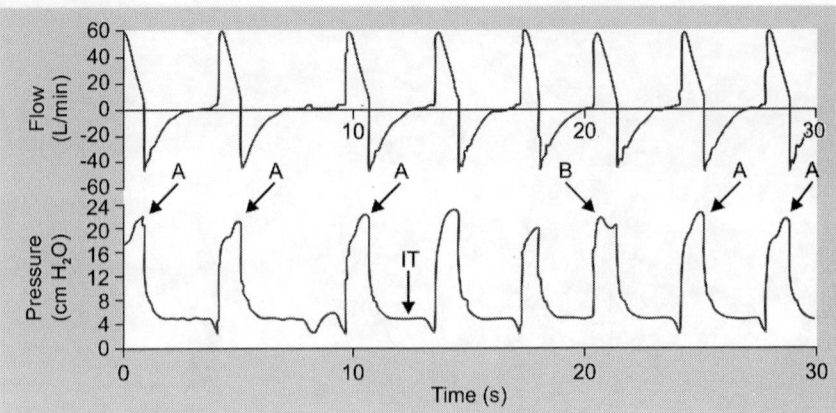

Fig. 38: Delayed cycling leading to pressure spike marked by A. Subsequent ineffective trigger also seen (IT).

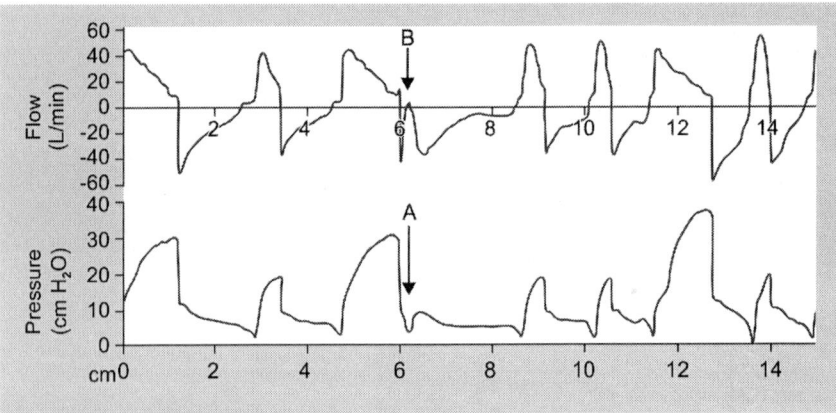

Fig. 39: Premature cycling seen as negative dip below positive end-expiratory pressure (PEEP) on pressure scalar (A).

inspiration and rapid decrease in flow (Fig. 38). Delayed cycling leads to insufficient expiratory time, air trapping, and subsequent failure of triggering. It should be corrected by decreasing inspiratory time and/or tidal volume.

Premature Cycling

Premature cycling is present when a patient is continuing to inhale after ventilator-assisted inspiration has terminated. This is seen on pressure-time scalar as a decrease in airway pressure at end of inspiration. Flow-time scalar will show an increase in air flow immediately after inspiration (Fig. 39). The timing of this event (just after inspiration) differentiates it from ineffective triggering.

Other Types of Asynchrony

Apart from the above described main types, there are few other conditions which are recognized to cause asynchrony. These include:

- *Expiratory asynchrony*: Insufficient expiratory time can lead to generation of auto-PEEP (already discussed previously).
- *Periodic breathing*: This asynchrony in seen in high PSV settings where high minute ventilation leads to CO_2 washout causing apnea followed by rise in CO_2 and this drive to breathe causes arousal from sleep.
- *Mode asynchrony*: It refers to inappropriate mode application leading to patient discomfort. With SIMV, for example, asynchrony can occur because of the different mandatory and spontaneous breath types. This is because the patient's inspiratory effort is often no different for the mandatory and spontaneous breaths and this lacks of adaptation to spontaneous and mandatory breaths precluded effective unloading of the respiratory muscles.

KEY MESSAGES

- Real-time pulmonary graphics do provide useful information regarding the breath-to-breath performance of the ventilator and its interaction with the baby.
- Some complications of mechanical ventilation, such as gas trapping and hyperinflation, may be detected by graphics before they are clinically apparent.
- Fine-tuning of ventilator settings based on pathophysiology and patient response allows for customization of settings.
- It can also decrease the frequency of blood gas analysis and radiography, reducing the cost of care and increasing the comfort of the patient.

SUGGESTED READING

1. Amato MB, Barbas CS, Medeiros DM, et al. Effect of a protective-ventilation strategy on mortality in the acute respiratory distress syndrome. N Engl J Med. 1998;338(6):347-54.
2. Cairo JM, Pilbeam SP. Mosby's Respiratory Care Equipment, 8th edition. St. Louis: Mosby Elsevier; 2009. pp. 364-400.
3. Chatburn RL, Volsko TA. Mechanical ventilators. In: Wilkins RL, Stoller JK, Kacmarck RM (Eds). Egan's Fundamentals of Respiratory Care, 9th edition. St. Louis: Mosby Elsevier; 2009.
4. Davis K Jr, Branson RD, Campbell RS, et al. Comparison of volume control and pressure control ventilation: is flow waveform the difference? J Trauma. 1996;41:808-14.
5. Gattinoni L, Pesenti A, Avalli L, et al. Pressure-volume curve of total respiratory system in acute respiratory failure: computed tomographic scan study. Am Rev Respir Dis. 1987;136(3):730-6.
6. Habashi NM. Other approaches to open-lung ventilation: airway pressure release ventilation. Crit Care Med. 2005;33(3 Suppl):S228-40.

7. Hill LL, Pearl RG. Flow triggering, pressure triggering, and autotriggering during mechanical ventilation. Crit Care Med. 2000;28(2):579-81.
8. Hubmayr RD. Perspective on lung injury and recruitment: a skeptical look at the opening and collapse story. Am J Respir Crit Care Med. 2002;165(12):1647-53.
9. Khilnani P. Respiratory function monitoring during mechanical ventilation in pediatric intensive care unit. Indian J Pediatr. 1998;65(3):409-18.
10. Marini JJ, Smith TC, Lamb VJ. External work output and force generation during synchronized intermittent mechanical ventilation. Effect of machine assistance on breathing effort. Am Rev Respir Dis. 1988;138(5):1169-79.
11. Neumann P, Wrigge H, Zinserling J, et al. Spontaneous breathing affects the spatial ventilation and perfusion distribution during mechanical ventilatory support. Crit Care Med. 2005;33:1090-5.
12. Pilbeam SP, Cairo JM. Mechanical Ventilation: Physiological and Clinical Applications, 4th edition. St. Louis: Mosby Elsevier; 2006.
13. Rappaport SH, Shpiner R, Yoshihara G, et al. Randomized, prospective trial of pressure-limited versus volume-controlled ventilation in severe respiratory failure. Crit Care Med. 1994;22:22-32.
14. Ranieri VM, Giuliani R, Cinnella G, et al. Physiologic effects of positive end-expiratory pressure in patients with chronic obstructive pulmonary disease during acute ventilatory failure and controlled mechanical ventilation. Am Rev Respir Dis. 1993;147(1):5-13.
15. Rossi A, Gottfried SB, Zocchi L, et al. Measurement of static compliance of the total respiratory system in patients with acute respiratory failure during mechanical ventilation. The effect of intrinsic positive end-expiratory pressure. Am Rev Respir Dis. 1985;131:672-7.
16. Roupie E, Dambrosio M, Servillo G, et al. Titration of tidal volume and induced hypercapnia in acute respiratory distress syndrome. Am J Respir Crit Care Med. 1995;152(1):121-8.

Care of the Patient on Ventilator

VSV Prasad, Praveen Khilnani

Survival of children admitted into the pediatric intensive care unit (PICU) is dependent on a multitude of factors. Some of the important factors are:

- Age of the child
- The disease profile
- Single/multisystem disease
- The stage of the disease process
- Underlying chronic major organ system disorders
- The efficacy of preadmission resuscitation
- Degree of derangement of physiological processes
- Nutritional status of the child
- Experience of the pediatric intensivist
- Quality of nursing personnel
- Availability of necessary technology, diagnostics and support staff.

In particular, the child who requires mechanical ventilatory support poses a challenge for the pediatric intensivist/pediatrician. The underlying pulmonary disease process dictates the need for the type and degree of respiratory support. Coexisting organ system dysfunction complicates the care of such patients. Survival of such critically ill children depends vastly on the quality of ancillary care and vigilance of the staff in the intensive care unit (ICU).

To address all issues pertaining to the care of the ventilated child would be exhaustive. This document highlights the basic principles of supportive care and is intended to stimulate those professionals to think and address these issues when embarking on providing level 3 care to children.

MAJOR ISSUES AND FACTORS IN THE CARE OF VENTILATED CHILDREN

- Respiratory care and pulmonary toilet
- Infection control procedures
- Sedation, analgesia and paralysis
- Feeding
- Skilled nursing

- Skin and bowel care
- Central nervous system (CNS) protection.

Respiratory Care and Pulmonary Toilet

Various important aspects of care of a patient on ventilator are discussed below.

Aerosol (Nebulizer or Inhaler) Therapy in Patients on Ventilator

An important therapy is the provision of bronchodilatory support in the form of beta-2 agonists. Nebulizer therapy needs to be provided particularly for those disease entities where bronchospasm contributes significantly to morbidity. Nebulization can either be performed in-line without disconnecting the ventilatory circuit or off-line, where the child is disconnected from the ventilator for a short period of time to perform the nebulization. Off-line therapy can be facilitated only when the child is in the weaning mode/or on a lower degree of ventilatory support. Beta-2 agonist therapy helps reduce airway resistance and helps clear secretions from the distal airways.

The size of the aerosol is expressed as mass median aerodynamic diameter (MMAD). The MMAD determines the rapidity with which the aerosol will settle in the airway. Aerosol gets deposited through the process of impaction, sedimentation and diffusion. In order to be maximally effective the aerosol particles should be 0.5–5 μm in size.

Technique of using nebulizer in mechanically ventilated patients:
- Suction the endotracheal tube if required to clear the airway secretions.
- Remove the heat and moisture exchanger (HME) filter as it acts as a barrier to drug delivery. Do not turn off the heat water humidifier as it can lead to drying of the airway secretions.
- Choose the nebulizer device (Jet vs Ultrasonic vs Mesh nebulizer)
- Place the drug solution (2.5 mg of salbutamol) in the nebulizer to optimum fill volume of 4–5 mL
- Place the nebulizer 15 cm from the Y piece in the inspiratory limb of the circuit.
- Select airflow of 6–8 L/min to power the jet nebulizer. Adjust minute ventilation to ensure constant tidal volume. Extra gas flow is not needed while using ultrasonic and mesh nebulizers.
- Attempt to achieve a longer inspiratory time, longer duty cycle (>0.3), lower inspiratory flow and a bias flow less than 2 L/min. However ventilator settings optimal for nebulization can lead to patient–ventilator dyssynchrony and a prescribed ventilatory pattern may not be practical.
- Observe nebulizer for adequate aerosol generation throughout its use.
- Disconnect nebulizer when all medication is nebulized or when no more aerosols are being produced. Store nebulizer under aseptic conditions.
- Reconnect HME and return to original ventilator and alarm settings.

Technique of using meter dose inhaler (MDI) in mechanically ventilated patients:

- Suction the endotracheal tube if required to clear the airway secretions.
- Remove the HME filter as it acts as a barrier to drug delivery. Do not turn off the heat water humidifier as it can lead to drying of the airway secretions.
- Shake pMDI and warm to hand temperature.
- pMDI spacer should be placed 15 cm from the Y piece in the inspiratory limb of the ventilator circuit.
- Coordinate MDI actuation with beginning of inspiration.
- Wait at least 20 sec between actuations; administer total dose (4 puffs of salbutamol).
- Monitor for adverse response.
- Reconnect HME.

Humidification

The addition of heat and moisture to inspired gases delivered to the patient during mechanical ventilatory support via an artificial airway is known as **humidification**. There is agreement among clinicians that heating and humidifying inspired gases is required. An endotracheal tube or tracheostomy tube bypasses the upper airway which normally heats and humidifies the inspired air. Cold and dry air can cause secretions to become thick and tenacious which can occlude the endotracheal or tracheostomy tube as well as cause mucosal injury to the airways. Excessive humidification is also a problem and can decrease mucociliary clearance, cause hyperhydration and loss of surfactant activity. Tracheal humidification can be provided by a heated water humidifier or a heat moisture exchanger (HME). Heated water humidifiers are used in ventilated patients and in self ventilating patients with thick secretions as preferred device. An appropriately sized HME is preferred in self ventilating patients with no or minimal oxygen keeping in mind the potential hazard of increased airway resistance and dead space. An HME must be removed from the patient circuit during aerosol treatments when the nebulizer is placed in the patient circuit.

Heated Humidifiers

These deliver more water to airways by heating the inspired gas. The temperature of gas that is delivered to the patient is regulated by a servo device that measures gas temperature at airway and adjusts the heater output of the humidifier. These are used when gases are being delivered via an artificial airway and mechanical ventilator. Heating the water causes a larger number of water molecules to gain sufficient kinetic energy to enter the gaseous state, thereby the vapor content of inspired gas is increased. Humidifiers are an important factor for bacterial colonization and development of ventilator acquired pneumonia, therefore extremely diligent care is required to take all precautions for infection control while following bundle care of a patient on the ventilator. Any visible soiling of circuit or humidification tubing must lead to a circuit change as well as humidifier replacement after sterilization.

Heat and Moisture Exchangers (HME's)

Placed on the distal end of the tracheal tube, HME's store a portion of the humidity from the expired volume and return this to the inspired air. They function as passive respiratory air humidifiers, which do not depend on a supply of external energy or source of water. Because their mode of operation is related to the nasal operating principle, they also are called "artificial noses". A HME can only return as much heat and humidity as has been stored reversibly from the previous breath. Therefore, the quantity of inspiratory humidity is determined by the moisture content of the expired air, which is defined by the patient temperature, and by the thermodynamic properties of the HME materials (specially designed paper, cellulose or polyurethane foams).

To improve the heat- and moisture-conserving qualities of the HME material, a hygroscopic coating, such as magnesium, calcium, or lithium chloride, is used. These compounds reversibly adsorb water molecules and thus increase the water retention capacity. After a few breaths HMEs are at almost full effectiveness and reach steady state within a few minutes. Subsequently, the moisture-returning properties of the HME depend only on ventilatory parameters, the most important of which is tidal volume, such that the moisture-returning performance decreases as the tidal volume increases. HMEs always result in an elevation of the inspiratory and expiratory airway resistances; this should be considered especially in cases that involve spontaneous respiration. The internal volumes of HMEs should be as small as possible so that they do not increase the effective dead space too much. A combination of HMEs and catheter mounts results in a further increase in the dead space, and therefore, must be considered critically, especially in cases that involve spontaneous respiration. If a catheter mount is necessary to add flexibility to the breathing system, the HME preferably should be connected directly onto the tracheal tube with the catheter mount behind it; otherwise, the humidification efficiency of the HME will be reduced by condensation in the catheter mount. Children should be ventilated with special HMEs that have a small internal volume.

Caution: HME sould be avoided in patients with thick, copious, or bloody secretions, patients with an expired tidal volume less than 70% of the delivered tidal volume (e.g. those with large broncho-pleuro-cutaneous fistulas or incompetent or absent endotracheal tube cuffs), patients with body temperatures less than 32°C, patients with high spontaneous minute volumes (>10 L/min) and during non-invasive ventilation.

Respiratory Care During Ventilation via Tracheostomy and Tracheostomy Care

Pediatric tracheostomies are less commonly performed (<3% patients) as compared to adult tracheostomies. It is classically done surgically. Percutaneous tracheostomies are rarely performed in children. There is lack of consensus on the timing of tracheostomy and the optimum decannulation protocol. Many patients with tracheostomy due to acute or chronic issues may require mechanical ventilation. It is essential for all care takers to be familiar with care of tracheostomy even though physiologically speaking it works similar to an endotracheal tube.

Care of new tracheostomy (Less than 7 days)

The initial 5–7 days after a tracheostomy are potentially hazardous as the track has not matured. Decannulation of the tube during this period can create a life threatening situation as reinsertion can be extremely difficult due to surgical inflammation, edema and bleeding. Nursing care in these first seven days is very different from that of an established stoma. Post surgery, a portable chest X-ray should be done immediately to confirm tube position and to rule out a pneumothorax and surgical emphysema. An emergency tracheostomy kit (having same size and one size smaller tracheostomy tube) should be kept bedside. Stay sutures should be taped to the anterior chest wall and labeled left and right. These stay sutures when gently retracted upwards helps in rapid identification of the newly created stoma, allowing fast replacement of the tube. Stay sutures should be removed at the time of the first postoperative tracheostomy tube change. Nurses should check that the tracheostomy ties are tight enough, ensuring that only one finger slips between the neck and tapes. Humidification and regular suctioning should be done to keep the tube patent.

Routine tracheostomy management

TRACHE care bundle approach (Hall et al.) can be used to remember the essential components of pediatric tracheostomy care:

T: Tapes: Keep the tube secure
R: Resus: Know the resuscitation process
A: Airway clear: Use correct suction technique
C: Care of the site: Stoma and neck
H: Humidity: Essential to keep tube clear
E: Emergency box: Have the box present

Chest Physiotherapy

Immobilization on the ventilator and supine positioning leads to atelectasis especially of the left lower lobe, due to the weight of the heart. Gravitation of posterior pharyngeal secretions around the endotracheal tube. Ciliary function gets suppressed with disease and sedation. This in turn leads to retention of secretions super added bacterial infection and nosocomial pneumonia. The central function of chest physiotherapy in pediatric respiratory disease is to assist in the removal of tracheobronchial secretions to remove airway obstruction, reduce airway resistance, enhance gas exchange with intention to reduce the work of breathing. Chest physiotherapy in conjunction with humidification and secretions control can improve a patient's respiratory status and speed up recovery. Its use is well established in acute atelectasis Neuromuscular disease, cystic fibrosis, bronchiectasis, post-abdominal surgery and in bed ridden immobile patients. There is very little hard evidence for the beneficial effect of chest physiotherapy.

In some patients on high FiO_2 with labile respiratory status, physiotherapy can worsen the status perhaps by increasing bronchospasm, inducing pulmonary hypertension, repositioning a foreign body, or destabilising a sick infant. Commonly available techniques of physiotherapy include positioning postural drainage, percussions and vibrations. After extubation one can use mobilisation and Incentive spirometry.

Pulmonary Toilet

Pulmonary toilet (clearance of secretions from the large airways) is necessary in certain forms of respiratory illnesses. In addition to debris in the airways from the underlying lung disease, bronchial secretions need periodic clearance from the larger airways and trachea since the natural mucociliary clearance is impaired. The procedure of disconnecting the patient from the ventilator, performing endotracheal suctioning (open suction) by the proper method and reconnecting the child back to the ventilator is fraught with many risks and dangers. In most patients on mild to moderate settings and physiological PEEP, a Manual hyperinflation is usually performed before and between suctioning to prevent hypoxemia. The patient is disconnected from the ventilator and is bagged with a resuscitator bag using slow deep inspiration, inspiratory hold and quick release to enhance expiration. This causes the recruitment of atelectatic segments and also mobilizes secretions.

In Patients with ARDS or severe pneumonia with high FiO_2 requirements and peak pressures or PEEP, a closed suctioning system with pediatric and neonatal catheter sizes (Figs. 1 and 2) is recommended where disconnection from ventilator is avoidable and therefore episodes of worsening hypoxemia and alveolar derecruitment due to loss of PEEP can be avoided. As far as infection rates are concerned, both open and closed suctioning methods have a similar incidence of infection risk.

Mucous plugging, mucolytic agents and saline

An adequate humidification of inspired gases will usually not lead to thick mucus plugging. Widespread indiscriminate use of mucolytic agents should be discouraged. N-Acetyl cysteine (mucomyst) can be used as aerosol only if thick secretions in patients with cystic fibrosis, bronchiectasis or other diseases. There are no randomized control trials, however, there have been

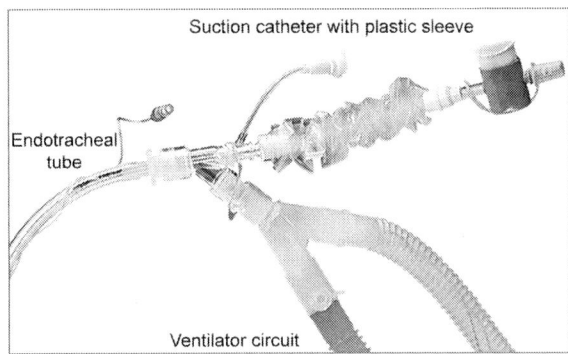

Fig. 1: Close suction system. (*For color version see Plate 3*)

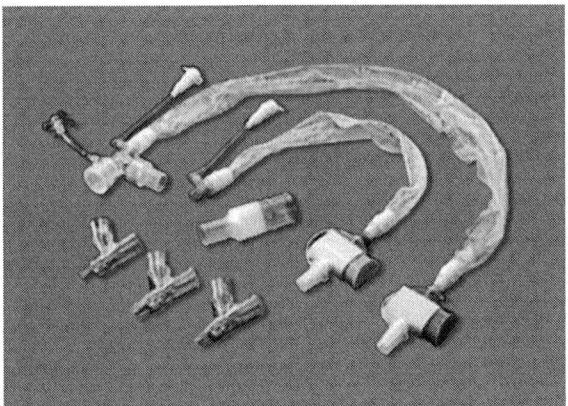

Fig. 2: Pediatric and neonatal close suction catheters. (*For color version see Plate 4*)

case reports in the use of N-acetylcysteine and deoxyribonuclease (DNase) in life-threatening situations of mucus plugs. Many centers use normal saline or 3% saline to facilitate loosening of thick secretions during suctioning. Many of the practices with widespread use are based on experience and expert opinion and may not have evidence-based support.

A thorough knowledge and a well-defined protocol need to be followed every time, endotracheal suctioning needs to be performed with due diligence. Disasters often happen in the PICU, purely due to iatrogenic reasons! Tube disconnection, dislodgement, displacement or accidental extubation could occur during process of suctioning with serious consequences. Poor knowledge, experience, improper planning, and pulmonary toileting are perfect recipes for untoward and disastrous consequences. A good knowledge of troubleshooting is important, if patient condition is deteriorating. Bag tube mask and reintubation equipment must be available as an emergency measure one should increase FiO_2 to 100% and take over the ventilation manually. One needs to follow DOPE protocol and emergently address displacement obstruction pneumothorax and equipment issues.

Infection Control Procedures

The ventilated child often demands maximal time, energy and resources to care for. Successful management depends on supportive care and effective troubleshooting. The sick patient invariably requires multiple intravenous lines, sometimes central venous access catheters, indwelling arterial lines, indwelling urinary catheters, and sometimes drains from various body cavities to allow drainage of fluid, etc. The child with multisystem disease is the most difficult to manage. All breaks in the skin and mucous membrane barriers pose the threat of ascending infection and sepsis.

Structured infection control protocols for the ICU help define clearly the methods to be adopted for placement/monitoring/and removal of such indwelling lines, catheters, etc. All staff in the PICU must be well versed with the infection control policies of the unit and the hospital and should strictly adhere to proper handwash techniques before every and each patient contact. In addition, following the proper aseptic process of adequate skin preparation, draping and disposal of materials after procedures is essential. During the period of mechanical ventilation of the child, prevention of ventilator-associated pneumonia (VAP) (see last section on bundle care approach), central line-associated bloodstream infections (CLABSIs), catheter-related bloodstream infection (CRBSI), catheter-associated urinary tract infections (CAUTIs), etc. are a major threat to the patient. Nosocomial infection rates dramatically increase with the degree of critical illness of the patient. Barrier nursing, body fluid contact precautions and the systematic segregation of biomedical waste and hygienic disposal are essential in the prevention of spread of nosocomial infection, and personal health of the staff working in the PICU. The institution of "bundled care" (e.g. VAP bundle, CRBSI bundle, etc.) has made structured care with checklists for sick children. The most important aspect of such maneuvers and interventions is a committed approach by all concerned, along with a cohesive team culture of both medical and nursing professionals to achieve and keep nosocomial infections rates as low as possible.

Sedation, Analgesia and Paralysis

Ventilated children unless there is underlying serious CNS pathology causing hypotonia/areflexia, invariably would require some form of sedation to keep the child calm and sedated. This is required to reduce anxiety in the child and prevent patient-ventilator dyssynchrony. Inadvertent movements of the ventilated child can cause disasters: accidental extubation, pneumothorax, etc. Analgesia is also required for all postoperative patients, and those requiring placement of invasive lines/catheters. Commonly used sedatives belong the benzodiazepine class of drugs and opiates. Midazolam is often the choice because of its shorter half-life, safety and virtually no hemodynamic side effects. Opiates commonly used in the PICU include morphine, fentanyl and pentazocine. Propofol anesthesia is sometimes used, and sometimes dissociative anesthetics such as ketamine are preferred in specific clinical settings. Drug doses need to be carefully calculated, and the mode of administration from continuous intravenous infusion to intermittent bolus dosing needs to be defined by the intensivist.

Muscle relaxation and paralysis is required in those ventilated patients where the risk of inadvertent movement of the patient would cause serious problems. Typically, the ventilated child requiring very high mean airway pressures on the ventilator, air-leak syndromes (pneumothorax, etc.) or those with pulmonary hypertension/pulmonary hypertensive crises require paralysis short term. The choice of muscle relaxants is often limited in children to: vecuronium, rocuronium, pancuronium or atracurium. Succinylcholine is rarely used in modern pediatric intensive care as safer alternatives are available.

A thorough understanding of these drugs, their indications, interactions with other drugs and risks are required. By default, all children requiring muscle relaxation *must have been already on adequate sedation with or without analgesia.*

Feeding

One of the greatest success stories in the arena of pediatric intensive care has been the realization and importance of feeding the critically ill child, particularly children on mechanical ventilatory support. Old schools of thought existed wherein feeding was deliberately withheld for prolonged periods of time. Current day pediatric intensive practice uses early feeding, preferably by the enteral route at the earliest possible time. Critical illness in children causes a highly catabolic state with a negative nutritional and nitrogen balance! Provision of enteral feeding with milk or other suitable formula is essential. Feeding is usually commenced once the child is hemodynamically stable and has adequate bowel function. Most PICUs use the nasogastric/orogastric route for administration of feeds. Less commonly used routes of feeding are through the jejunum or stomach. For short-term ventilatory support, nasogastric/orogastric feeds are preferred. In those children with serious CNS injury/CNS impairment, wherein protective airway reflexes have been lost/impaired, or the possibility of oropharyngeal/gastric content aspiration into the trachea is a serious threat, preference is given for the establishment of a surgical gastrostomy (with or without a Nissen/Thal's procedure) or surgical jejunostomy.

The benefits of early and adequate enteral nutrition in the sick child have been well documented and researched. Of importance is the fact that feeding preserves gut mucosal integrity and prevents bacterial/toxin translocation into the bloodstream.

Skilled Nursing

Positive outcomes of children admitted in the PICU are dependent on a high quality of skilled nursing care. Medical/physician support is obviously important, but the commitment and skill of a trained ICU nurse is vital in the care of patients. Skill sets of pediatric critical care nursing need to be reviewed periodically and quality assurance maintained. Motivation, pride, and the feeling of a sense of belonging to the unit are highly essential for successful pediatric intensive care. A poorly trained/inadequately trained nurse can spell disaster in the ICU! Proper and careful selection of nursing staff and ongoing training and teaching are mandatory in any PICU.

Skin and Bowel Care

Often overlooked in the PICU is proper care of the skin of the sick child. Indwelling intravenous lines, central lines often extravasate, and early recognition of the problem by nursing staff is important to prevent cellulitis/ sepsis and sometimes gangrene! Children on mechanical ventilatory support are often nursed immobile for extended periods of time. During this period, dependent skin is liable to become devitalized due to poor blood supply and prolonged pressure from the concerned body part. Decubitus ulcers, with their attendant risks and complications invariably happen. Frequent change of position to change the pressure points on the mattress, proper bathing, and skin hygiene are essential. Entry points for indwelling lines and catheters need to be protected and managed carefully to prevent ascending sepsis.

Sick children, particularly those on opiates, etc. develop constipation and impaction of feces. Prevention of these problems is important and bowel cleansing as necessary by artificial stool softeners or enemas. Bowel hygiene prevents bacterial translocation and reduces the risk of sepsis.

Central Nervous System Protection

Children requiring mechanical ventilatory support and those with CNS disorders/head injury are at risk for brain injury. Monitoring the CNS is an extremely important task in the PICU. Clinical monitoring alone may not suffice in many circumstances. Intermittent or continuous electroencephalogram (EEG) monitoring may be required in high-risk patients. Early detection of raised intracranial pressure and urgent management is crucial. Subclinical seizures and nonconvulsive status epilepticus can cause silent and unrecognizable irreversible brain injury. Ensuring adequate cardiac output and the maintenance of an optimal cerebral perfusion pressure, with appropriate management of intracranial hypertension and seizures will prevent injury to the brain during the critical phase of the child's illness.

Parent/Family Counseling

Often overlooked and sometimes taken for granted is the "quality of parent and family counseling" throughout the stay of the sick child in the PICU. There are no strict guidelines that are too applied to the form of counseling, but the continuous availability of a qualified pediatric intensivist/house staff in the ICU, along with regular scheduled counseling sessions of all parents of admitted children is mandatory to successful care of critically ill children. Every family is different, and the approach has to modify and individualized keeping in mind their socioeconomic background, their education levels, and language to be utilized for counseling. Proper documentation in writing along with audiovisual recording of sessions is important to avoid future conflict and confusion with the family. Audiovisual documentation also serves the purpose of medicolegal protection of health care professionals involved in the care of such sick children.

Patience, unhurried discussions, empathy and compassion are required to see the family through a very stressful period in their child's life.

VENTILATOR-ASSOCIATED PNEUMONIA/EVENT: BUNDLE CARE APPROACH

Pneumonia Types

The 2005 American Thoracic Society/Infectious Diseases Society of America (ATS/IDSA) guidelines distinguish the following types of pneumonia:

- Hospital-acquired (or nosocomial) pneumonia (HAP) is pneumonia that occurs 48 hours or more after admission and did not appear to be incubating at the time of admission.
- Ventilator-associated pneumonia is a type of HAP that develops more than 48–72 hours after endotracheal intubation.
- Health care-associated pneumonia (HCAP) is defined as pneumonia that occurs in a nonhospitalized patient with extensive health care contact, as defined by one or more of the following:
  - Intravenous therapy, wound care, or intravenous chemotherapy within the prior 30 days
  - Residence in a nursing home or other long-term care facility
  - Hospitalization in an acute care hospital for 2 days or more days within the prior 90 days
  - Attendance at a hospital or hemodialysis clinic within the prior 30 days.

Respiratory Sampling

Lower respiratory tract sampling is indicated for all patients who are suspected of having VAP and have an abnormal chest radiograph. There are a variety of methods available to sample material from the airways and alveoli, including nonbronchoscopic (i.e. blind) and bronchoscopic techniques.

Nonbronchoscopic lower respiratory tract sampling includes tracheobronchial aspiration or mini-bronchoalveolar lavage (BAL):

- Tracheobronchial aspiration is performed by advancing a catheter through the endotracheal tube until resistance is met and then applying suction.

- Mini-BAL is performed by advancing a catheter through the endotracheal tube until resistance is met, infusing sterile saline through the catheter, and then aspirating.

Bronchoscopic sampling is performed using either BAL or a protected specimen brush (PSB). The decision about whether to perform nonbronchoscopic or bronchoscopic sampling ultimately depends upon a case-by-case determination of the benefits of a narrow antibiotic regimen versus the risks of bronchoscopy.

Microscopic Analysis

Gram's satin, total leukocyte count (TLC), differential leukocyte count (DLC) and culture.

Ventilator-associated Pneumonia

It refers to pneumonia that develops at least 48 hours after the initiation of mechanical ventilation. It is probably caused by aerodigestive tract colonization, followed by aspiration of contaminated secretions into the lower airways. Many of the risk factors for VAP increase the risk of colonization and aspiration, while most of the interventions to prevent VAP reduce colonization and aspiration. Clinical pulmonary infection score (CPIS) is often used to determine severity of infection and to diagnose VAP. It takes into account fever, white blood cell (WBC) count, tracheal secretions, PaO_2/FiO_2 ratio and chest radiograph.

Role of the Ventilator Circuit in Ventilator-associated Pneumonia

The ventilator circuit appears to have only a small effect on the development of VAP, assuming that reasonable infection control practices are followed. This view is supported by several pieces of evidence:
- Aspiration of contaminated secretions is the predominant cause of nosocomial pneumonia, not inhalation of aerosols containing bacteria
- The microorganisms that colonize the ventilator circuit originate in the patient. This suggests that the patient contaminates the circuit, rather than the circuit contaminating the patient
- Changing the ventilator circuit more frequently does not decrease the frequency of VAP.

Bottom line: Ventilator circuits need not be changed routinely for infection control purposes unless visibly soiled.

Passive versus active humidification: Active and passive humidification are strategies to warm and humidify inspired gases during mechanical ventilation. Such warming and humidification is necessary because the endotracheal tube bypasses the area of the respiratory tract in which these processes normally occur in spontaneous breathing individuals. Active humidification occurs when a humidifier in the ventilator circuit warms and humidifies the inspired gas. Passive humidification uses a device called an artificial nose (or HME filter) to trap the patient's exhaled warm humidity. Some artificial noses also serve as filters, decreasing circuit contamination.

Although active and passive humidification are associated with similar rates of VAP, there are other important differences that should be considered:

- Passive humidifiers are cheaper than active humidifiers
- Passive humidifiers are less effective than active humidifiers, which may lead to a greater risk of airway occlusion
- Passive humidifiers have higher resistance to flow, which may be problematic in spontaneous breathing modes (e.g. pressure support ventilation)
- Passive humidifiers increase dead space volume, which can be problematic during low tidal volume ventilation.

Bottom line: Active humidifiers do not need to be changed at regular intervals. Passive humidifiers can be safely used for at least 48 hours in most patients and even longer (e.g. up to 7 days) in some populations. Patients who require the more frequent changes include those with obstructive airways disease, copious airway secretions, or frequent clogging with secretions. When frequent clogging is an issue, use of an active humidifier instead of a passive humidifier should be considered.

Heated versus unheated circuit: Heat minimizes condensation, which is a source of ventilator circuit contamination. However, trials have failed to find evidence that a heated circuit reduces the rate of VAP.

Bottom line: Use it.

Closed versus open suction: Tracheal secretions are removed during mechanical ventilation by passing a suction catheter through the endotracheal tube. With a closed suction system, the suction catheter is part of the ventilator circuit and, therefore, the patient can be suctioned without being disconnected from the ventilator. With an open suction system, the patient is disconnected from the ventilator and then the suction catheter is passed through the endotracheal tube.

Use of a closed or open suction system does not appear to affect the frequency of VAP.

Bottom line: It is better to use closed suction. When closed suctioning systems are used, the suction catheters should be considered part of the ventilator circuit and not changed routinely. The maximum duration of time that closed suction catheters can be used safely is unknown.

Nebulizer versus inhaler: Nebulizers can be incorporated into the ventilator circuit and used to deliver medications. However, they frequently become contaminated and might contribute to the development of VAP.

Use of a metered-dose inhaler probably eliminates this risk. Like a nebulizer, a metered-dose inhaler delivers aerosolized medication directly into the ventilator circuit. However, metered-dose inhalers do not become contaminated because they are not part of the ventilator circuit. Metered-dose inhalers are also less expensive, easier to use, and deliver a dose more reliably than nebulizers.

In conclusion provision of comprehensive clinical support to the ventilated child improves outcomes, and the ancillary care sometimes is as important as or more important than providing ventilatory care alone.

KEY MESSAGES

- *Elevation of the head of the bed*: The head of the bed is elevated to 30–45° (unless contraindicated).
- *Sedation level assessment*: Unless the patient is awake and comfortable, sedation is reduced/held for assessment at least daily (unless contraindicated).
- *Oral hygiene*: The mouth is cleaned with chlorhexidine gluconate (≥1–2% gel or 0.1–0.2% liquid) 6 hourly (as chlorhexidine can be inactivated by toothpaste, a gap of at least 2 hours should be left between its application and tooth brushing). Teeth are brushed 12 hourly with standard toothpaste.
- *Subglottic aspiration*: A tracheal tube (endotracheal or tracheostomy) which has a subglottic secretion drainage port is used if the patient is expected to be intubated for >72 hours. Secretions are aspirated via the subglottic secretion port 1–2 hourly.
- *Tracheal tube cuff pressure*: Cuff pressure is measured 4 hourly, maintained between 20 cm H_2O and 30 cm H_2O (or 2 cm H_2O above peak inspiratory pressure) and recorded on the ICU chart.
- *Stress ulcer prophylaxis*: Stress ulcer prophylaxis is prescribed only to high-risk patients according to locally developed guidelines.
- *Minimizing transport out of the ICU*: Patients who are transported out of the ICU have an incidence of VAP that is three to four times that of patients who are never transported out of the ICU.
- Avoiding the need for reintubation.
- Noninvasive instead of invasive mechanical ventilation whenever possible.
- *Positive end-expiratory pressure (PEEP)*: The application of PEEP may decrease the incidence of VAP. A possible mechanism is that the positive tracheal pressure opposes aspiration of pharyngeal secretions around the cuff of the endotracheal tube.
- *Weaning protocols*: Weaning protocols are recommended by many organizations, in order to reduce the duration of ventilation.
- Addressing multiple issues and evaluating the patient as a whole can go a long way in improving pediatric survivals. Audit or quality improvement tool is a continuous process of re-evaluating a unit's performance and

such tool requires proper mentoring, discipline and culture of an organization and unit to improve upon existing practices.

- Patient outcomes of ventilated children are dependent heavily on multiple factors, apart from the nature of illness or stage of illness alone.
- Care of the all ventilated patient essentially involves close clinical monitoring and gas exchange (oxygenation and carbon dioxide), troubleshooting of ventilator and circuit issues, patient positioning, physiotherapy, humidification, aerosol therapy, suctioning, skin and eye care.

SUGGESTED READING

1. Ari A. Aerosol therapy in pulmonary critical care. Respir Care. 2015;60(6):858-74; discussion 874-9.
2. C. Doherty, R. Neal et al. Multidisciplinary guidelines for the management of paediatric tracheostomy emergencies. Anaesthesia. 2018;73:1400–17.
3. Dhand R. Aerosol delivery during mechanical ventilation: from basic techniques to new devices. J Aerosol MedPulm Drug Deliv. 2008;21(1):45-60.
4. Dhanani J, Fraser JF, Chan HK, et al. Fundamentals of aerosol therapy in critical care. Crit Care. 2016;20(1):269.
5. Fink JB. Aerosol delivery to ventilated infant and pediatric patients. Respir Care 2004;49(6):653–65.
6. Gupta S, Sinha S. Care of the ventilated infant. Paediatr Child Health. 2009;19(12):544-9.
7. Hall A, Bates J et al. Implementation of the TRACHE care bundle: improving safety in paediatric tracheostomy management. Arch Dis Child. 2017;102(6):563-5.
8. Ramakrishnan M. Care of the ventilated patient. In: Khilnani P (Ed). Practical Approach to Pediatric Intensive Care, 3rd edition. New Delhi, India: Jaypee Brothers Medical Publishers (P) Ltd.; 2015. pp. 443-5.
9. Watters KF. Tracheostomy in infants and children. Respir Care. 2017;62(6): 799–825.

Weaning from Ventilator

Sanjay Wazir, Kumar Ankur, Praveen Khilnani

NEONATE

Despite the growing use of noninvasive ventilation (NIV) in neonatal intensive care units (NICUs) across the globe, mechanical ventilation (MV) use is quite common with almost 75–83% of extremely low birth weight (ELBW) babies requiring invasive ventilation during the course of stay in NICU. MV although is lifesaving in such tiny babies is not without its attendant risks including mortality and neurodevelopmental handicap.

Weaning is not equivalent to pulling out endotracheal tube (ETT) but a process of slowly decreasing the amount of ventilatory support, with the patient gradually assuming a greater proportion of overall ventilation. While there is a relative consensus as to when MV should be initiated in a particular child, the management of babies during recovery from respiratory failure remains largely subjective and is predominantly determined by institutional or individual practices or preferences. This can lead to babies either being left on the ventilator too long, or extubated too hastily, thus requiring repeated reintubation. Only two-thirds of the ELBW babies can be successfully extubated exposing rest to periods of hypoxia, hypercapnia and trauma, infection and atelectasis during the reintubation attempts.

In physiologic terms, effective spontaneous breathing is dependent on a delicate balance between the loads imposed on the respiratory system and its capacity. The inability to tolerate extubation may be the result of poor effort, increased load on the respiratory muscles, and/or decreased inspiratory drive. Weaning attempts that are repeatedly unsuccessful usually indicate either incomplete resolution of the underlying illness or the development of new problems. Causes of extubation failure in neonates are presented in Table 1. Factors increasing the infant's respiratory workload must be examined and optimized.

Weaning Strategies

- *Decrease the most potentially harmful parameter first*: Once the infant has "stabilized" clinically and blood gas values suggest that ventilatory needs are decreasing, the general principle should be to decrease the

Table 1: Common causes of extubation failure in neonates.	
↑ *Respiratory load*	↓ *Respiratory capacity*
Increased elastic load	**Decreased respiratory drive**
• Unresolved lung disease	• Sedation
• Secondary pneumonia	• CNS infection
• Left-to-right shunt (PDA)	• PVH/PVL
• Abdominal distension	• Hypocapnia/alkalosis
• Hyperinflated lungs	
Increased resistive load	**Muscular dysfunction**
• Thick/copious airway secretions	• Muscular catabolism and weakness
• Narrow/occluded endotracheal tube	(malnutrition)
• Upper airway obstruction	• Severe electrolyte disturbances
	• Chronic pulmonary hyperinflation
	(BPD)
Increased minute ventilation	**Neuromuscular disorders**
• Pain and irritability	• Diaphragmatic dysfunction
• Sepsis/hyperthermia	• Prolonged neuromuscular blockage
• Metabolic acidosis	(in renal failure, concomitant use of
	aminoglycoside and phenobarbitone)
	• Myotonic dystrophy
	• Cervical spinal injury

(BPD: bronchopulmonary dysplasia; CNS: central nervous system; PDA: patent ductus arteriosus; PVH/PVL: periventricular hemorrhage/periventricular leukomalacia)

most potentially harmful parameter first, e.g. in case of synchronized intermittent mandatory ventilation (SIMV) mode of ventilation, one should reduce the peak inspiratory pressure (PIP) as this is one responsible for the barotrauma more than other variables.

- Limit changes to one parameter alone at one time so that if the process fails we know which parameter was responsible.
- Avoid changes of large magnitude—limit changes to 1–2 in PIP and rate changes to less than 10 at one time depending on the mode being used.
- Document response to all the changes

Mode of Ventilation and Weaning

- *Assist-control (AC)*:
  - Decrease PIP but provide adequate VT (4 mL/kg)
  - Decrease back-up rate to 25–30
  - May increase trigger sensitivity to condition respiratory muscles
  - Extubate directly from assist-control or switch to SIMV
  - Birth weight (BW) < 1,000 g: Mean airway pressure (MAP) < 7 cm H_2O and FiO_2 < 0.30, BW > 1,000 g: MAP > 8 cm H_2O and FiO_2 < 0.30
- *SIMV*:
  - Decrease PIP but provide adequate VT (4 mL/kg)
  - Decrease rate

- Extubate when stable at low rate (i.e. 15 bpm) or combine with pressure support ventilation (PSV)
- PIP < 14 cm H_2O, positive end-expiratory pressure (PEEP) < 50 cm H_2O, rate < 20, FiO_2 < 0.30
- *SIMV plus PSV:*
  - Add PSV when SIMV rate below 30/min
  - Adjust level of PSV to give adequate VT (4 mL/kg), reduce SIMV slowly
  - Extubate when stable at low SIMV rate (i.e. 15 bpm)
  - BW < 1,000 g: MAP < 7 cm H_2O and FiO_2 < 0.30, BW > 1,000 g: MAP > 8 cm H_2O and FiO_2 < 0.30.
- *High-frequency oscillatory ventilation (HFOV):*
  - Decrease both mean airway pressure and amplitude.
  - As the patient improves, and as amplitude decreases, the patient will do more spontaneous breathing.
  - When achieving most of the CO_2 elimination with spontaneous breathing, and the mean airway pressure has decreased sufficiently, patient can be extubated. General guidelines for extubation.
    - Patient < 1,000 g: Mean airway pressure < 8 cm H_2O and FiO_2 < 0.25
    - Patient > 1,000 g: Mean airway pressure < 9 cm H_2O and FiO_2 < 0.3

Available data do not clearly document superiority of one mode over another in terms of their effect on lung injury, but there is good evidence, as well as a sound physiologic rationale, for using modes that support every breath of the patients. For example, with SIMV, the spontaneous breaths in excess of the set intermittent mandatory ventilation (IMV) rate are not supported, resulting in uneven tidal volumes and potentially a high work of breathing, especially true during weaning, when the number of unsupported breaths increases, issue is most important in extremely small infants with correspondingly narrow ETT, because resistance to flow is inversely proportional to the fourth power of the radius. Consequently, in order to achieve adequate alveolar minute ventilation, a relatively large VT is required for the limited number of mechanical inflations provided by the ventilator. Despite these considerations, many clinicians still prefer SIMV for weaning from MV, based largely on tradition and the belief that fewer mechanical breaths are inherently less damaging. Another misconception is that supporting every breath does not provide the infant with an opportunity for respiratory muscle training with compliance of the respiratory system, determines the VT. During weaning, as ventilator peak inflation pressure is decreased, the infant gradually assumes a greater proportion of the work of breathing and in the process achieves training of the respiratory muscles. The major disadvantage of SIMV can be mitigated by the use of pressure support (PS) for the spontaneous breaths.

Clinical data: Comparing patient triggered ventilation (PTV) versus SIMV, there are two small trials suggesting that weaning is faster in the PTV mode than SIMV. One trial comparing SIMV + PS versus SIMV alone also showed shorted duration of weaning in the SIMV + PS group. In pressure versus volume ventilation Cochrane review which included six studies on the secondary outcome of duration of intermittent positive pressure ventilation (IPPV), suggested that volume ventilation resulted in 1.5 days less on ventilator than the pressure limited group. Effect however was not significant for the less than 1,000 g babies. Twenty six center, randomized, noncrossover, controlled clinical trial comparing HFOV with SIMV showed age at successful extubation was significantly lower for infants assigned to high-frequency oscillatory ventilation. In conclusion, using other modes than the conventional SIMV mode may result in faster weaning but user friendliness to the new mode must be the prime reason for using a particular mode.

What should the newborn be extubated to?
There are three options while removing from the ventilator:
1. Nasal intermittent mandatory ventilation (NIMV)
2. Continuous positive airway pressure (CPAP)
3. Head box oxygen.

Cochrane review of extubation to CPAP versus head box showed benefit of extubating to CPAP with NNT being 5. The appropriate duration of treatment with nasal continuous positive airway pressure (NCPAP) however, remains uncertain, as does the method of its weaning. Cochrane review comparing extubation to NIMV versus CPAP has shown decreased reintubation rates with use of NIMV after extubation. Nasal intermittent positive pressure ventilation (NIPPV) delivery was synchronized in all trials using the Infant Star ventilator with Star Synch abdominal capsule. Ventilator settings applied after extubation varied between studies. IMV rates varied between 10 and 25 per minute, and PIP from that used preextubation to 2 to 4 cm water above that used preextubation. A recent abstract presented at Pediatric Academic Societies (PAS) meeting 2012, PAS a multinational trial of nonsynchronized NIMV versus CPAP, and showed no difference in the outcome. Hence, in our setting where we have nonsynchronized ventilation during nasal ventilation present data do not show superiority of one over the other and postextubation care would depend on the expertise of the caregiver.

OTHER PRACTICES

Postnatal steroids: Endotracheal intubation is used to provide IPPV for a number of neonatal conditions. The presence of a foreign body in contact with delicate upper airway mucosa can lead to injury. This may take the form of laryngeal edema, vocal cord injury or subglottic stenosis, all of which may present clinically as upper airway obstruction (UAO) after extubation. This may in turn lead to increasing respiratory distress requiring reintubation of the trachea. Factors that may increase the likelihood of damage include repeated passage of an endotracheal tube, prolonged intubation and the presence of a large tube relative to the size of the glottis.

In a high-risk population, the equation of treating six infants with dexamethasone in order to prevent one reintubation seems to favor treatment. The use of exogenous surfactant, increased use of antenatal steroids and the trend to extubate early to NCPAP have reduced the duration of endotracheal intubation. In addition, an increasing number of survivors at 22–24 weeks forms a new population in whom this treatment may have a different safety/efficacy profile. Dexamethasone reduces the need for endotracheal reintubation of neonates after a period of IPPV. In view of the lack of effect in low risk infants and the documented and potential side effects, it appears reasonable to restrict its use to infants at increased risk for airway edema and obstruction, such as those who have received repeated or prolonged intubations.

Caffeine: A systematic Cochrane review has indicated a relative risk of failed extubation of 0.48 for infants exposed to methylxanthines before extubation, and on that basis, caffeine is virtually always administered before extubation in ELBW infants. A higher dose of 20 mg/kg is more beneficial in extubation than a smaller dose.

Postextubation X-ray: This idea was borne out of high incidence of PEA to the tune of 40% in 1970s which resulted in almost one-third getting intubated again. But now the humidification and ventilation techniques have changed significantly in the last three decades and 1990s study have shown an incidence of 2.5% PEA. None of the babies with PEA required reintubation but some babies who required CPAP manifested with increased FiO_2 requirements and work of breathing. Hence, X-ray is required only in patients with increasing FiO_2 requirements.

Chest physiotherapy: Cochrane review on this topic showed no clear benefit of periextubation active chest physiotherapy. Active chest physiotherapy did not significantly reduce the rate of postextubation lobar collapse. Applicability of the results of the review to current practice may be compromised due to advancements in neonatal care which have occurred over the interval since the earlier trials were performed.

Nebulized racemic epinephrine: There is no evidence either supporting or refuting the use of inhaled nebulized racemic epinephrine in newborn infants. Similarly there is no evidence for the practice of saline nebulization after extubation.

"Some common causes of extubation failure are worth mentioning such as severe or multiple episodes of apnea, hypoxemia, hypercapnia, upper airway obstruction due to edema of the epiglottic or subglottic area or stenosis if it was a prolonged or traumatic intubation. Risk factors for extubation failure include lower gestational age (<26 weeks), prolonged ventilation

(>10–14 days), previous extubation failure, heavy sedation (e.g. morphine, fentanyl), Multiple reintubations: Upper airway problems, Evidence of residual lung injury such as Bronchopulmonary dysplasia (BPD), pulmonary interstitial emphysema. Additional risk factors include extubation from high ventilatory settings, extubation from high FiO_2 or hemodynamically significant PDA.

Weaning and extubation from MV remain an inexact science. Current practice in most units is a trend toward NIV and if that is not feasible then using MV for as short a time as possible. Alternate primary modes of ventilation apart from the conventional SIMV are likely to result in faster weaning. There is a strong evidence base for using caffeine and distending airway pressure after extubation. Gradually lower the ventilatory settings, as the lung pathology resolves. This will be appreciated by improvement in tidal volume and SPO_2 and decrease in FiO_2 and decrease in respiratory distress."

WEANING A CHILD FROM THE VENTILATOR

Weaning is the transition from ventilatory support to completely spontaneous breathing, during which time the patient assumes the responsibility for effective gas exchange while positive PS is withdrawn. Note that spontaneous breathing is a prerequisite for weaning to begin and decreasing ventilator support is not the sole criterion of successful weaning.

Weaning process and its pace will vary widely depending upon the primary indication for intubation and MV as follows:

Airway (upper or lower) related problems, cardiopulmonary issues such as primary lung parenchyma related problems or secondary lung problems due to cardiogenic etiologies (low cardiac output states), depressed central nervous system or neuromuscular weakness, chronic ventilation or simply postoperative ventilation.

Practical approach to weaning from MV for respiratory causes (most common indication) will be discussed.

Mechanical ventilation for respiratory conditions essentially has three phases:

1. *Acute phase* of mechanical ventilator support includes primary lung recruitment, once it is achieved ventilator support is titrated to achieve nontoxic level of FiO_2 and PIP to <35 cm H_2O.
2. *Maintenance phase* refers to that period spent waiting for improvement in primary disease process that led to need for intubation. Usually, only FiO_2 and PEEP are actively adjusted during this period.
3. *Weaning phase* is that period when patient start triggering ventilator with spontaneous breathing effort, ventilator rate is gradually decreased and peak pressure to maintain tidal volume and oxygenation are decreased. Patient eventually tolerates spontaneous breathing trial (SBT) and extubated from ventilator.

Standard indices for assessing patient weaning ability include:

- Resolution of primary indication for intubation and stable respiratory status.
- $FiO_2 < 50\%$ and decreased PEEP to < 7cm H_2O
- Respiratory rate < 60 for infants, <40 for preschool and school aged children, <30 for adolescents.
- No acidosis or hypercapnia ($PCO_2 > 60$)
- PaO_2/FiO_2 (P/F) ratio > 270, $SpO_2 > 94\%$ with $FiO_2 < 0.5$, peak pressure < 20
- Hemodynamically stability with exception of dopamine ≤ 5 ug/kg/min.
- Improved Glasgow coma scale (GCS), muscle power
- Optimum fluid balance (no fluid overload) and normal electrolytes.

Following indices are also available with limited pediatric data:

Rapid shallow breathing index (RSBI = f/VT), *CROP index* (Dynamic compliance × Maximal negative inspiratory pressure × (PaO_2/PAO_2)/ Respiratory rate).

RSBI ≤ 8 breaths/min/mL/kg body weight and CROP index ≥ 0.15 mL/kg body weight/breaths/minute were good predictors of successful extubation in adults but not in pediatric studies.

TECHNIQUES OF WEANING

The most common approach to weaning infants and children is gradual reduction of ventilator support.

Weaning with IMV or SIMV occurs by reducing the ventilator rate. With PSV, the inspiratory pressure is initially set to provide the required support and then reduced gradually. PS is often combined with IMV/SIMV during weaning. Volume support (VS) and volume-assured pressure support (VAPS) are special forms of PS available in certain ventilators that guarantee a minimal tidal volume per assisted breath. Weaning with VS is semiautomatic, where the PS level required to maintain a certain tidal volume is reduced automatically as respiratory mechanics improve. Extubation occurs from a low level of ventilator support or after an extubation readiness test (ERT).

Positive end-expiratory pressure (PEEP) and FiO_2 may be weaned based on acceptable oxygenation (SpO_2, 89–92) and if pressure limited ventilation is used PIP may be weaned slowly as long as measured expired (or delivered) tidal volume is in acceptable range 5–6 mL/kg.

Spontaneous Breathing Trials and Extubation Readiness Tests

Once the patient has been brought to minimal settings of MV and physician feels patient is ready for extubation, spontaneous breathing trial can be given with either of CPAP ≤ 5 alone, CPAP with minimal PS, T-piece or flow inflating bag (C-circuit-anesthesia bag) for 30–120 min. Trials with either of strategy has shown similar results. Patient should be followed for below mentioned signs/symptoms and laboratory criteria, if these develop, SBT should be

Box 1: Suggested criteria for failure during 2 hours on CPAP < 5 cm H_2O or T-piece.

Clinical criteria:
- Anxious look
- Diaphoresis
- Nasal flaring
- Increasing respiratory effort
- Tachycardia (increase in HR > 40 bpm)
- Cardiac arrhythmias
- Hypotension or hypertension
- Apnea

Laboratory criteria:
- Increase of $PetCO_2$ > 10 mm Hg
- Decrease of arterial pH < 7.32
- Decline in arterial pH > 0.07
- PaO_2 < 60 mm Hg with an FiO_2 > 0.40 (P/F O_2 ratio < 150)
- SpO_2 declines > 5%

(CPAP: continuous positive airway pressure)

aborted. Decision to abort SBT is mainly clinical based on close monitoring (Box 1).

Readiness for Extubation

After passing SBT, if patient is sufficiently awake with intact airway reflexes, is hemodynamically stable and has manageable secretions, extubation can be performed.

Steroids before extubation decrease the chances of stridor because of UAO which contribute to 30-40% of extubation failure. Studies using steroid has not shown decreased chances of reintubation after steroid administration. A recent Cochrane review on the role of steroids concludes "using corticosteroids to prevent (or treat) stridor after extubation has not proven effective for neonates, children or adults. However, given the consistent trend toward benefit, this intervention does merit further study".

If used it should be started 24 hours prior to extubation in the dose of 0.15 mg/kg/dose for 5-6 doses.

Leak test to assess UAO—if an audible leak (to the ear, not the stethoscope) can be heard at < 25 cm H_2O in a patient with the head in neutral position, this is probably good news. However, extubation should not be delayed if the test is negative and all other conditions for extubation are favorable. Many patients, particularly those with numerous secretions and/or prolonged intubated, will have a "seal" around their ETT which will be coughed out once the ETT is removed.

Failed Extubation

Despite the best efforts some patients will fail extubation. Besides medical measures such as nebulization, suctioning, positioning, diuresis or steroids, NIV should be considered as a valid option to be tried before reintubation.

KEY MESSAGES

- For newborns as a basic principle following prerequisites should be met for weaning from mechanical ventilation.
  - No s/o encephalopathy—alert, active.
  - Off sedation and good respiratory effort.
  - SpO_2—as per target with FiO_2 requirement ≤ 0.40.
  - Maintaining tidal volume with minimal settings.
  - Consider for caffeine before extubation if premature.
  - After extubation electively consider for nasal ventilation (CPAP or NIMV).
- Despite all the weaning protocols available in literature, none of the protocols have been shown superior to other in pediatric patients.
- With good clinical monitoring, low ventilator settings, low secretions, optimum fluid and electrolyte status, good neurological status most children will extubate successfully.

SUGGESTED READING

1. Baumeister BL, el-Khatib M, Smith PG, et al. Evaluation of predictors of weaning from mechanical ventilation in pediatric patients. Pediatr Pulmonol. 1997;24(5):344-52.
2. Davis S, Worley S, Mee RB, et al. Factors associated with early extubation after cardiac surgery in young children. Pediatr Crit Care Med. 2004;5(1):63-8.
3. Farias JA, Retta A, Alia I, et al. A comparison of two methods to perform a breathing trial before extubation in pediatric intensive care patients. Intensive Care Med. 2001;27(10):1649-54.
4. Faustino EVS, Gedeit R, Schwarz AJ, Asaro LA, Wypij D, et al. Accuracy of an extubation readiness test in predicting successful extubation in children with acute respiratory failure from lower respiratory tract disease. Crit Care Med. 2017;45(1):94-102.
5. Fioretto JR, Ribeiro CF, Carpi MF, et al. Comparison between noninvasive mechanical ventilation and standard oxygen therapy in children up to 3 years old with respiratory failure after extubation: A pilot prospective randomized clinical study. Pediatr Crit Care Med. 2015;16(2):124-30.
6. Gizzi C, Moretti C, Agostino R. Weaning from mechanical ventilation. J Matern Fetal Neonatal Med. 2011;24 Suppl 1:61-3.
7. Greenough A, Prendergast M. Difficult extubation in low birth weight infants. Arch Dis Child Fetal Neonatal Ed. 2008;93(3):F242-5.
8. Khemani RG, Hotz J, Morzov R, et al. Pediatric extubation readiness tests should not use pressure support. Inten Care Med. 2016;42(8):1214-22.
9. Kurachek SC, Newth CJ, Quasney MW, et al. Extubation failure in pediatric intensive care: A multiple-center study of risk factors and outcomes. Crit Care Med. 2003;31(11):2657-64.
10. Laudato N, Gupta P, Walters HL, et al. Risk factors for extubation failure following neonatal cardiac surgery. Pediatr Crit Care Med. 2015;16(9):859-67.
11. Mahle WT, Nicolson SC, Hollenbeck-Pringle D, et al. Utilizing a collaborative learning model to promote early extubation following infant heart surgery. Pediatr Crit Care Med. 2016;17(10):939-47.

12. Newth CJ, Venkataraman S, Willson DF, et al. Weaning and extubation readiness in pediatric patients. Pediatr Crit Care Med. 2009;10(1):1-11.
13. Sinha SK, Donn SM. Weaning newborns from mechanical ventilation. Semin Neonatol. 2002;7(5):421-8.
14. Thiagarajan RR, Bratton SL, Martin LD, et al. Predictors of successful extubation in children. Am J Respir Crit Care Med. 1999;160(5 Pt 1):1562-6.
15. Venkataraman ST, Khan N, Brown A. Validation of predictors of extubation success and failure in mechanically ventilated infants and children. Crit Care Med. 2000;28(8):2991-6.
16. Venkataraman ST. Weaning and extubation in infants and children: religion, art, or science. Pediatr Crit Care Med. 2002;3(2):203-5.
17. Winch PD, Staudt AM, Sebastian R, et al. Learning from experience: Improving early tracheal extubation success after congenital heart surgery. Pediatr Crit Care Med. 2016;17(7):630-7.

16

Extracorporeal Membrane Oxygenation (ECMO)

Praveen Khilnani, Romit Saxena

Extracorporeal membrane oxygenation (ECMO) provides continuous cardiopulmonary support on a long-term basis, typically on the order of days to weeks, as adjunctive management of severe respiratory and cardiac failure.

Extracorporeal membrane oxygenation is a modification of conventional cardiopulmonary bypass used to support heart and lungs for extended periods of time till the underlying disease process is treated. Use of a semipermeable membrane oxygenator to prevent direct contact of blood and gas is well established.

Extracorporeal membrane oxygenation is a complex technique and requires a dedicated team, appropriate equipment, institutional commitment and thorough preparation. Potential complications are significant and its use is advocated only in patients who have substantial risk of death. Rationale was to minimize ventilator-induced lung injury while allowing additional time to treat the underlying disease process and to permit recovery from acute injury.

Persistent pulmonary hypertension of the newborn (PPHN) is a complication of several respiratory diseases characterized by an elevation in pulmonary vascular resistance with resultant right-to-left shunting of blood and severe hypoxemia in the neonatal period. PPHN carries a high rate of morbidity and mortality, particularly in limited-resource settings (low-income and/or developing country). Echocardiography remains the gold standard for diagnosis of PPHN. Modern therapies such as inhaled nitric oxide (NO), high-frequency oscillatory ventilation, ECMO, and/or other pulmonary vasodilators agents can reduce the mortality rate of PPHN.

Historically, ECMO was first used by Dr Bartlett (a pediatric surgeon) in 1975 in Michigan, USA on a baby named Esperanza with meconium aspiration syndrome (MAS). The baby girl was named as Esperanza (meaning, hope in Spanish) who survived during the times when many full-term newborn babies with PPHN (triggered my meconium aspiration and others with diaphragmatic hernia in the perioperative period) were dying despite the use of conventional ventilation (pressure controlled time cycled ventilation) with 100% oxygen, high pressures leading to air-leak syndromes multiple chest tubes in various neonatal intensive care units (NICUs) in the world. Vasodilators like tolazoline to treat pulmonary hypertension would also not help due to issues with concomitant systemic hypotension (due to nonavailability of any other pulmonary vasodilator with minimal systemic effects.

The first successful neonatal extracorporeal membrane oxygenation case (1975) is important in the development of extracorporeal life support (ECLS), but the case report was never published. It was only recently published in ASAIO journal in 2017. This is the report of that case with commentary on the evolution of ECMO since 1975.

She is a 43-year-old woman now doing well!

In 1975 selective pulmonary vasodilators were not available. Later Paul–Bunnel built a jet ventilator to use to reduce barotrauma in general for respiratory distress syndrome (RDS) (hyaline membrane disease). Surfactant use was also not prevalent at that time period for RDS.

That jet ventilator found use in neonates with PPHN with good results. Later in late 80s Sensormedics developed high-frequency oscillatory ventilator (HFOV) (3100 A), the first high-frequency ventilator in Colorado popularized in early '90s for PPHN babies to mainly reduce barotrauma. Use of HFOV was beginning to show improvement of results. Nitric oxide and sildenafil (selective pulmonary vasodilators) were almost unknown to the neonatologists barring the pediatric cardiac anesthesiologists who would use it selectively on cardiac babies with life-threatening persistent pulmonary hypertension pre- and postoperatively. Over the next decade especially in late '90s and early 2000, NO and sildenafil became available (sildenafil mainly for erectile dysfunction was also found to be a specific selective pulmonary vasodilator also leading to its use in PPHN).

Extracorporeal membrane oxygenation involved ligation of right carotid artery (postcannulation) in earlier years leading to concerns regarding right-sided ischemic lesions in post-ECMO newborns upon follow-up MRIs and clinical neurodevelopmental deficits. Some pediatric surgeons were routinely repairing the carotid trunk post-decannulation in patients who survived ECMO.

Extracorporeal membrane oxygenation for influenza has been performed in neonatal and pediatric populations, with overall survival to discharge of 50%. Recent reports of successful ECMO support in older H1N1 influenza patients with severe respiratory failure raise curiosity as to the role of extracorporeal support for adolescents and adults.

During the 2009 Australia and New Zealand outbreak, the majority of H1N1 influenza cases receiving ECMO support were over 18 years of age, with a median age of 36 years. At the time of the most recent report, 32% of the cohort remained alive in the hospital, 47% had survived to discharge home, and 21% had died. ECMO utilization was estimated at 2.6 per million population, or potentially 800 or 1,300 cases if extrapolated to the US and European populations.

Adult experience: In 1986, Gattinoni reported a series of 43 patients managed with membrane lung support with low-flow extracorporeal CO_2 removal ($ECCO_2R$) combined with low frequency "rest-ventilation". The survival was 48.8%. Morris reported a randomized, controlled clinical trial of pressure-controlled inverse ratio ventilation and $ECCO_2R$ which showed no difference in survival between the two arms (42% vs 33%), however overall survival was significantly higher than in the previous decade.

Given the negative results from these trials, enthusiasm for the use of ECMO in adult respiratory failure waned in the 1980s, and ECMO research continued primarily in neonatal pediatric and cardiac populations. Advances in overall intensive care unit (ICU) care, ventilator management and ECMO technology render these early trial results not applicable to current practice.

However, CESAR did demonstrate that protocolized care including ECMO in an expert acute respiratory distress syndrome (ARDS) center yielded higher survival than the best standard care in tertiary ICUs in the UK.

Experience with ECMO in 2009 influenza A (H1N1) ARDS was reported by the Australia and New Zealand Extracorporeal Membrane Oxygenation (ANZ ECMO) Influenza Investigators.

METHODS OF EXTRACORPOREAL MEMBRANE OXYGENATION SUPPORT

Components utilized in ECMO include (1) pump, (2) oxygenator, and (3) vascular access to circuit with the patient's native circulation. Currently, the most efficient systems utilize a small centrifugal pump and a low-resistance polymethylpentene oxygenator. Based on type of access, there are two primary forms of ECMO:

- Venovenous (VV)
- Venoarterial (VA).

The artificial lung is used in series (VV) or in parallel (VA) with the native lungs, depending on the indications

In VV ECMO, venous blood is withdrawn through a large bore venous cannula (21–25 Fr). Oxygen is added and CO_2 removed, and oxygenated blood is returned to the venous circulation close to the right atrium. VV ECMO is accomplished through either two single lumen catheters, typically placed via the right internal jugular and femoral veins, or one bicaval dual lumen catheter (VVDL, 27–31 Fr) placed via the right internal jugular vein. This technique offers respiratory support with reduced hemodynamic effects, a low risk of ischemia from embolic phenomena or reduced extremity flow, and is utilized in the majority of adult patients with acute respiratory failure.

Venoarterial ECMO provides both respiratory and cardiac support. Blood is withdrawn from the venous circulation, oxygen is added and CO_2 removed, and returned to the patient's arterial circulation. Depending on the age and condition of the patient, a variety of access choices are available. In the adult, femoral venous and femoral arterial cannulation is preferred. A number of additional potential complications exist compared to VV ECMO. Ischemic complications (arterial ischemia of the extremity or other organs) may accompany arterial cannulation. VA ECMO directs oxygenated blood retrograde through the aorta; if flow is insufficient, it may not reach the proximal circulation, and thrombotic or air emboli may be perfused into the systemic circulation.

Extracorporeal membrane oxygenation as a treatment modality in adult respiratory failure did not gain universal popularity due to no difference in outcomes when compared to conventional ventilator management. In the same period, however, neonates especially those with PPHN had improvement in outcomes secondary to ECMO, although premature babies at less than 35 weeks' gestation had an unacceptably high incidence of intracranial hemorrhage. Since then, ECMO as a rescue treatment modality for infants over 35 weeks' gestation and children has grown and become increasingly popular in ICUs. Since 2009 there was outbreak of H1N1 influenza leading to severe hypoxemic respiratory failure where ECMO technology showed promising result in improving mortality, leading to resurgence of use of ECMO both in adults and pediatric age groups. Currently ECMO is considered as a valid alternative if there is a failure of conventional therapies.

Robert Bartlett in Michigan (USA) was the first physician to use neonatal ECMO successfully in 1972 in a case of meconium aspiration syndrome. The ECMO has been revolutionized since then. From VA ECMO, which has been the norm for all reversible pathologies, physicians are shifting toward VV ECMO for respiratory pathology not needing cardiac support, which is more physiological in application for noncardiac conditions. The size of the circuits has been miniaturized since then, besides further development of biocompatible oxygenators and coated circuits to reduce the complications of consumptive coagulopathy and thrombocytopenia. The shift from roller pump ECMO machines, which are mainly gravity dependent for achieving flow to magnetically driven centrifugal ECMO pumps, has made noticeable change to the practice. The advances ensuing further reduction in size of the components resulted in compactness of the entire system, making it much more friendly to use for transport as mobile ECMO. All these innovations have benefited our patients remarkably, leading to improvement in their outcomes

INDICATIONS OF EXTRACORPOREAL MEMBRANE OXYGENATION

The ECMO can be used for rescuing patients following respiratory or cardiac conditions. Sometimes, it could be a combination of both.

Cardiac indications have been limited to children with intractable cardiac failure after cardiothoracic surgery, but the use has been increased in patients with severe viral myocarditis, toxic myocardial depression and intractable arrhythmias. Patient outcomes depend mainly on the etiology of the cardiac failure. Overall, there has been an increase in the number of these indications resulting in better outcomes, which is probably due to increased experience.

Most recently, ECMO has been used as a tool for resuscitation on patients with cardiopulmonary arrest and some centers have used ECMO for support of donor abdominal organs. The prediction of mortality in pediatric patients is more difficult due to the coexistence of multiple organ failure. Matching for diagnosis and severity of illness, ECMO-treated patients had a 74% survival versus 51% survival in non-ECMO-treated patients. This study shows that when used appropriately, survival in some patients is enhanced by ECMO.

Determining that a patient is unresponsive to "maximal medical therapy and considering the use of ECMO remains difficult and controversial". Most criteria have evolved from the neonatal ECMO experience.

RESPIRATORY EXTRACORPOREAL MEMBRANE OXYGENATION

Eligibility criteria for respiratory ECMO: Reversible respiratory failure is an absolute basic requirement to consider ECMO in any patient. Sometimes, the "irreversibility factor" might be unclear at the time of initiation of ECMO, but might become evident at a later stage. It emphasizes the fact that ECMO is only a support mechanism to help the patient, while allowing the underlying disease process to heal.

The patient should have been treated with maximal conventional support for the optimal time period before considering ECMO. When the conventional therapy is not working, patient should be offered ECMO. The dialogue between treating physician and ECMO physician is of paramount importance to select the right patient and treat them with ECMO at the right time, avoiding undue delay. Cost remains a major issue in our country, however considering the significant mortality benefit, it is a therapy worthy of serious consideration, if the primary problem is a reversible one.

Patient should not have any contraindication for anticoagulants like heparin. There should not be any intracerebral bleed or intraventricular bleed greater than grade 2 (in premature term newborns or infants).

Respiratory Extracorporeal Membrane Oxygenation Indication

Clinical indications of ECMO for respiratory conditions in pediatrics are as follows:

- Severe ARDS, refractory to maximal conventional treatment stands out as the major factor for which we consider respiratory ECMO. The etiology of ARDS might differ. It could be secondary to bacterial pneumonias, malaria, tuberculosis or viruses. In recent days, the efficacy of ECMO in supporting patients with H1N1 has been very well-established.
- Meconium aspiration syndrome

- Severe bronchiolitis
- Inhalation pneumonia (postburns)
- Post-traumatic lung contusions
- Acute chest syndrome (sickle chest)
- Status asthmaticus
- Persistent air leaks
- Reactive pulmonary hypertension in neonatal period (reversible).
- Congenital diaphragmatic hernia (CDH)
- Near drowning, etc.

Respiratory Extracorporeal Membrane Oxygenation Selection Criteria

Presence of any two criteria from the following, observed over a period of 4–6 hours after using maximum medical resuscitation measures may help us in selecting the patients. These criteria provide us with guidance. The overall assessment of an experienced physician in evaluating the progression of the disease is more important in selecting the right patient who will be benefited by ECMO.

The respiratory ECMO selection criteria are as follows:

- Partial pressure of O_2 in arterial blood (PaO_2)/fraction of inspired oxygen (FiO_2) ratio of <75%.
- Oxygen index of >40 for 4–6 hours
- Murray's score 2 of >3.0
- Alveolar-arterial (A-a) gradient > 600 mm Hg
- Lung compliance < 0.5 cc/H_2O/kg
- Ventilation index > 40 for 4 hours.

Exclusion Criteria

- Irreversible disease—malignancy with poor outcome
- Patient on ventilator for >10 days (lung fibrosis is likely to set in). Significant intracranial bleed.
- Patient in gross multiple organ failure (relative).
- Severe central nervous system (CNS) injury including encephalitis, persistent vegetative state where the neurological outcome is expected to be dismal.

CARDIAC EXTRACORPOREAL MEMBRANE OXYGENATION

Cardiac Extracorporeal Membrane Oxygenation Indications

Reversible cardiac failure includes:

- Acute reversible refractory cardiac failure situations
- Preoperative stabilization
- Failure to weaning from cardiopulmonary bypass

- Low cardiac output syndrome (postoperatively)
- Myocarditis (postviral, poisonings like scorpion sting, etc.)
- Intractable arrhythmias
- Postcardiac arrest
- Reversible pulmonary hypertension.

It is indicated in irreversible cardiac diseases only as a bridge to ventricular assist devices like Berlin heart or those awaiting urgent heart transplantation. In countries such as India and Africa, since pediatric heart transplant facilities are underdeveloped, only reversible cardiac conditions such as postcardiac surgery operative low cardiac output or myocarditis would be applicable indications for cardiac ECMO.

Extracorporeal Membrane Oxygenation Selection Criteria for Cardiac Support

Strict criteria for the usage of ECMO in pediatric cardiac failure are not available. None of the published severity of illness markers or clinical parameters has been proven to universally predict outcome, but may remain of assistance when trying to identify patients who might be benefited by extracorporeal life support.

Presence of any two criteria from the following, observed over a period of 4–6 hours after maximum conventional management might be helpful in selecting the patients who will be benefited by ECMO. Following are the criteria for the selection of ECMO for cardiac support:

- *Refractory arrhythmias*
- *Cardiogenic shock with high-inotropic requirements (more than 20 points as per inotropic score)*
- *Lactate level > 50 mg/dL or 5 mmol/L or rising liter or central venous oxygen saturation ($ScvO_2$) < 60%*
- *pH less than 7.15 with oliguria (<1 mL/kg/h) in spite of intra-aortic balloon pulsation (IABP) and inotropic supports in selective group of patients*
- *Cardiac index < 2 L/min.*

There is a miscellaneous group of disorders like septic shock, poisoning due to beta blockers, calcium channel blockers overdose, etc. which are refractory to maximal conventional management that might be benefited by VA ECMO, allowing time for recovery.

There is renewed interest in the understanding and practice of ECMO in India. It is feasible to do it in selective ICUs, geared up to accept the challenges, work in teams and achieve the benefits. Figure 1 shows the currently published international extracorporeal life support organization (ELSO) registry data of pediatric and adult, which is showing survival ranging from 55% to 64% in adults and 65% to 85% in pediatric age group depending upon cardiac or respiratory indication.

Extracorporeal membrane oxygenation for cardiopulmonary resuscitation (ECPR) is being carried out at many western hospitals with pediatric

Table 1: Current status of ECMO (as reported by ESLO, January, 2019).			
	Total runs	*Survived ECLS*	
Neonatal:			
Pulmonary	3,1591	27,779	87%
Cardiac	8,252	5,684	68%
ECPR	1,864	1,315	70%
Pediatric:			
Pulmonary	9,487	6,797	71%
Cardiac	11,377	8,155	71%
ECPR	4,361	2,628	60%
India, 2017			
Pediatric cardiac ECMO		25/34 (73.4%)	
Pediatric respiratory ECMO		21/52(40.4%)	

(ECLS: extracorporeal life support; ECMO: extracorporeal membrane oxygenation; ECPR: extracorporeal cardiopulmonary resuscitation)

survivals as good as 54–63%. Few centers in India have begun participation in ELSO registry and an Asian chapter also has recently been formed (Table 1).

TECHNIQUE OF EXTRACORPOREAL MEMBRANE OXYGENATION

The two basic types of ECMO are (1) venoarterial (VA) and (2) venovenous (VV).

This terminology describes the direction of blood flow. The outflow is always venous, but the inflow can be arterial or venous. Outflow of blood in VA and VV ECMO is from the right atrium through a catheter placed through the right internal jugular vein. In older patients, other venous sites have been used. In VA mode, after oxygenation in the ECMO circuit, the blood is returned to the patient through an arterial cannula, which is placed in the ascending aorta through the right common carotid artery (Figs. 1 and 2). A cannula can also be placed directly into the right atrium and the aorta through a sternotomy. Patients with profound left ventricular failure need a left atrial or ventricular catheter to obtain decompression of the left heart. The artery that was cannulated is permanently ligated. The effect of this is unknown. Some centers have begun repairing the artery at decannulation. Repairs had an early patency rate of 90% in some centers. Patients with normal cardiac function, as well as those with severe pulmonary disease, may be candidates for VV ECMO support.

Cannulation is done at the bedside under deep sedation and analgesia. A double lumen venous cannula has been used in neonates; and in adults, the blood is returned to the distal iliac vein of the inferior vena cava. The

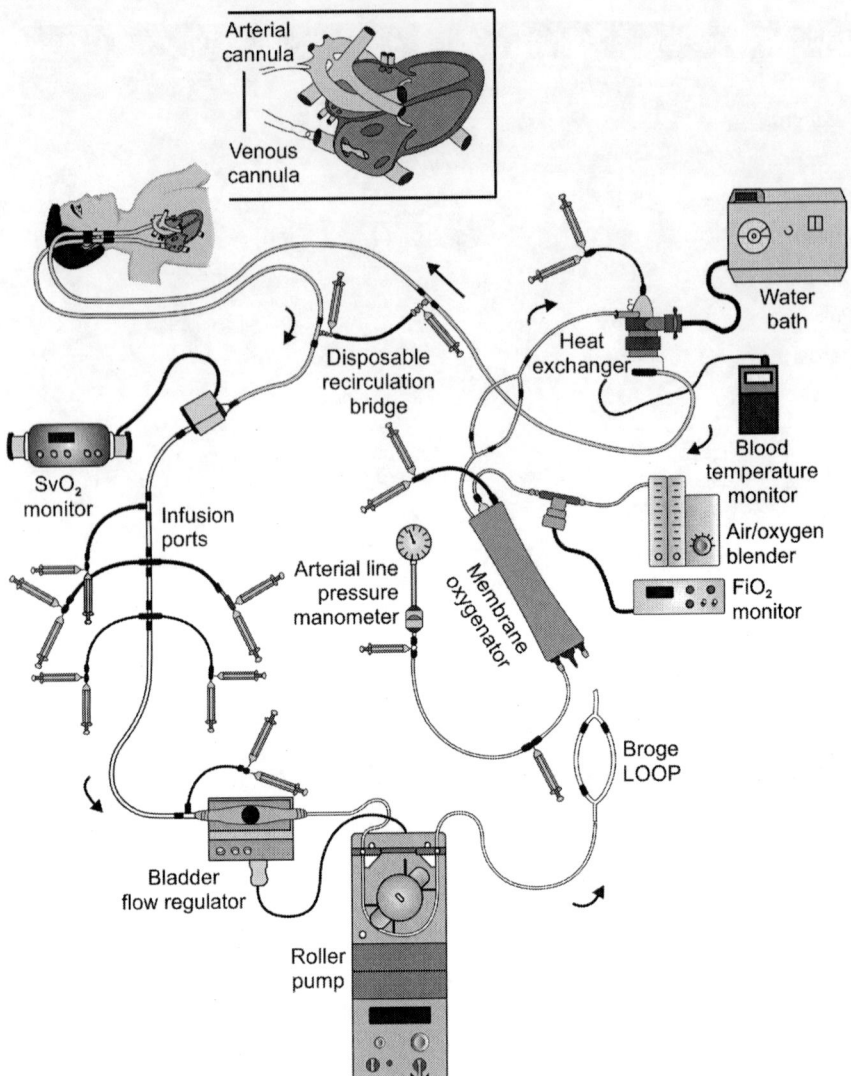

Fig. 1: Schematic diagram of a patient on extracorporeal membrane oxygenation (ECMO) circuit.

blood first enters a small bladder that is attached to a servoregulated box connected to a roller pump. Inadequate blood return triggers an alarm on the bladder box, which in turn, shuts the pump off. When the bladder refills, the pump restarts. This process prevents excessive negative pressure, which otherwise might result from a kinked cannula or hypovolemia and more importantly, prohibits the formation of air bubbles. After exiting the bladder, the blood is actively pumped by a roller pump into a membrane oxygenator. The oxygenator consists of a hollow silicon envelope placed inside a silicone sleeve. The blood flows on the outside of the coiled envelope and the gas flows

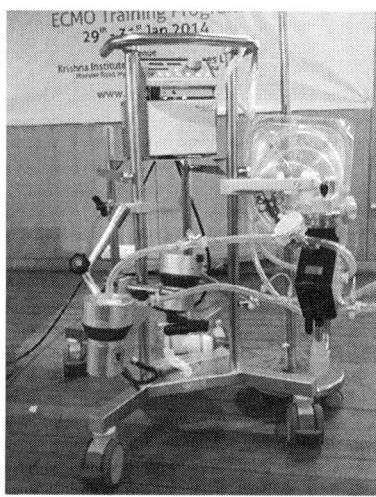

Fig. 2: Extracorporeal membrane oxygenation (ECMO) equipment in pediatric intensive care unit (PICU). (*For color version see Plate 4*)

in a countercurrent direction inside the membrane. The size of the membrane is chosen according to patient size. There is an effective gas exchange here. Next, the blood flows into a heat exchanger and then, it is infused back into the patient.

The ECMO circuit is designed with a bridge that allows the child and the circuit to be isolated from one another. The blood is heparinized, and the heparin effect is measured by activated clotting time (ACT), which is maintained at 180–220 seconds. ACT can be measured at the bedside.

MANAGEMENT OF EXTRACORPOREAL MEMBRANE OXYGENATION

Patient management is supportive and all principles of pediatric critical care apply. ECMO management is under following broad headings: initiation and decannulation

- *Initiation*:
  - Fluids/RRT/nutrition:
  - Sedation/analgesia:
  - Ventilator management
  - CO_2 removal by sweep gas flow
  - Antibiotics
  - Anticoagulation and monitoring for clots
  - Weaning ECMO flows
- *Decannulation*:
  - Post-ECMO care: Ventilation
  - CMV or HFOV

Initiation of Extracorporeal Membrane Oxygenation

Under sedation and neuromuscular blockade an initial bolus of heparin (100–200 units) is given just prior to the cannulation after which a heparin infusion is started and continued throughout the duration of the ECMO. The flow is initially started low by 50 mL/kg/min and gradually increased by 50 mL increments. Infants need 100–200 mL/kg/min for adequate perfusion and oxygenation, although there are patients who may need more. Pediatric patients usually need 90 mL/kg/min to achieve the same goals.

In VA ECMO, as the flow is increased, the left ventricular output decreases and the arterial waveform becomes less pulsatile. Stored blood is used to prime the circuit, which may be acidotic and calcium depleted. Using tromethamine (THAM) or bicarbonate in the priming fluid can correct acidosis. It is also recommended to measure the electrolyte concentration of the stored blood. Patients will need intermittent blood products transfused. Fresh frozen plasma may be needed intermittently to replenish clotting factors.

The ECMO circuit also sequesters platelets, and counts of 80,000–100,000 are maintained routinely.

Adequacy of nutrition is maintained by initiation of hyperalimentation and early enteral feeds are not a contraindication. Diuretics may be needed to prevent fluid retention.

Renal replacement therapy with hemofiltration or hemodiafiltration can be effectively instituted in ECMO circuit.

Ventilator management: While on a ventilator, patients are placed on relatively nontraumatic settings to promote lung healing. A peak inspiratory pressure (PIP) of 18–20 mm H_2O, with a positive end-expiratory pressure (PEEP) of 4–5 mm H_2O, is generally used. The ventilator rates are set at 6–12 breaths per minute and the FiO_2 is 25–30%. Sometimes, older children are managed with a PEEP of 10–12 mm H_2O to prevent loss of functional residual capacity. Tolerate pCO_2 55–65, SpO_2 > 88%. Time of "rest" depends on process (generally 3–5 days minimum for ARDS).

Suctioning may be performed as needed with a closed suction system. One should avoid manual bagging to avoid alveolar derecruitment.

Resolution of air leak occurs in 48–72 hours. Patients with barotrauma and air leak may benefit from high-frequency ventilation, in addition to ECMO. Typically, neonates benefit from low mean airway pressure and lung rest, and pediatric patients benefit from maintenance of functional residual capacity with higher PEEP. For CO_2 removal sweep gas flow in the ECMO circuit can be regulated.

Antibiotics: As a part of treatment for sepsis, appropriate antibiotics need to be continued based on cultures and clinical status, however routine use of prophylactic antibiotics is not recommended.

> **Box 1:** Extracorporeal membrane oxygenation management summary.
> - After cannulation and establishing ECMO flow
> - Change ventilation to minimal setting rate of 5–8 and PEEP to prevent atelectasis.
> - Monitor vitals
> - Monitor ACTs, and
> - Daily Na K Ca KFT chest X-ray
> - Pre- and post-ECMO gases
> - Patient ABG, SpO_2
> - Strict IO,
> - Urine output,
> - Sedation as necessary
> - Monitor for block/clots in circuit
> - CO_2 control by sweep gas flow
> - Cardiac output and oxygenation by ECMO flow (in VA ECMO)
> - Oxygenation by ECMO flow in VV ECMO
> - Wean ECMO flow… Decannulation when condition improves

Anticoagulation

Since blood is heparinized, the heparin effect is measured by ACT, which is maintained at 180–220 seconds. Thromboelastogram (TEG) is now available at many centers for coagulation monitoring.

Weaning Extracorporeal Membrane Oxygenation Flows and Decannulation

When the underlying process improves, the patient is weaned to low ECMO flows (50–100 mL/kg/min) and optimal ventilator settings. A decision to decannulate is made after the patient maintains adequate oxygenation and perfusion in these settings for 2–4 hours. This weaning of flow can be achieved in slow reductions of flow rate by increments of 10–20 mL/kg/min every 1–2 hours, up to a flow rate of 50–100 mL/kg/min. During the process of weaning, blood gases and the mixed venous saturations should be frequently monitored. A more rapid weaning rate can be achieved by decreasing the flow in larger increments over shorter time intervals. Once a flow rate of 50–100 mL/kg/min has been achieved, the patient is monitored for a few hours. If deterioration is seen, high flow is re-established for 24 hours before a repeat trial is performed.

The summary of ECMO management has been described in Box 1.

COMPLICATIONS OF EXTRACORPOREAL MEMBRANE OXYGENATION

Mechanical Complications

The most common mechanical problems are oxygenator failure, tubing rupture or leak, cannula kinking, power failure, air in the circuit and accidental decannulation.

Patient Complications

Bleeding from heparinization is a common complication. Intracranial hemorrhage is catastrophic. Daily head ultrasounds are performed on infants with open fontanels. As any other site can be involved just as easily, a high index of suspicion is needed.

Since infection is also problematic, frequent surveillance cultures are ordered on all ECMO patients. Prophylactic antibiotics are not used to treat infection. Embolization is another risk, especially with VA ECMO; and can consist of a clot, air or particulate matter. A bubble trap is added to the arterial side of the circuit in an attempt to reduce this risk. Sensorineural hearing loss is a long-term complication with a reported incidence rate as high as 24%. Additionally, there is the possibility of catastrophic technical mishaps like catheter rupture, kinking of cannulae, power disruption and accidental decannulation.

OUTCOMES

Newborns

Infants with MAS have had the highest survival rate (71%) compared with other diagnoses analyzed (26.3%; p < 0.001). The most common diagnosis associated with prolonged ECMO support in neonates is congenital diaphragmatic hernia (CDH; 69%). Nonsurvivors were more likely to experience complications on ECMO, and multivariate analysis showed that the need for inotropes while on ECMO support was independently associated with mortality. Neonates requiring prolonged ECMO support have a 24% survival to discharge. Many of these cases involve CDH. Complications are common with prolonged ECMO, but only receipt of inotropes was shown to be independently associated with mortality.

Pediatric

In one study from Germany, by 31 December 2014, over 900 patients had been treated, the vast majority for respiratory failure, and over 650 patients had been transported during ECMO. The median ECMO duration was 5.3, 5.7, and 7.1 days for neonatal, pediatric and adult patients, respectively. The survival to hospital discharge rate for respiratory ECMO was 81%, 70%, and 63% in the different age groups, respectively, which is significantly higher than the overall international experience as reported to the ELSO registry (74%, 57%, and 57%, respectively).

H1N1 Adult Outcomes

One hundred eighty adult patients, randomized controlled trial, intention to treat ECMO showed improved survival at 6 months (63% vs 47%) (Peek

GJ, et al. CESAR trial collaboration Lancet, 2009). 80 ECMO referrals, H1N1, propensity-matched controls, showed improved survival (76% vs 53%) ECMO when compared to conventional ventilator management (Noah MA, Peek GJ, Finney SJ, et al. JAMA 2011).

Extracorporeal Life Support Organization Registry Analysis

Data was collected from 170 centers participating in the ELSO registry. Relationships between in-hospital mortality and risk factors were assessed using logistic regression. Survival was defined as being discharged from the hospital.

Six hundred sixty-two eligible records were reviewed. Mortality occurred in 303 (46%) infants. Congenital diaphragmatic hernia patients, cardiac failure with associated, and pulmonary failure including RDS had the highest odds of mortality in this cohort. Birth weight (BW) < 3 kg, ECPR, hemofiltration, and dialysis were all independent predictors of mortality.

SETTING UP AN EXTRACORPOREAL MEMBRANE OXYGENATION PROGRAM

Evidence shows better outcomes in high-volume centers with rapid turnover of patients. Skills have to be maintained in low volume centers by attending review courses, simulation and water labs. As the number of patients requiring ECMO in any bigger city is going to be a fraction of ventilated cases, at present, we would like to recommend it as standard of care in high-volume cardiothoracic centers. Though ECMO is a multidisciplinary specialty, invariably, one tends to need some help from surgeons, more so from cardiac surgeons. One will need echocardiographic guidance in the form of regular assessment of cardiac function and watching parameters for resolution of pulmonary hypertension. The ELSO has published guidance on establishing ECMO centers. Though they are universally applicable, minor modifications to suit the sociocultural and economic climate in resource-limited countries may be necessary.

EXTRACORPOREAL LIFE SUPPORT ORGANIZATION GUIDELINES REGARDING EXTRACORPOREAL MEMBRANE OXYGENATION CENTERS

1. The ECMO centers should be located in tertiary centers with a tertiary level NICU, pediatric ICU, and/or adult ICU.
2. The ECMO centers should be located in geographic areas that can support a minimum of six ECMO patients per center per year. The cost-effectiveness of providing fewer than six cases per year combined with the loss or lack of clinical expertise associated with treating fewer than this number of patients per year should be taken into account when developing a new program.

3. The ECMO centers should be actively involved in the ELSO including participation in the ELSO registry.

General Structure

The ECMO center should be located in a tertiary level ICU with the following components:

- There should be a single physician ECMO program director with responsibility for the overall operation of the center. While there may be several associate directors with specific interests or focus in limited areas of ECMO care, the primary medical director should be responsible for assuring appropriate specialist training and performance, directing quality improvement meetings and projects, assuring proper and valid data submission to ELSO, and should also be responsible for the credentialing of other physicians who care for ECMO patients or who manage the ECMO circuit.
- There should be an ECMO coordinator with responsibility for the supervision and training of the technical staff, maintenance of equipment, and collection of patient data.
- The multidisciplinary ECMO team should have quality assurance review procedures in place for annual ECMO evaluation internally.
- Formal policy and procedures outlining the indications and contraindications for ECMO, clinical management of the ECMO patient, maintenance of equipment, termination of ECMO therapy and follow-up of the ECMO patient should be available for review.
- Appropriate laboratory space for training and continuing medical education should be available.

INDIAN SCENARIO AND FUTURE OF EXTRACORPOREAL MEMBRANE OXYGENATION

In India, many centers have started acquiring ECMO technology, however cost remains a major issue. Survival benefit with appropriate early institution in selected patients is the real motivating factor. With portability of the equipment and availability of personnel and proper training of ECMO specialist (intensivist or anesthesiologist or a surgeon), round the clock critical care nurses and perfusionists, it can be accomplished in tertiary centers with round the clock critical care and ancillary services. Hospital administrative commitment and support is of prime importance for success of any ECMO program.

KEY MESSAGES

- Presently, ECMO is viewed as an invasive procedure with significant risks, and should be used only after careful evaluation of risks/benefits and discussion with the family.

- It continues to represent an important support option in select critically ill infants and children. In the future, with increased experience, this procedure will become an even safer, more effective alternative to many less efficacious conventional therapies.

SUGGESTED READING

1. Bairdain S, Betit P, Craig N, et al. Diverse Morbidity and Mortality Among Infants Treated with Venoarterial Extracorporeal Membrane Oxygenation. Cureus. 2015;7(4):e263.
2. Bartlett RH. Esperanza: The First Neonatal ECMO Patient. ASAIO J. 2017;63(6): 832-43.
3. Coughlin JP, Drucker DE, Cullen ML, et al. Delayed repair of congenital diaphragmatic hernia. Am Surg. 1993;59(2):90-3.
4. Cruz-Blanquel A, Espinosa-Oropeza A, Romo-Hernández G, et al. Persistent pulmonary hypertension in the newborn: therapeutic effect of sildenafil. Proc West Pharmacol Soc. 2008;51:73-7.
5. Domico MB, Ridout DA, Bronicki R, et al. The impact of mechanical ventilation time before initiation of extracorporeal life support on survival in pediatric respiratory failure: a review of the Extracorporeal Life Support Registry. Pediatr Crit Care Med. 2012;13(1):16-21.
6. Extracorporeal Life Support Organization. (2019). ECLS Registry Report: International Summary. [online] Available from https://www.elso.org/Registry/ Statistics/InternationalSummary.aspx [Last accessed November, 2019].
7. Guner YS, Khemani RG, Qureshi FG, et al. Outcome analysis of neonates with congenital diaphragmatic hernia treated with venovenous vs venoarterial extracorporeal membrane oxygenation. J Pediatr Surg. 2009;44(9):1691-701.
8. Keszler M, Subramanian KN, Smith YA, et al. Pulmonary management during extracorporeal membrane oxygenation. Crit Care Med. 1989;17(6):495-500.
9. Khilnani P, Pooboni S, Jaya Kumar I, et al. INSPIRED Multicenter data summary of Pediatric respiratory and cardiac ECMO from India. INSPIRED (Indian network of Specialist Pediatric intensivists for research Education and data). J Pediatr Crit Care. 2017;4(2):93-5.
10. Marsh TD, Wilkerson SA, Cook LN. Extracorporeal membrane oxygenation selection criteria: Partial pressure of arterial oxygen versus alveolar-arterial oxygen gradient. Pediatrics. 1988;82(2):162-6.
11. Mehta U, Laks H, Sadeghi A, et al. Extracorporeal membrane oxygenation for cardiac support in pediatric patients. Am Surg. 2000;66(9):879-86.
12. Nakwan N. The Practical Challenges of Diagnosis and Treatment Options in Persistent Pulmonary Hypertension of the Newborn: A Developing Country's Perspective. Am J Perinatol. 2010;35(14):1366-75.
13. Ortiz RM, Cilley RE, Bartlett RH. Extracorporeal membrane oxygenation in pediatric respiratory failure. Pediatr Clin North Am. 1987;34(1):39-46.
14. Peek GJ, Mugford M, Tiruvoipati R, et al. Efficacy and economic assessment of conventional ventilatory support versus extracorporeal membrane oxygenation for severe adult respiratory failure (CESAR): A multicentre randomised controlled trial. Lancet. 2009;374(9698):1351-63.
15. Prodhan P, Bhutta AT, Gossett JM, et al. Extracorporeal membrane oxygenation support among children with adenovirus infection: a review of the Extracorporeal Life Support Organization registry. ASAIO J. 2014;60(1):49-56.

16. Prodhan P, Stroud M, El-Hassan N, et al. Prolonged extracorporeal membrane oxygenator support among neonates with acute respiratory failure: a review of the Extracorporeal Life Support Organization registry. ASAIO J. 2014;60(1):63-9.

17. Roberts N, Westrope C, Pooboni SK, et al. Venovenous extracorporeal membrane oxygenation for respiratory failure in inotrope dependent neonates. ASAIO J. 2003;49(5):568-71.

18. Schumacher RE, Barks JD, Johnston MV, et al. Right-sided brain lesions in infants following extracorporeal membrane oxygenation. Pediatrics. 1988;82(2):155-61.

19. Sigalet DL, Tierney A, Adolph V, et al. Timing of repair of congenital diaphragmatic hernia requiring extracorporeal membrane oxygenation support. J Pediatr Surg. 1995;30(8):1183-7.

20. Zabrocki LA, Brogan TV, Statler KD, et al. Extracorporeal membrane oxygenation for pediatric respiratory failure: Survival and predictors of mortality. Crit Care Med. 2011;39(2):364-70.

How to Choose a Ventilator?

Praveen Khilnani, Kumar Ankur, Naresh Lal

In the last two decades the role of mechanical ventilation in the neonatal intensive care unit (NICU) has been rapidly evolving. Prior to the early 1970s, neonates either died without access to appropriate ventilators, or they were supported in the first days of life with pediatric volume ventilators and a large preset tidal volume (VT) (approximately 18 mL/kg). The ongoing clinical management was based principally on subjective assessment of optimal chest rise, breath sounds, color, and maintaining normal blood gas values. Nearly three decades following the advent of the microprocessor, several advances in neonatal ventilator technology have ushered in a number of proposed improvements to the neonatal ventilator.

Published information on the value and effectiveness of individual devices and features is limited. Improved patient outcomes due to technology innovation are difficult to demonstrate.

Broadly, there are two types of ventilators available in market:
1. Cradle to grave ventilators
2. Dedicated neonatal ventilators.

Cradle to grave ventilators (newborn to adult ventilators) are promoted by manufacturers as ventilator suitable for patients with all age groups. Though many clinicians are fancied with this notion, these ventilators are not at par with dedicated neonatal ventilator in mechanics. Dedicated neonatal ventilators such as Drager Babylog 8000 plus has lower ventilator-imposed expiratory resistance, better trigger response time and more accurate VT measurements than ventilators common for all ages. However, these are reasonable option in less busy centers, as these ventilators will be utilized more often across different age groups than dedicated neonatal ventilators and hence will be more cost effective.

Selection of a neonatal ventilator for your unit should be based upon:
- Technical features and skill and ability of clinician to utilize technology to its best
- Level of expertise of nursing and resident staff to understand mechanics and troubleshooting

- Type and age group of patients being treated
- Budget of purchase and maintenance cost
- After sale service.

TECHNICAL SPECIFICATIONS OF A VENTILATOR

Conventionally ventilators are categorized in pressure control ventilators and volume control ventilation. In contrast to adult ventilation, pressure control ventilation has been more popular in neonates. In following paragraphs there is a brief discussion of various modes of ventilation, one might be looking for in a ventilator (details of individual modality is covered elsewhere).

Early neonatal pressure ventilators were relatively inexpensive and simple to operate. Mechanical breaths were machine-triggered, intermittent flow, time-cycled, and pressure controlled and is known as continuous mandatory ventilation (CMV). There was no flow of gases for spontaneous breaths in between the mechanical breaths. Subsequently, intermittent mandatory ventilation (IMV) provided continuous flow, intermittent pressure-controlled breaths. Continuous flow of gases in circuit allowed spontaneous breaths in between mechanical breaths. However, there is no synchrony between ventilator driven breath and spontaneous breaths. Hence, there is potential for mechanical breaths to be delivered out of phase with the neonate's spontaneous respiratory effort, resulting in the patient fighting the ventilator. To improve patient-ventilator synchrony and patient comfort, neonates require sedation and/or neuromuscularly paralysis.

Patient triggered ventilation is further sophistication, where machine senses patient's efforts and delivers mechanical breath in synchrony with patient's breath. However, technical limitations of detecting and responding rapidly to small patient efforts in neonates challenged scientists till '90s. Respiratory monitoring during ventilation has grown more comprehensive and sophisticated. Today most neonatal ventilators incorporate small, lightweight, hot-wire or variable orifice flow sensors that can accurately and precisely measure flow and pressure changes at the proximal airway and provide patient-triggered ventilation in even the smallest of patients. Flow-triggering with a sensor placed at the proximal airway is currently preferred for neonatal ventilation over pressure-triggering or flow sensor placed more distally (close to machine). A proximal flow sensor is necessary not only for triggering, but for accurate VT measurement and airway graphic display.

The most widely used forms of patient-triggered ventilation in the NICU are what have been referred to as "assist/control" and "synchronized intermittent mandatory ventilation" (SIMV). These forms of patient-triggered ventilation are preferred because premature neonates often have unpredictable breathing patterns.

In pressure support ventilation (PSV), the patient controls the start of inspiration, the start of expiration, the inspiratory time, the breathing frequency, and the minute volume, so the patient has complete control of the breath, which enhances patient comfort and patient-ventilator synchrony. It is important to note that to use PSV the neonate must have sufficient respiratory drive, though some of the newer PSV modes have an apnea backup mode.

Recently with improved volume monitoring capabilities and lung mechanics measurements has generated interest in volume targeted ventilation. Most of the currently available neonatal-capable ventilators allow setting the VT as low as 2–3 mL and, remarkably, with great precision and accuracy. PSV has evolved to employ adaptive targeting: for example, "volume support" (on the Servo-I ventilator, Maquet, Solna, Sweden) or "pressure support volume guarantee" (on the VN500, Drager, Lubeck, Germany), which is a mode that automatically adjusts the inspiratory pressure to maintain a minimum preset VT target. Adaptive pressure control involves volume-targeted breaths that automatically adjust inspiratory pressure based on VT measurements to target a minimum inspiratory or expiratory VT.

Neurally adjusted ventilatory assist (NAVA) is a novel form of ventilation, which uses the electrical activity of the diaphragm (EAdi) to determine the timing and magnitude of inspiratory pressure delivery during spontaneous breathing. The EAdi signal is obtained with a 5.5 French esophageal catheter placed at the level of the diaphragm. When positioned properly, the EAdi signal can accurately and reliably trigger and cycle a positive-pressure breath, independent of air leak. Additionally, the magnitude of the inspiratory pressure assist is a product of the EAdi signal and the preset NAVA level. However, NAVA requires frequent bedside attendance and requires intact respiratory drive of infant. Although many of the difficulties associated with flow sensors at the airway might be bypassed with this new EAdi method, new issues such as proper sensor placement and higher cost might develop instead.

High frequency ventilation is a mode of ventilation where mechanical breaths are given at very high rates (300–900/minutes) with a very small VT (1–2 mL/kg). This mode of ventilation has been shown to be superior to conventional ventilation and lung protective. However, this mode requires more careful monitoring and frequent adjustments in ventilator parameters.

While a tremendous amount of resources have gone into the design and testing of these devices and modalities, the question remaining is, have these advances actually improved outcomes for neonates? Current-generation ventilators have added a new level of complexity and expense to neonatal care. We are an equipment-centered profession. The more complex the device, the more we dive into its intricacies and master its details. There is a great desire to constantly modernize our technology and stay current. It is not uncommon for clinicians to be seduced by new advanced features found on neonatal ventilators. However, increased complexity of technology may increase risk to patients. These risks include misunderstanding and misapplication by clinicians. But in reality many of these features are never used in clinical practice. Further, improvements to neonatal ventilators have not come without a cost. Thus, the seasoned clinician is left wondering if the costs and risks of novel ventilators and ventilation modes outweigh the clinical benefit to patients.

In my opinion, SIMV, if used appropriately with judicious selection and frequent adjustment of ventilator settings may clinically be as effective as newer modes and may be less complicated and is easy to understand and practice by resident and nursing staff. Newer ventilators with complex modes of ventilation should be resorted to only if required expertise can be assured round the clock.

One should choose a ventilator based on what is his requirement and not by the fact that which machine has maximum number and/or most recent of modes. One should list his specification needs and then pick the machine which fulfills all the requirements within the stipulated budget rather than throwing unnecessary money on an unnecessary functions. Critical points to be looked into while purchasing a neonatal ventilator are (Box 1):

- There should be patient trigger mode/modes
- Sensing mechanism should be close to endotracheal tube (ETT); not at machine end
- Heated wire anemometer is preferred

Box 1: Prototype specification for a basic neonatal ventilator.

Modes of ventilations:
- Pressure control modes
  - CPAP mode
  - IMV
  - SIMV
  - Pressure support ventilation (can be optional)
    - Volume guarantee (can be optional)
    - High frequency ventilation (optional)
    - Provision of nebulization during uninterrupted mechanical ventilation

Flow sensor:
- Heated wire anemometer (preferred)
- Should be distal [close to endotracheal tube (ET) end]

Circuits and humidifiers:
- Should provide a humidifier with temperature display of distal end at circuit
- Humidifier should have both nasal and ET modes options
- Should be compatible with most commercially available ventilator circuits and humidifier

Ventilatory controls (should have following controls with described ranges):
- *Inspiratory time*: 0.1 sec to 1 sec
- *Respiratory frequency*: 1–150 breaths/min
- *Inspiratory flow*: Auto-adjusting
- *Tidal volume*: Lower limit 2 mL; upper limit 150 mL or more

Contd...

Contd...

- Peak pressure limit up to 60–70 mbar
- CPAP/PEEP limit 0–20 mbar
- *FiO₂*: 21–100%
- *Triggering*: Preferably flow triggering

Measure parameters (should display following parameters):
- PIP
- PEEP
- MAP
- Respiratory rates
- Inspiratory time
- Expiratory time
- I/E ratio
- Tidal volume
- Minute ventilation
- FiO_2
- Compliance
- Resistance
- Leak
- Spontaneous breaths (%)

Alarms:
- Low gas supply/pressure (for O_2 as well as air)
- Low battery
- Low FiO_2
- FiO_2 sensor inoperable
- High/low PIP
- High/low PEEP
- High/low tidal volume
- High/low minute ventilation
- Apnea
- Leak in circuit
- Hose/tubings kinking/obstruction
- Inverse ratio ventilation

Waveforms and loops display:
- Pressure, flow, and volume waveform
- Pressure-volume and flow-volume loops

Battery operations:
- Operating time at least 1 hr
- Alarm for power failure

Power requirements: 100–240 volt

Other specifications (optional):
- Ability to print data in tabulated format as well as ability to print waveforms
- Ability to export data to external device (USB device, hard disk, computer)
- Ability to retrieve and save breath to breath data of all measured parameters in excel format
- Connectivity to other devices (with ethernet, dicom, etc.)

Spares and warranty

(CPAP: continuous positive airway pressure; IMV: intermittent mandatory ventilation; MAP: mean airway pressure; PEEP: positive end-expiratory pressure; PIP: peak inspiratory pressure; SIMV: synchronized intermittent mandatory ventilation; I:E: inspiratory expiratory)

- Modes of ventilation depend upon unit's expertise and budget. Minimum requirement is continuous positive airway pressure (CPAP) and SIMV.
- Spares and after sale service (try to have annual maintenance contract (AMC)).

KEY FEATURES OF COMMONLY AVAILABLE NEONATAL VENTILATORS

Dragger Babylog 8000 Plus

- *Control principle*: Continuous flow, pressure-limited, time-cycled
- *Modes*: CPAP/IMV/SIMV/PSV/HFV/volume guarantee
- *Trigger*: Hot wire anemometer; flow/volume trigger
- *Trigger delay*: Approximately 30 ms
- *High frequency ventilation (HFV)*: Flow interrupter (not a strong oscillator; can oscillate infant up to 2 kg).

SLE 5000

Modes: CPAP, CMV, SIMV, PSV, SIMV + PSV, high frequency oscillation (HFO), HFO + CMV
Trigger: Hot wire flow sensor technology; flow /volume trigger
High frequency ventilation: Can oscillate patient up to 15 kg.

Stephanie

Modes: CPAP, IMV, SIMV, A/C, PSV SIMV-PSV, SIMV-PAV, minute volume guarantee (MVG), synchronized nasal intermittent positive pressure (SNIPPV)
Trigger: Flow/volume trigger
High frequency ventilation: Can ventilate patient up to 25 kg.

COMMONLY AVAILABLE VENTILATORS

There are three fundamentally different modes of ventilation available in the pediatric intensive care unit (PICU) and the neonatal intensive care unit (NICU): (1) "pressure ventilators", (2) "volume ventilators", and (3) "high frequency ventilators". They all serve to support adequate ventilation and oxygenation, but each has its own particular niche. There are different types of ventilators available in the market. It is obviously impossible to provide a detailed description of every ventilator in common use. These ventilators will be described with brief salient features.

Volume Ventilators

Historically, volume ventilators (time cycled, volume regulated, volume limited) were used in anesthesia (a bellows of defined VT pumped at a given rate) and as pediatric and adult intensive care evolved. Initially these ventilators were not used in the NICU due to the difficulty achieving consistent small volumes (5–7 mL/kg in a 1,200 g infant). Current volume ventilators are able to deliver small volumes consistently. In the past, triggering was inconsistent and increased the work of breathing. The latest generation (Baercub, Vela, Draager, Siemens 300 and Servo I) has resolved these problems. In the NICU their use has been primarily in large infants with chronic lung disease [partly because SIMV (synchronized intermittent mandatory ventilation)] was only available on volume ventilators until recently or preoperatively (a tradition likely related to familiarity of operating room personal with volume ventilators). Their use in the acute NICU settings has extended into the micropremie population.

Pros: Stable minute ventilation with known tidal volume. Simple models are available for use outside hospital setting. Control or SIMV modes are available. Home ventilators currently available are typically "volume ventilators".

Cons: Tidal volume is maintained at the expense of peak airway pressure. If lung compliance falls by 50% [i.e. ETT slipping downright mainstem] then to maintain VT, peak airway pressure doubles, possibly increasing the risk of volutrauma or barotrauma. Since these ventilators do not have constant flow, to breathe spontaneously the infant always has to trigger open a valve to allow airflow. Large leaks around the ETT can be problematic due to difficulty maintaining VT and "triggering" (patient cycling) of the ventilator causing frequent alarming.

Pressure Ventilators

These are the most frequently used ventilators in the NICU. Traditional "pressure ventilators" are constant flow, time cycled, pressure limited devices (Sechrist ventilator). Constant flow implies that there is a constant flow of gas past the top of the ETT. Pressure limited means that once the preset PIP has been reached, it is maintained for the duration of the inspiratory cycle. Time cycled implies that breaths are given at fixed intervals, independent of the infant's respiratory efforts. Newer "pressure ventilators" can sense infant's breaths and synchronize with them.

Pros: The constant flow permits the infant to easily take spontaneous breaths. Pressure limitation prevents sudden changes in PIP (peak inspiratory pressure) as compliance changes (i.e. on a pressure ventilator if compliance falls by 50% PIP does not change—though VT drops, for example ETT slipping downright mainstem). Leak around the ETT is compensated in a pressure ventilator by achieving preset pressure with whatever volume it has to pump.

Cons: Variable VT as lung compliance changes, should lung compliance worsen then VT will drop (if the ETT plug VT drops to zero, but the ventilator does not sense it). Should improve compliance (following surfactant for example) this may result in overdistention. If the child is exhaling during a nonsynchronized ventilator breath, then the breath is ineffective.

High Frequency Ventilators

This is a radical innovation in ventilator design. The rate in "high frequency" is the Hz (range 3–15 Hz) (i.e. 180–900 breathe/minute). Since the VT generated by these ventilators approximates dead space, simple pulmonary mechanics are not applicable.

Pros: May allow gas exchange when conventional ventilation has failed.

Cons: Unclear which patients will respond and there is some risk involved in "just trying". Switching ventilators on an unstable patient who is on conventional ventilation may result in clinical deterioration. The high airway pressures often seen with HFV can be transmitted to the heart (particularly with compliant lungs) and result in impaired cardiac output requiring inotropes and/or volume boluses. High-frequency oscillatory ventilation (HFOV) makes turning patients, taking X-rays, or performing ultrasounds more complex due to the heavy, nonflexible tubing. Stopping HFOV for suctioning or administering nebulized medications may negate its benefit.

How to choose a ventilator?

Requirements will vary from unit to unit:

- Small unit <6 beds or large unit
- Tertiary or quarternary care (whether trauma cases, involved in heart surgeries, transplant, complex surgeries)
- *If small set up*: Whether combined NICU or PICU
- Ventilation facility recommended in the PICU and the NICU.

CPAP setup:

- *Conventional ventilator*: Standard modes [CMV, assist/control (A/C), SIMV "pressure", "volume ", pressure support, trigger, graphics, alarms]
- Noninvasive ventilator bilevel positive airway pressure (BIPAP)
- High frequency ventilator.

What should I be looking for?

- Cost
- Hidden cost of additional modules
- Low maintenance machine
- Machine should be user friendly, play with it for a week or so before buying
- Biomedical support in hospital
- Good after sale service
- Friendly representative who does not disappear after sale
- User list.

APPROXIMATE COST OF SOME COMMONLY AVAILABLE VENTILATORS

- Servo I: 10 lac
- Sensormedics oscillator 3100A and 3100B: 13–18 lac
- SLE 5000: 15 lac

- Engström: 8–9 lac
- Sechrist: 6–9 lac
- Puritan Bennett: lac
- Drager Babylog: 10–15 lac
- BIPAP (NIV): 1–3 lac
- Bubble CPAP: ₹ 80,000 to 1.5 lac

MONITORED PARAMETERS AVAILABLE IN ALL NEWER VENTILATORS

Exhaled tidal volume, spontaneous exhaled tidal volume, exhaled minute volume, spontaneous exhaled minute volume, PIP, MAP, PEEP, FiO$_2$, total breath rate, I:E ratio, etc. Inspiratory hold function is available for static lung compliance measurement and display. Comprehensive alarm package includes high pressure, low pressure, low minute volume, low/high O$_2$ inlet pressure, apnea alarm, and high breath rate.

Variable apnea backup ventilation is available whenever apnea is detected.

Specific Ventilators

Note: Each ventilator manufacturer has utilized specific names for mode functions of their specific machine that may not be identical with other machines. Generally speaking most manufacturers aspire for providing a universal ventilator for all age groups, not yet achieved, however with increased sophistication in technology; pulmonary graphics facility is now available in most modern ventilators. Each user should familiarize oneself with manual knobs or touch screen, to start and set up the ventilator, achieve the initial settings of modes (A/C, pressure regulated volume control (PRVC) or SIMV), rate (frequency), FiO$_2$, VT, PIP, PEEP, pressure support, inspiratory time (or I:E ratio), flow rate as well as setting of various ranges of alarms.

Engström Ventilator (Fig. 1)

The Engström Carestation (EC) is a critical care ventilator that is flexible and physically adaptable to a variety of work environments. A wide selection of performance options gives the user full control of the system configuration. The Engström Carestation is a complete system featuring patient monitoring, patient ventilation, and the capability of interfacing with central monitoring. These can be used in all age group from 0.5 to 7 kg, 1–15 lb for neonates, 5–200 kg, 10–440 lb for pediatric and adult.

Features:

- Simplified user interface
- Paramagnetic O$_2$ sensing
- Noninvasive ventilation (optional)
- Secure access to central stations

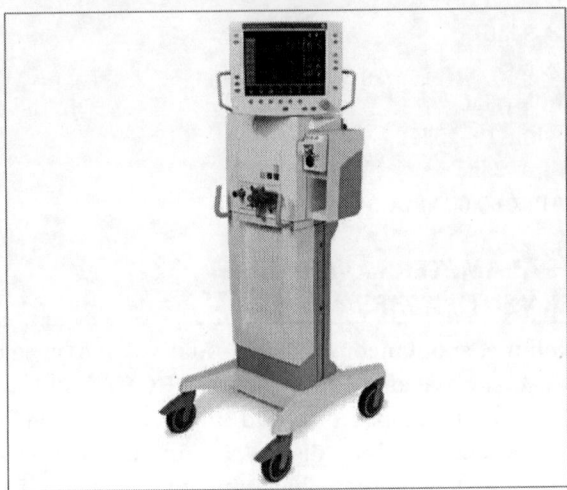

Fig. 1: Engström ventilator. (*For color version see Plate 5*)

- Sophisticated power management control with battery backup
- Auxiliary pressure sensor
- Airway resistance compensation.

Integrated ventilation and monitoring:
- Advanced ventilation
- *INview™ Suite*: SpiroDynamics[R] and FRC INview
- Plug and play modules
- Patient Spirometry™
- Gas monitoring with metabolics and energy expenditure
- Optional use of proximal Neo Flow Sensor with neonatal ventilation.

Aerogen Aeroneb® Pro:
- Built-in advanced nebulization system
- Operated in-line or independently for infants through adults

Modes of ventilation:
- Volume controlled ventilation (VCV)
- Pressure controlled ventilation (PCV)
- Pressure controlled ventilation, volume guaranteed (PCV-VG)
- Synchronized intermittent mandatory ventilation, volume controlled (SIMV-VC)
- Synchronized intermittent mandatory ventilation, pressure controlled (SIMV-PC)
- Synchronized intermittent mandatory ventilation, pressure controlled, volume guaranteed (SIMV-PCVG) (optional)
- BiLevel airway pressure release ventilation (APRV capable)
- BiLevel with volume guaranteed (BiLevel-VG) (optional)

- Noninvasive ventilation (NIV) (optional); nCPAP available with neonatal option
- Constant positive airway pressure/pressure support ventilation (CPAP/PSV)
- Apnea backup available in SIMV-VC, SIMV-PC, BiLevel, SIMV-PCVG, BiLevel-VG, and CPAP/PSV (institutionally selectable defaults)
- Volume guarantee-pressure support (VG-PS) available with neonatal option.

Drager Babylog 8000 (Fig. 2)

This ventilator is specifically designed for infants up to 10 kg (22 pounds). It is capable of both volume and pressure ventilation. A flow sensor at the Y piece close to the patient accurately measures VT and senses air flow initiated by the patient allowing triggering of the ventilator cycle. The sensor is able to compensate for small ETT leaks. High frequency ventilation can be delivered at 5–20 Hz.

Controls (as listed by the manufacturer):

- *Conventional ventilation*: Continuous flow, pressure-limited, time-cycled
- *Triggered ventilation*: SIMV, SIPPV, PSV1, leak adapted
  - *Trigger*: Flow/volume trigger, leak adapted
  - *Trigger delay*: Approximately 40–60 ms
- *High frequency ventilation*: CPAP + HFV, IMV + HFV
  - Frequency 5–20 Hz
- *Volume guarantee ventilation*: SIMV + VG, SIPPV + VG, PSV + VG
- *Oxygen mixer loss (bleed flow)*: 0 (zero) L/min.

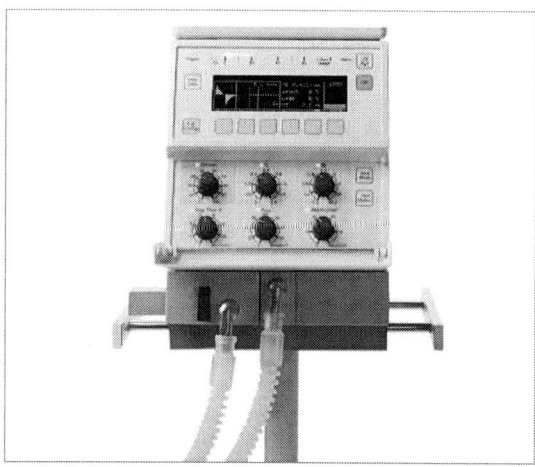

Fig. 2: Drager Babylog 8000. (*For color version see Plate 5*)

Settings:

- *Inspiratory oxygen concentration*: 21–100 volume% oxygen
- *Peak inspiratory pressure*: 10–80 mbar
- *PEEP/CPAP*: 0–25 mbar
- *Maximal frequency*: 200 bpm
- *Inspiratory time*: 0.1 to 2 seconds
- *Expiratory time*: 0.2 to 30 seconds
- *Inspiratory flow*: 1–30 L/min
- *Base flow (VIVE)*: 1–30 L/min.

Monitoring:

- *Flow monitoring*: At the Y-piece, integrated
- *Volume monitoring*: At the Y-piece, integrated
- *Lung function monitoring*: Compliance, resistance C20/C
- *Method*: Linear regression analysis
- *FiO$_2$ monitoring*: Integrated
- *Real-time curves*: Flow and pressure, integrated
- *Inspiratory oxygen concentration*: 21–100 volume% oxygen
- *Peak pressure*: to 99 mbar
- *Mean airway pressure*: to 99 mbar
- *Graphic trends*: 6 parameters, integrated
- *Logbook*: Record of up to 100 alarms.

Drager Babylog 8000 Plus, Evita XL, Evita 2 Dura (Fig. 3)

The Babylog 8000 plus is designed for harmonious ventilation of small children and the smallest preterm babies. It has an advanced upgrade platform that has allowed it to keep pace with all new forms of treatment and clinical advances. Sensitive synchronization with gentle but precise support

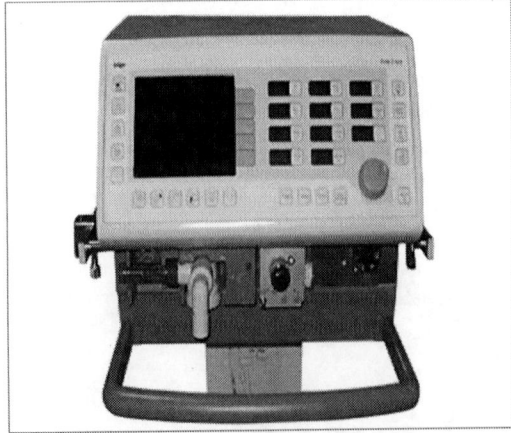

Fig. 3: Drager Babylog 8000 Plus. (*For color version see Plate 5*)

for spontaneous breathing reduces the work of breathing and makes the ventilation process much more comfortable for patients. All of the above features of Babylog 8000 are available in Babylog plus.

Drager Evita XL is a newer model useful for pediatric, neonatal as well as adult age group. The Drager Evita 2 Dura Ventilator is used for adult and pediatric patients. Options include DC monitoring plus, ventilation plus, neo flow. Its features include modes such as, Invasive - volume-controlled modes assist/control - SIMV PSV - mandatory minute ventilation (MMV) and pressure-controlled modes, assist/control SIMV (PSV), CPAP, BIPAP/PCV.

Sechrist Ventilator (Old and Newer Versions) (Figs. 4A and B)

This is continuous flow of a pressure cycled time of cycled ventilator. It has been commonly used for neonates with standard CPAP availability. Newer models are becoming available. The greatest advantage is absence of a demand valve to trigger ventilator cycle. Pressure support is not available in older models.

Siemens Servo-I (Maquet) (Table 1 and Fig. 5)

These ventilators support neonatal and pediatric patients through multiple ventilation modes and sensitive triggering responses. The pressure support

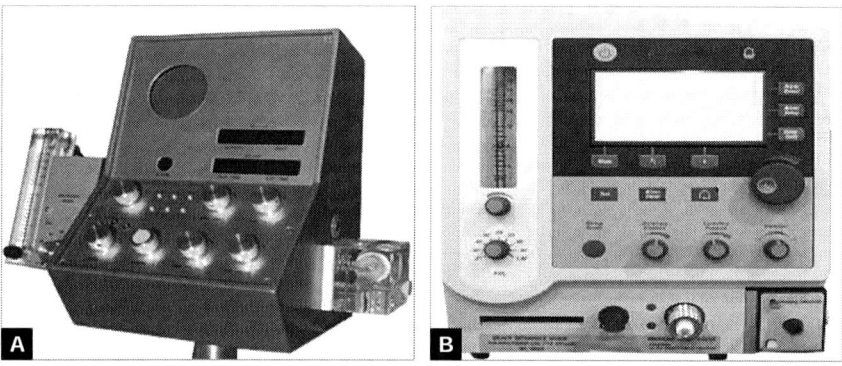

Figs. 4A and B: Sechrist ventilator: (A) Old and (B) New. (*For color version see Plate 6*)

Table 1: Patient weight ranges served by each configuration.			
Configuration	Weight range (normal modes)	Weight range (NIV PC + PS infant)	Weight range (NIV nasal CPAP)
Servo-I (infant)	0.5–30 kg	3–30 kg	0.5–10 kg
Servo-I (adult)	10–250 kg	Not applicable	Not applicable
Servo-I (universal)	0.5–250 kg	3–30 kg	0.5–10 kg

(CPAP: continuous positive airway pressure; NIV: noninvasive ventilation; PC: pressure controlled; PS: pressure support)

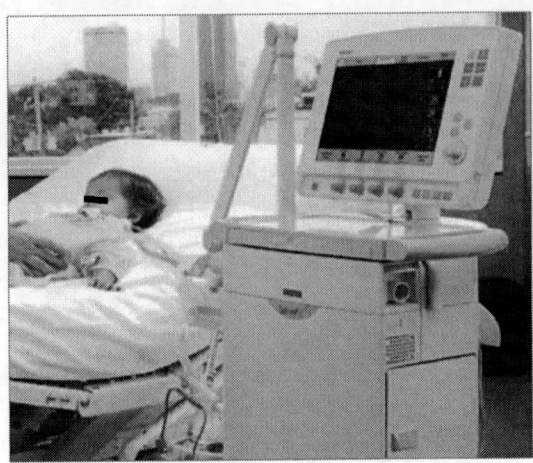

Fig. 5: Siemens Servo-I (Maquet).

mode of Servo-I infant reduces the work of breathing and responds instantly to the child's changing needs.

Treatment parameters and ranges can be flexibly customized and are automatically set, even when changing from one mode to another. The system can be upgraded to Servo-I universal standard for all patient categories.

Product Benefits
- Automode for fully adaptive patient interaction
- Lung recruitment for an even wider perspective of ventilation
- *Methodology and modes*: The ability to explore different treatment strategies
- Transportation with no loss of treatment quality
- New generation of ventilators.

Technical Specifications

Inspiratory tidal volume (mL): 5–350 (Optional—together with volume-related ventilation modes)

Inspiratory minute volume (L/min): 0.3–20 (Optional—together with volume-related ventilation modes)

Apnea, time to alarm (s): 5–45

Automode trigger timeout (s): 3–7

Pressure level (cm H_2O): 0–(80–PEEP)

PEEP (cm H_2O): 0–50

PEEP in NIV (cm H_2O): 2–20

CPAP pressure (cm H_2O): 2–20

CMV frequency (breaths/min): 4–150

SIMV frequency (breaths/min): 1–60

Breath cycle time, SIMV (s): 0.5–15

P_{High} *(cm H_2O)*: (PEEP +1)–50
T_{High} *(s)*: 0.2–10
T_{PEEP} *(s)*: 0.2–10
PS above P_{High} *(cm H_2O)*: 0–(80–P_{High})
PS above PEEP (cm H_2O): 0–(80–PEEP)
PS above PEEP in NIV (cm H_2O): 0–(32–PEEP)
Back-up pressure above PEEP (cm H_2O): 5–(80–PEEP)
NIV back-up rate (breaths/min): 4–40
O_2 concentration (%): 21–100
I:E ratio: 1:10–4:1
T_{Insp} *(s)*: 0.1 – 5
NIV back-up T_{Insp} *(s)*: 0.3–1
T_{Pause} *(s)*: 0–1.5
T_{Pause} *(% of breath cycle time)*: 0–30
Flow trigger sensitivity level (fraction of bias flow): 0–100%
Press. trigger sensitivity (cm H_2O): –20–0
Inspiratory rise time (% of breath cycle time): 0–20
Inspiratory rise time (s): 0–0.2
Inspiratory cycle off (% of peak flow): 1–70
Inspiratory cycle off in NIV (% of peak flow): 10–70
Nebulizer time (min): 5–30
Parameter: Setting range
Oxygen breaths: 100% for 1 minute
Servo Ultra Nebulizer (optional): Nebulizer on/off

Puritan Bennett™ 840 Ventilator (Fig. 6)

The Puritan Bennett™ 840 ventilator provides a solid foundation on which to build your ideal ventilation solution. With the addition of optional advanced

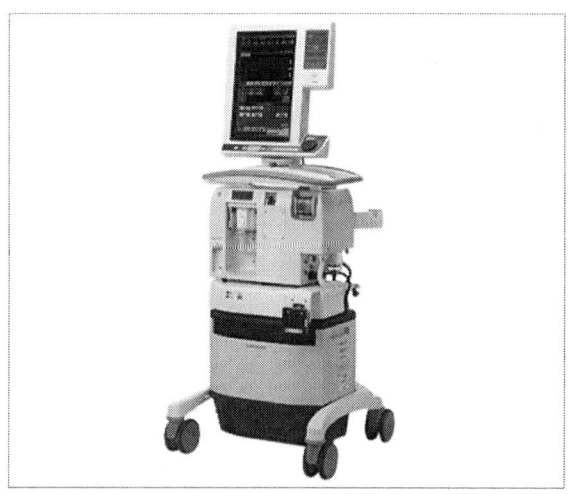

Fig. 6: Puritan Bennett™ 840 ventilator. (*For color version see Plate 6*)

technology upgrades, this ventilator can meet the specific needs of practically every patient type—from neonatal patients weighing as little as 300 g to adult patients weighing as much as 150 kg.

- *Puritan Bennett™ 840 neonatal ventilator:*
  - *Tidal volume*: 2–315 mL
  - *Patient weight*: 300 g to 7 kg
- *Puritan Bennett™ 840 pediatric-adult ventilator:*
  - *Tidal volume*: 25–2,500 mL
  - *Patient weight*: 7–150 kg
- *Puritan Bennett™ 840 universal ventilator:*
  - *Tidal volume*: 2–2,500 mL
  - *Patient weight*: 300 g to 150 kg

Puritan Bennett™ 840 ventilator settings:

Ideal body weight (IBW): 0.3 to 7.0 kg with NeoMode 2.0 (0.66 to 15 lbs), 7–24 kg (15–53 lbs), 25–150 kg (55–330 lbs)

Modes: Assist/control, SIMV, or spontaneous (SPONT), Bi-level software options: NeoMode 2.0, leak compensation, tube compensation, Bi-level, volume ventilation plus (volume control plus and volume support), Proportional Assist™* Ventilation Plus (PAV™*+), respiratory mechanics and trending.

Mandatory breath types: Volume control (VC), pressure control (PC) or volume control plus with volume.

Ventilation plus option spontaneous breath types: Pressure supported (PS), volume supported (VS), proportional assist (PA), none, vent type: Invasive or noninvasive

Pressure support (P_{SUPP}): 0–70 cm H_2O

Rise time (%): 1–100%

Expiratory sensitivity ($_{ESENS}$): 1–80%; 1–10 L/min with PAV™* +

Tidal volume: 25–2,500 mL, 2–315 mL with NeoMode

Respiratory rate (f): 1.0–100/min, 1–150/min with NeoMode

Peak inspiratory flow (V_{MAX}): 3–150 L/min for IBW >24 kg; 3–60 L/min for IBW ≤24 kg, 1–30 L/min with NeoMode

Flow pattern: Square or descending ramp

Plateau time (T_{PL}): 0.0 to 2.0 seconds

Inspiratory pressure (P_I): 5–90 cm H_2O

Constant during rate change: Inspiratory time (T_I), I:E ratio or expiratory time (T_E)

Inspiratory time (T_I): 0.2–8.0 seconds

I:E ratio: ≤1:2.99–4.00:1

Expiratory time (T_E): $T_E ≥ 0.2$ second

Trigger type: Pressure (P_{TRIG}) or flow (V_{TRIG} flow-by flow triggering)

Pressure sensitivity (P_{SENS}): 0.1 to 20 cm H_2O below PEEP

Flow sensitivity (V_{SENS}): 0.2 to 20 L/min, 0.1 to 10 L/min with NeoMode

PEEP: 0–45 cm H$_2$O

Apnea ventilation: Apnea mandatory type-volume control (VC) or pressure control (PC)

Applications	
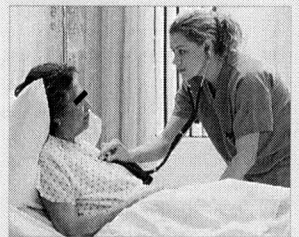 **Fig. 7:** Long-term care.	*Long-term care (Fig. 7):* • Small footprint • Easy to setup and use • Central monitoring capable • Multiple connectivity options
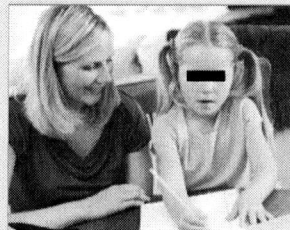 **Fig. 8:** Home care.	*Home care (Fig. 8):* • Simplified full color touch screens • On-screen help function • Safe and effective alarms • Hot swappable battery with fast recharge
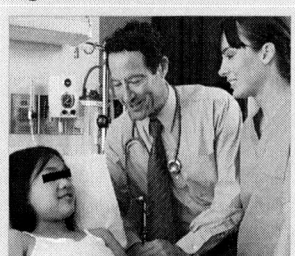 **Fig. 9:** Hospital care.	*Hospital (Fig. 9):* • Exceptional clinical capability • Invasive or noninvasive use • Customizable patient presets • Event log and trend screens
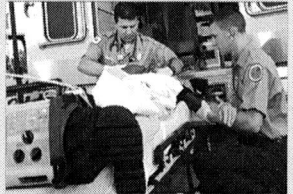 **Fig. 10:** Emergency preparedness.	*Emergency preparedness (Fig. 10):* • Fast setup with presets • Rugged construction • Quickset alarm function • Up to 10 hours on integrated battery
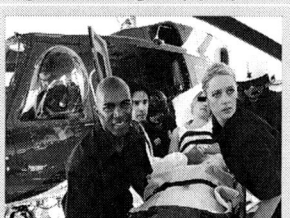 **Fig. 11:** Transport care.	*Transport (Fig. 11):* • Oxygen efficient • Air transport rated • Built-in oxygen monitor with alarms (optional)

Sensor Medics 3100A (High Frequency Oscillator Ventilator) (Figs. 12A and B)

It is high-frequency oscillatory ventilator (HFOV) with active inhalation/exhalation driven by a moving piston and diaphragm. The SensorMedics 3100A HFOV was first approved for use in 1991 and is the only HFOV approved for early intervention in the treatment of neonatal respiratory failure. The scope of application was broadened in 1995 to include selected pediatric patient failing conventional mechanical ventilation. The 3100A provides the ultimate in lung protection by inflating the lung with a continuous distending pressure and superimposing very small pressure and volume swings.

Numerous publications, including clinical, animal and bench studies have reported improved benefits and outcomes associated with the use of HFOV. There are over 3,500 SensorMedics HFOVs in use worldwide today. The 3100A is the standard of care in more than 90% of level III nurseries and 75% of the PICUs in the US.

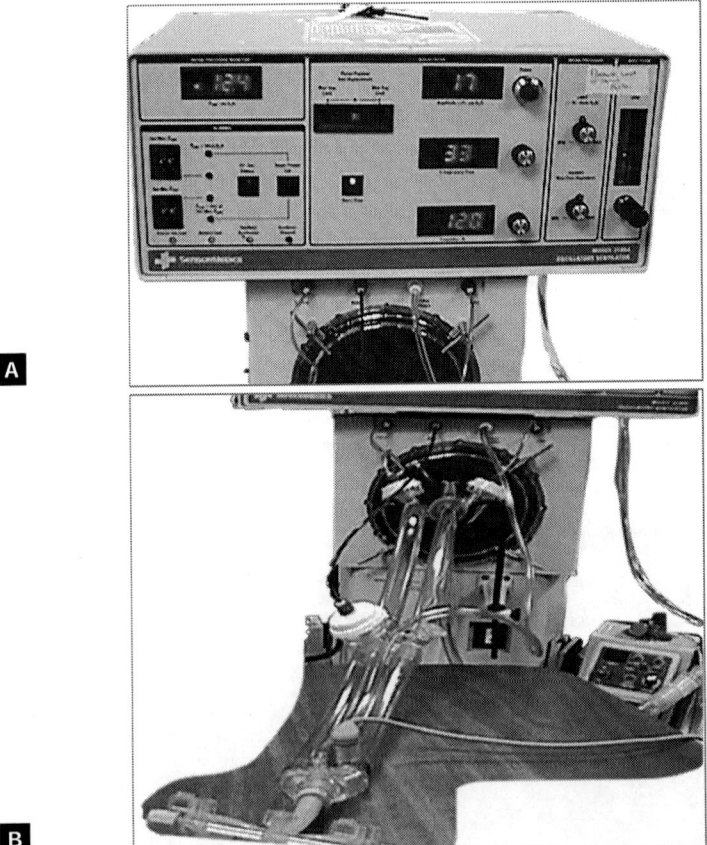

Figs. 12A and B: SensorMedics 3100A (high frequency oscillator ventilator). (*For color version see Plate 7*)

It requires special stiff non-compliant ventilator circuit. It can be utilized for a wide weight range of infants. Some preliminary work using it in smaller infants suggests that it may result in less barotrauma than conventional ventilation. It is used extensively in western countries in severe acute respiratory distress syndrome (RDS) and meconium aspiration to avert the need for extracorporeal membrane oxygenation (ECMO). Model 3100B is also available for >35 kg and adult age group.

Purpose: The high frequency oscillator is used for patients with RDS and for those patients that have failed conventional mechanical ventilation.

Description: High-frequency oscillatory ventilation improves gas exchange by continuous alveolar recruitment with the use of increased mean airway pressure (MAP) and active exhalation. After each patient use the ventilator is to be set up, calibrated, and a performance check out performed. The use of the oscillator is to be used on the order of the attending physician.

Indications:
- Respiratory distress syndrome, rescue
- Respiratory distress syndrome, prophylaxis
- Failure of conventional mechanical ventilation.

Hazards:
- Barotrauma
- Decreased venous return
- Intraventricular hemorrhage
- Hypocapnea
- Decreased cardiac output
- Hypotension
- Persistent pulmonary hypertension of the newborn (PPHN).

Personnel: Respiratory therapists and technicians (Table 2).
- *Procedure*: Obtain order and take vent to bedside.
- Plug into power and gas sources. Turn on the ventilator.
- Set the "limit" and "adjust" knobs to "max".
- Set the MAP with the "bias flow" knob at 5–10 cm H_2O above the prescribed MAP. *Note*: Flows may be as low as 6–10 lpm.
- Use the "adjust" knob to set the prescribed MAP.
  Note: If the patient requires a MAP greater than the "bias flow" allows, repeat steps 3–5.
- Set the "power" at 3.00.
- Set FiO_2.
- Set the high and low pressure alarms at ± 3 cm H_2O of the MAP.
- Place the patient on the ventilator.
- Adjust the "power" for adequate chest excursion.
- Recommend a chest X-ray within 30–60 minutes.
- Monitor per protocol.

Table 2: Controls and settings of sensorMedics oscillator.

Controls and settings	
Bias flow	0–40 L
Mean airway pressure (mPAW)	3–45 cm H$_2$O
Maximum mean pressure limit	10–45 cm H$_2$O
Amplitude (delta-P)	>90 cm H$_2$O
Frequency	3–15 Hz
Percent inspiratory time	30–50%
Piston centering adjust	Applies electrical counter force to piston coil to maintain piston centering
Pressure measurement	
Range	±130 cm H$_2$O
Displays	
Mean airway pressure, amplitude (delta-P), bias flow, piston displacement, frequency, percent of inspiratory time	
Alarms	
Safety (dump valve open): mPAW > 50 cm H$_2$O, mean airway pressure < 20% of set maximum PAW *Warnings:* High or low mean airway pressure *Caution:* Oscillator over heated, battery low, sources gas low, power failure, oscillator stopped, 45 second alarm silence	

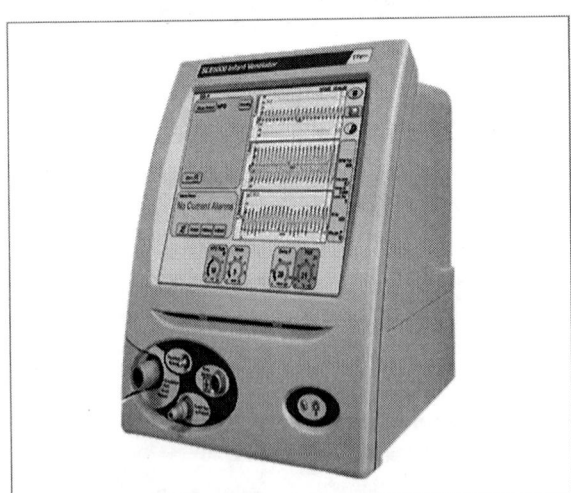

Fig. 13: SLE5000 ventilator. (*For color version see Plate 8*)

SLE5000 Ventilator (Fig. 13)

Modes include: CPAP, CMV+ targeted tidal volume (TTVplus), patient triggered ventilation (PTV), PSV, SIMV+ TTVplus + PSV, HFO, HFO + CMV.

The SLE5000 also has:

- The ability to preset parameters in all modes of operation
- Powerful HFO with active expiration to cover a wide range of patients
- Full color, total touch-screen operation
- Integral flow monitoring measuring lung mechanics and displaying of loops and waveforms
- Trending of measured parameters
- Standard patient circuit for all modes including HFO
- Unique, patented valveless technology
- Integral battery with up to 60 minutes operating capability
- Software based, allowing for upgrading to versions with new or improved functions
- Very quiet operation HFOV, yet with the performance to successfully provide HFO to both the smallest preterms and the largest infants
- Same patient circuit is used for conventional and HFO ventilation, minimizing risk of lung derecruitment
- Proximal hot wire flow sensor technology ensures sensitivity to even the tiniest of patient breathing efforts, and control of tidal volumes as small as 2 mL
- Volume targeting capability to limit and monitor delivered tidal volumes as part of the lung protective strategy
- Color display of respiratory waveforms and key respiratory parameters, in addition to 24-hour trending data
- Simple upgrade capability to keep up to date with latest software and modality enhancements
- Easy to set up, easy to use, easy to train, easy to clean
- Can be used with the SLE INOSYS, nitric oxide system.

KEY MESSAGES

- A ventilator with pressure control, volume control, wide range of VT from neonate to adult, pressure support, SIMV, assist-control, CPAP, noninvasive ventilation capability (leak compensation), built in high/low pressure alarm, low tidal volume alarm, apnea alarm, power failure alarm with backup battery, low/high oxygen alarm, good humidification and warming system is desirable.
- Graphics, though optional are becoming a standard feature in most ventilators.
- Although all these ventilators have mostly proven satisfactory in use, most intensive care units will tend to use one make, so that nursing and medical staff can become familiar with the controls and monitors.
- Microprocessor technology makes it easy to adapt all these machines to encompass new ventilatory modes, but since there is no clear evidence that any one mode is superior to another it would also seem wise to

restrict the problems of patient care and monitoring that are specific to each mode.

■ Company that provides cost efficient product, hands on training, good after sales service and a maintenance contract should be chosen for purchase of a ventilator. It is also suggested that a user list be requested so the buyer can talk to the users and practical issues and with different ventilators can be discussed with current users. Following are integral to choosing ventilator:

- Know your unit needs
- Expected patient population neonate/pediatrics
- Budget
- One vent (with essential features) and one CPAP may be good to start in small mixed unit
- Good after sale service is a must.

SUGGESTED READING

1. Najaf-Zadeh A, Leclerc F. Noninvasive positive pressure ventilation for acute respiratory failure in children: a concise review. Ann Intensive Care. 2011;1(1):15.
2. Vignaux L, Piquilloud L, Tourneux P, et al. Neonatal and adult ICU ventilators to provide ventilation in neonates, infants, and children: a bench model study. Respir Care. 2014;59(10):1463-75.

Index

Page numbers followed by *f* refer to figure, *fc* refer to flow chart, and *t* refer to table